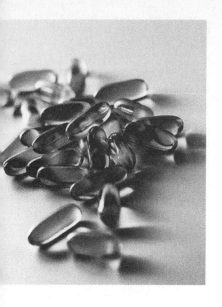

Introduction to the

Pharmaceutical

Sciences

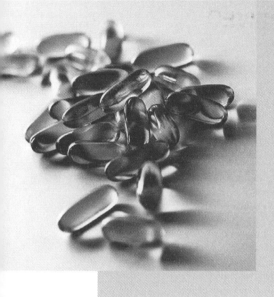

Introduction to the Pharmaceutical Sciences

Nita K. Pandit, PhD

Professor of Pharmaceutics
Department of Pharmaceutical Sciences
College of Pharmacy
Drake University
Des Moines, Iowa

Acquisitions Editor: David B. Troy
Managing Editor: Andrea M. Klingler
Marketing Manager: Marisa O'Brien
Production Editor: Eve Malakoff-Klein
Designer Coordinator: Doug Smock
Compositor: Nesbitt Graphics, Inc.
Printer: Courier Corporation—Kendallville

Library of Congress Cataloging-in-Publication Data

Pandit, Nita K.
    Introduction to the pharmaceutical sciences / Nita K. Pandit.— 1st ed.
        p. ; cm.
    Includes bibliographical references and index.
    ISBN-13: 978-0-7817-4478-2
    ISBN-10: 0-7817-4478-4
    1. Pharmacology. 2. Pharmacokinetics.   I. Title.
    [DNLM: 1. Pharmacokinetics.   2. Pharmacology.   QV 38 P189i 2007]
RM300.P26 2007
615'.7—dc22

                                                                2005034266

                                        06   07   08   09
                    1   2   3   4   5   6   7   8   9   10

Foreword

In recent years, the use of drugs to treat acute and chronic diseases has significantly increased, to the extent that it is now a major factor driving healthcare policy and economics. This has come about primarily because of the scientific revolutions that have occurred in biology and in the physics and chemistry of materials. The greater understanding of molecular biology has led to improved strategies for diagnosing and treating disease, including more rational approaches to the discovery of chemical entities with greatly enhanced therapeutic potency and selectivity. Technologic advances arising from the materials revolution have led to improved approaches for the design, analysis, and manufacture of safe, effective, and convenient means of delivering drugs to the patient. These changes, as one might expect, have had a significant effect on two professional groups: the pharmacy profession, which provides the last step in the control of quality in the dispensing of drug products and in their appropriate use by patients, and the pharmaceutical industry, which is responsible for the discovery and development of new safe and effective medications.

With the advances noted above, pharmacists now play a greater role in the pharmacotherapeutic use of drugs, in addition to their traditional role in the dispensing of prescriptions. This has led to a major change in the curricula of schools of pharmacy, with much greater emphasis on the clinical use of drugs, e.g., the rational choice of drugs, appropriate dosing of patients, bioavailability, and drug–drug interactions. With this, however, has come less emphasis in the curriculum on the theoretical underpinning of drug therapies presented in pharmaceutical science–related courses, which provides a basis for understanding the factors that lead to the safe and effective use of drugs by patients. How to maintain a balance between the basic and clinical aspects of the curriculum remains a major challenge.

The pharmaceutical industry also faces extraordinary challenges in meeting the healthcare needs of a worldwide society. More adequate treatments of major diseases, including cancer, cardiovascular diseases, diabetes, and neurologic diseases, and of infectious diseases of worldwide proportions, such as influenza, AIDS, various parasitic diseases, and tuberculosis, are needed badly. Other major challenges include the development of vaccines and the addressing of an increasing general tendency for microorganisms to develop resistance to many of the important anti-infective drugs now in use. To meet these needs, it is necessary to have a highly efficient drug discovery and development process, conducted over the shortest time possible and at minimal cost. However, despite great progress in a number of areas, today's "pipeline" of drug candidates with high potential for success is not what it should be.

One possible cause of such failure, in my opinion, is the unfortunate disconnect that often occurs between the drug discovery and drug development processes. Although some efforts have been made in recent years to bridge this gap, newly obtained drug candidates are often sent into development with little consideration given to those molecular characteristics that might lead to poor druglike properties. Furthermore, those involved in the formulation and processing of drugs into drug products often lack an appreciation of the many critical biological issues that determine efficacy, toxicity, and drug disposition. This often arises from an inadequate understanding of the scientific principles underlying all aspects of drug discovery and development and of the important roles played by the different disciplines contributing to the success of the program.

Consequently, I believe that any effort to provide a better understanding of the interdisciplinary nature of drug therapy on the part of pharmaceutical educators, and of the drug development process by the pharmaceutical industry, is critical and valuable. An enhanced mutual respect for the work done by various individuals involved in filling and advancing the pipeline will follow, further helping to bring important drugs to the market in a less costly and more timely manner, with the ultimate result of better professional service to patients.

With this in mind, the appearance of this first edition of *Introduction to the Pharmaceutical Sciences,* with its timely presentation in textbook form of the science underlying the discovery and development of therapeutic agents, is most welcome. Here, for the first time, we have a comprehensive treatise devoted to the pharmaceutical sciences written entirely from the perspective of one author with extensive experience in various aspects of both the pharmaceutical industry and pharmaceutical education. This uniquely organized presentation provides a clear and concise discussion of topics ranging from the underlying fundamentals of therapeutic targets and drug molecule properties, *in vitro* and *in vivo,* to issues such as formulation, manufacturing, clinical trials, and the regulatory process. Specifically designed as a textbook rather than a compilation of multi-authored chapters, this book can serve as an excellent pedagogic vehicle for professional students in pharmacy who will be directly involved in the pharmacotherapeutic use of drug products by patients, providing them with a clear and concise way to see the connections between the science and practice of pharmacy. In addition, this material, and the way it is presented, can serve as an excellent text for students considering a career in the pharmaceutical sciences, as well as for scientists already in the pharmaceutical industry seeking to broaden their understanding of drug development. Its stress on the multidisciplinary nature of the drug development process can be an excellent starting point for those who, in the future, will be working to meet critical societal needs in the treatment, cure, and prevention of disease.

George Zografi, PhD
School of Pharmacy
University of Wisconsin—Madison

Preface

If the study of all these sciences, which we have enumerated, should ever bring us to their mutual association and relationship, and teach us the nature of the ties which bind them together, I believe that the diligent treatment of them will forward the objects which we have in view, and that the labor, which otherwise would be fruitless, will be well bestowed.

—*Plato* (c. 427–347 BCE)

Introduction to the Pharmaceutical Sciences is an introductory text that provides a simple, integrated, and coherent overview of pharmaceutical science concepts for the beginner or nonspecialist. It introduces and explains fundamental principles that underlie all of the pharmaceutical science disciplines, reveals the connections between them, and highlights their pharmaceutical and therapeutic applications. As scientists, we are rarely encouraged to look up from our own specialty areas and narrow research interests to appreciate the "big picture" into which our discipline fits. It is no wonder that our students often have difficulty understanding how their pharmaceutical science courses relate to each other and to their future pharmacy careers. This book takes a big picture look at the pharmaceutical sciences and shows students these links and associations.

The pharmaceutical sciences are a collection of related disciplines that study the discovery, development, and use of drugs to treat diseases. Traditionally, the pharmaceutical sciences have been separated into specialty areas such as pharmacology, medicinal chemistry, pharmacokinetics, and pharmaceutics. The lines between these individual disciplines are blurred, however, when pharmacists and pharmaceutical scientists have to solve real problems in the workplace. Pharmacists must be able to integrate their knowledge of the pharmaceutical sciences to solve a patient's drug therapy problem. Pharmaceutical scientists must use an interdisciplinary approach to new drug discovery and development as they participate in project teams with scientists from many disciplines.

My colleagues and I at Drake University had a vision that this philosophy of integration could be the basis of a new course called "Introduction to Pharmaceutical Sciences" for first-year pharmacy students. Such a course was developed and has been taught at Drake since 1998. Because a detailed search of the market failed to identify a suitable textbook, I decided to create a manuscript to fill the needs of our course. The course and the manuscript have evolved over the years, and both have received strong student support. Students in subsequent years of the pharmacy program continue to tell us how important this first course was in their curriculum, and how much better the manuscript is compared with other pharmaceutical science texts. It is this first-hand experience that convinces me that an integrated and introductory course in the pharmaceutical sciences is valuable to students and helps them see the importance of pharmaceutical sciences in drug therapy. The manuscript has undergone many changes on the basis of input from a variety of sources, and has resulted in this text.

This book targets first-year pharmacy students, junior-level science undergraduates, and readers who have had at least 2 years of college-level science and math. My assumption is that readers have a basic background in general chemistry, organic chemistry, biology, and algebra. Some knowledge of introductory biochemistry and calculus is helpful but not required. Physiological concepts are introduced as needed.

The text could be used for a one-semester or a full-year course, depending on the desired depth of coverage. All topics may not be necessary for a one-semester course, and selection of material could depend on the primary course objectives and subsequent curriculum. A full-year course may use the entire book with detailed discussion and additional readings as desired. Graduate students may be able to grasp and learn all the content in a one-semester course.

The course could be taught by one faculty member because the content is presented at an introductory level. However, the book is written so that a team-taught approach works just as well, with two to three faculty teaching different parts of the course. In such an instance, it is very important that the faculty team members are aware of what is being taught by their teammates, and that there is close communication among them.

Although this book is written as a text so that it can be used in formal courses, I have adopted a broad view of the population for whom it is intended. Based on my work experience in the pharmaceutical industry, I know that this book could be very valuable to junior scientists in research and development, and to other professionals in the pharmaceutical industry who need a simple overview of the pharmaceutical sciences.

Strategy

The pharmaceutical sciences share many common concepts in organic, general, and physical chemistry; physiology; biochemistry; cell and molecular biology; genetics; engineering; and mathematics. These concepts form the basis of the book, and the connection to different aspects of the pharmaceutical sciences and drug therapy is revealed as the book progresses.

I strongly believe that students who understand the language of the pharmaceutical sciences, its fundamental concepts, and the links between concepts are better able to grasp material that they encounter later in more advanced courses. They appreciate and learn the content of these specialty disciplines with more motivation and less memorizing because everything makes sense. For a pharmacy student, an understanding of the basic concepts of the pharmaceutical sciences will be followed by courses in pharmacology, pharmaceutics, pharmacokinetics, and medicinal chemistry. For graduate students, this book will provide a broad context in which to study and investigate problems in their chosen pharmaceutical specialty.

It is important to state what this book is not intended to be. It is not meant to be an encyclopedia of the pharmaceutical sciences, a "how-to" book of experimental techniques, or a book for the specialist in any one of the pharmaceutical science disciplines. Because I wish to emphasize the concepts underlying this field, discussion of special topics and details of any one discipline are generally limited. There are several other courses and excellent books that fill these needs.

I have aimed for simplicity, clarity, and brevity in my writing so that the book is easy to read. My philosophy has been "less is more." Historical development of theories and hypotheses has been mostly omitted. Need-to-know concepts are emphasized; good-to-know content and material that will be taught later in pharmacy curricula or that are not directly relevant have been minimized.

Organization

The book is intended to be self-contained and easy-to-read. One of the advantages of a single-author book is that the theme, style, and nomenclature remain consistent.

Material in the chapters progresses logically, and readers are frequently asked to refer to previous chapters as concepts are further developed and reinforced. The reader is also told when a concept being discussed will be used later. To provide coherence and readability, individual statements are not referenced to the primary literature; however, every attempt has been made to ensure that statements reflect generally accepted scientific views.

Chapter 1, the Introduction, sets the stage for the book by outlining the scope of the pharmaceutical sciences and stimulates readers by posing some questions about drug design, delivery, disposition, and action. It then gives a glimpse of the applications of these concepts in therapy and drug development.

I have grouped the remaining chapters into sections based on pharmaceutical principles rather than traditional disciplines. **Basic Principles** (Chapters 2–5) presents the chemical, biological, and physical principles that form the foundation of the pharmaceutical sciences. Chapters on Ionization, Solubility and Lipophilicity, Rates of Pharmaceutical Processes, and Membranes and Tissues give simple but clear explanations of these concepts. An example of the integrated approach is illustrated in the discussion of kinetic principles in Rates of Pharmaceutical Processes, in which I approach these concepts in relation to drug stability, pharmacokinetics, and enzyme-catalyzed reactions. Membranes and Tissues introduces cell structure concepts with emphasis on biomolecules and properties and behavior of membranes.

Drug Structure and Design (Chapters 6–8) introduces drug targets (receptors, enzymes), the influence of drug structure on its ability to reach and bind to the intended target, and how new drugs are discovered and optimized. The chapters in this section are Drugs and Their Targets, Drug Discovery and Optimization, and Transport Across Biological Barriers. An example of an integrated approach is illustrated in the discussion of transport mechanisms, in which connections to intestinal absorption, renal excretion, the blood–brain barrier, and drug efflux of chemotherapeutics are shown. In this section, I frequently refer readers back to earlier information on ionization, lipophilicity, and membrane properties.

Drug Delivery (Chapters 9 and 10) presents the importance of dosage forms and routes of administration in drug therapy. In Drug Absorption, I discuss the rates and mechanisms of oral and nonoral absorption of drugs. Drug Delivery Systems deals with the principles (such as dissolution and stability) underlying dosage form design, and introduces students to the challenges of controlled delivery and delivery of macromolecular drugs. As before, these chapters use concepts discussed in the Basic Principles section.

Drug Disposition (Chapters 11–14) focuses on the fate of the drug after administration and examines how drug and membrane properties influence where a drug goes, how quickly it travels, and what happens when it gets there. Again, concepts in Basic Principles are used. Each chapter name indicates its primary focus: Drug Distribution, Drug Excretion, and Drug Metabolism. The chapter on Plasma Concentration–Time Curves brings together discussions from Drug Delivery and Drug Disposition and introduces readers to pharmacokinetics. I also introduce concepts of pharmacodynamics to set the stage for the next section.

Drug Action (Chapters 15–17) picks up on earlier information on drug targets, presents the major types of receptors and enzymes, and examines how a drug modulates the behavior of its target. In Ligands and Receptors, I discuss principles of cellular communication and introduce the ligand and receptor classes involved. Emphasis again is on molecular properties and interactions; concepts presented in earlier chapters are referred to extensively. Mechanisms of Drug Action focuses on theories of agonism and antagonism, and shows the similarities between the behavior of receptors and that of enzymes in their interactions with drugs. Dose–Response Relationships examines drug action quantitatively and presents principles of drug efficacy and safety. This discussion sets the stage for the next section.

Drug Therapy (Chapters 18–20) brings together all earlier discussions and shows their importance in treating patients. Therapeutic Variability examines the absorption, distribution, metabolism, and excretion characteristics and pharmacodynamic and compliance factors that affect an individual's drug response based on pharmaceutical science principles. Drug Interactions discusses the pharmaceutical, pharmacokinetic, and pharmacodynamic basis for drug interactions with other drugs or foods. I emphasize again the pharmaceutical science principles behind these interactions. Pharmacogenomics introduces the reader to genetic factors that underlie interindividual variability, and gives students a glimpse of the future when new drugs are developed using a pharmacogenomic approach and therapy is determined on the basis of the genetic makeup of an individual.

The final section is **Special Topics** (Chapters 21 and 22). Biopharmaceuticals is an important chapter that deals with biopharmaceuticals and related therapeutic agents (therapeutic proteins, antibodies, vaccines, and genes) and highlights similarities and differences between them and small molecule drugs. I felt that a separate chapter was needed for this topic. Drug Discovery, Development, and Approval outlines the industrial drug development process and subsequent regulatory considerations, including clinical trials and postmarketing considerations. This section again provides an opportunity to take fundamental pharmaceutical principles and show their important applications to drug therapy.

Features

The text contains words set in bold purple type; these represent **Key Terms** that form the language of the pharmaceutical sciences. These terms are explained and defined when they first appear.

Key Concepts are summarized at the end of each chapter so readers know what they should have learned from a particular chapter. A list of **Review Questions** is posed at the end of each chapter. These are broad questions that test understanding of the concepts rather than the details. All chapters include a list of **Additional Readings** at the end to which a reader can turn for further information on a topic.

Drug examples have been included so readers can appreciate the practical importance of a particular concept. Many of the extensive examples or illustrations are set apart in boxes so they do not interrupt the flow of the text. Some drug examples appear in the text if appropriate. As the book progresses and readers have mastered more of the fundamentals, more such examples are included in the text.

I hope that the availability of this text will make it easier for faculty to develop and teach a truly integrated course in the pharmaceutical sciences. I hope further that this book will be used in other degree programs so that students in chemistry, biology, or premedical programs can appreciate the applications of pharmaceutical sciences and see this area as a career opportunity. Lastly, I want to emphasize that this book is a "work in progress"; feedback and comments from our students will continue to be considered. In addition, I welcome advice from readers on how to improve this book.

Nita K. Pandit, PhD

Acknowledgments

The inspiration to write a book comes from my two mentors at the School of Pharmacy, University of Wisconsin. My PhD advisor, Professor Ken Connors, infected me with his enthusiasm for writing and showed me how good writing is done. My profound gratitude also goes to Professor George Zografi, who has supported me throughout my career and who wrote the foreword to this book.

As with any book, this text has benefited from contributions of many people. My students at Drake have been my primary audience, and I thank them for their input and patience as the course and the book evolved. My colleagues at Drake have actively participated in the development and teaching of the course, and I am grateful for their ideas, suggestions, and support.

The book has also improved as a result of extensive reviews provided by faculty members from many institutions. These have been very valuable in making the book suitable not just to the needs of Drake students, but to students, teachers, and readers elsewhere.

I wish to particularly thank the wonderful people at Lippincott Williams & Wilkins, whose enthusiasm, commitment, professionalism, and patience made this a rewarding endeavor.

Reviewers

Val J. Watts, Ph.D.
Associate Professor
Department of Medicinal Chemistry & Molecular Pharmacology
Purdue University and Indiana University School of Medicine—Lafayette
West Lafayette, IN

Jane Alcorn
Assistant Professor of Pharmacy
College of Pharmacy and Nutrition
University of Saskatchewan
Saskatoon, Saskatchewan
Canada

Audra L. Stinchcomb, Ph.D.
Associate Professor
Department of Pharmaceutical Sciences
College of Pharmacy
University of Kentucky
Chief Scientific Officer and Founder
AllTranz
Lexington, KY

Eric L. Barker, PhD
Associate Professor
Department of Medicinal Chemistry & Molecular Pharmacology
Purdue University School of Pharmacy
West Lafayette, IN

Bill Bowman, Ph.D.
Assistant Professor of Pharmaceutical Science
Midwestern University, Glendale
College of Pharmacy
Glendale, AZ

Victoria F. Roche, Ph.D.
Senior Associate Dean
Professor of Pharmacy Sciences
School of Pharmacy and Health Professions
Creighton University
Omaha, NE

Renu Chhabra, Pharm.D.
Senior Health Promotion Officer
Division of Drug Information
Center for Drug Evaluation and Research
Food and Drug Administration
Rockville, MD

Philip G. Kerr, PhD
Lecturer in Medicinal Chemistry
School of Biomedical Sciences
Charles Sturt University
Wagga Wagga, NSW
Australia

Michalakis Savva, Ph.D.
Assistant Professor
Arnold & Marie Schwartz College of Pharmacy
Division of Pharmaceutics
Brooklyn, NY

Ann M. Lynch, R.Ph., Pharm.D.
Assistant Professor of Pharmacy Practice
Massachusetts College of Pharmacy and Health Sciences
Worcester, MA

Michelle L. Hilaire, Pharm.D., C.D.E.
Clinical Assistant Professor of Pharmacy Practice
University of Wyoming School of Pharmacy
Fort Collins Family Medicine Residency Program
Fort Collins, CO

Amanda Ballentine, Pharm.D.
Department of Pharmacy Healthcare Administration
College of Pharmacy
University of Florida
Gainesville, FL

Karim Iskander
Department of Pharmacology
Baylor College of Medicine
Houston, TX

Contents

Introduction

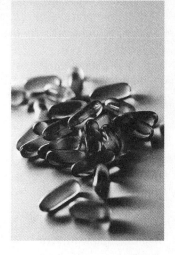

The pharmaceutical sciences are a group of interdisciplinary areas of study involved with the design, action, delivery, disposition, and use of drugs. This field draws on many areas of the basic and applied sciences, such as chemistry (organic, physical, and analytical), biology (anatomy and physiology, biochemistry, molecular biology), mathematics, physics, and chemical engineering, and applies their principles to the study of drugs.

The pharmaceutical sciences are further subdivided into several specific specialties, for example:

- **Pharmacology**: the study of the biochemical and physiological effects of drugs on organisms.
- **Pharmacodynamics**: the study of the cellular and molecular interactions of drugs with their receptors.
- **Pharmaceutical toxicology**: the study of the harmful or toxic effects of drugs.
- **Pharmacokinetics**: the study of the factors that control the concentration of drug at various sites in the body.
- **Medicinal chemistry**: the study of drug design to optimize pharmacokinetics and pharmacodynamics, and synthesis of new drug candidates.

- Pharmaceutics: the study and design of drug formulation for optimum delivery, stability, pharmacokinetics, and patient acceptance.
- Pharmacogenomics: the study of the inheritance of characteristic patterns of interaction between drugs and organisms.

As new discoveries advance and extend the pharmaceutical sciences, subspecialties continue to be added to this list. Importantly, as knowledge advances, boundaries between these specialty areas of pharmaceutical sciences are beginning to blur. Many fundamental concepts are common to all pharmaceutical sciences. In this book, we will focus on these shared fundamental concepts to understand their applicability to all aspects of pharmaceutical research and drug therapy.

What Is a Drug?

A drug can be defined as a chemical substance that interacts with a part of the body to alter an existing physiological or biochemical process. A drug can decrease or increase an existing function of an organ, tissue, or cell, but cannot impart a new function to them. For example, drugs are available to decrease blood pressure, decrease acid formation in the stomach, increase urine production, and increase bone density. Some therapies, such as vaccines and gene therapy, are not drugs in the traditional sense but are also used in management of diseases.

An ideal drug is one that:

- Has a desirable pharmacological action;
- Has few or no side effects;
- Reaches its intended location in the right concentration at the right time;
- Remains at the site of action for the necessary period of time;
- Is rapidly and completely removed from the body when it is no longer needed.

All these goals cannot be achieved when developing a new drug, but need to be considered and optimized during the research and development process. The success of a new drug depends on how close the drug comes to meeting these objectives.

How Do Drugs Work?

The site of action of a drug is the location in the body where the drug performs its function. For example, a drug may act in the brain, heart, eye, or kidney. Within these organs, the drug may act on a particular component of the organ, such as a certain type of cell. The action may be extracellular, in which the drug performs its function outside the cell, or intracellular, in which the drug has to enter the cell to work. Alternatively, the action may be on the cell surface, at the cell membrane.

Drugs work by interacting with target molecules in our bodies and altering their activities in a way that is beneficial to our health. In some cases, the effect of a drug is to stimulate the activity of its target, whereas in other cases the drug blocks target activity. In most cases, a drug temporarily attaches (binds) to the target before exerting its action. Drug targets are usually biological molecules, such as proteins, protein complexes, or nucleic acids, that play a role in a disease process. One type of drug target is a receptor, generally a protein on the cell membrane, that can bind with a specific type of molecule (such as a drug) to alter the cell's function. Other drug targets include enzymes and nucleic acids.

Pharmacodynamics is the study of biochemical and physiological effects of a drug, its mechanisms of action, and correlation of these actions with the chemical structure and blood levels of drug. Pharmacodynamics may also be defined as a description of interactions that occur between a drug and its receptor, and succeeding events that lead to pharmacological action of the drug.

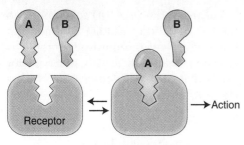

Drug **A** binds to receptor
Drug **B** cannot bind to receptor

Figure 1.1. A simplified diagram illustrating the lock-and-key concept of drug–receptor binding. Drug A has a structure that is complementary to the receptor and therefore can bind to it. The structure of Drug B is not compatible with the receptor, and thus no binding occurs.

A simplified analogy often used to describe drug–receptor interactions is that of a *lock and key*—the receptor is a lock that only a certain drug (key) can fit into and open; this is illustrated in Figure 1.1. Ideally, the key should not fit any other lock, and different keys should not open this lock. Some keys can fit in the lock, but not perfectly. Consequently, these imperfect keys cannot open the door. Yet by fitting into the lock, these keys prevent the original key from fitting into the lock and opening the door; they therefore block the door from opening. Such compounds also work as drugs by preventing or decreasing an existing action.

Most drugs, however, are not as specific as a key. Few drugs interact exclusively with their intended target. Many drugs bind to more than one type of receptor and influence physiological or biochemical processes that were not targeted. This leads to undesirable side effects of drugs, or toxicity.

How Are Drugs Designed?

A good drug must be able to pass through barriers our body puts in its path, and to interact with certain components of the body but not with others. It must be able to withstand, for an ade-

quate time, the action of protective mechanisms designed to decompose it and eliminate it; however, the body must eventually be able to deactivate and eliminate the drug. The molecular structure of a drug uniquely defines all its properties and ultimately controls its behavior in the body. Successful drug design depends on a thorough understanding of the chemistry of the drug, and of the interaction of the drug with numerous molecules it encounters in the body. Navigating the physiological minefield of the body to reach its target and exert its effect is a challenge only a well-designed drug can meet.

In the past, most drugs were discovered through a search of natural sources such as plants and microorganisms. Subsequently, trial and error approaches resulted in discovery and development of many important drugs. This process, called **random screening**, still has a place in drug discovery and is used by pharmaceutical companies to identify *lead compounds*. These lead compounds are then synthetically modified to give new compounds with improved properties.

Today, increased knowledge about cell and protein structure and physiological mechanisms has led to **rational drug design** for identifying potential drugs. The process starts with an understanding of fundamental biochemical and physiological aspects of a disease. If altering the action of a particular drug target can treat the disease, then the detailed structure and function of the target are studied. Once these are known, chemical compounds are synthesized with structures that allow them to bind to and alter the behavior of the desired target.

Much of this is done through computer simulations and computational techniques such as molecular modeling. If this rationally designed compound is found to have desired biological activity, then its structure is successively modified and refined. The goal is a compound that comes as close as possible to the characteristics of an ideal drug.

How Are Drugs Administered?

A drug can exert its intended action only when it reaches its intended target at the site of action. This means a drug that acts on the heart must reach appropriate receptors in the heart, and a drug that acts on the brain must reach its receptors in the brain. It is often inconvenient or impossible to apply a drug directly at its site of action; instead, drugs must be given at an administration site far removed from the site of action. For accuracy and convenience of dosing, the drug is almost always incorporated into a dosage form or drug delivery system (such as tablets, patches, inhalers). Delivery systems can also be designed to provide *controlled* or *sustained* release of drug.

The method and form of administration must consider the body's protective barriers, the drug's physical and chemical properties, and patient acceptance. Most drugs are given orally because patients prefer this administration method. After oral dosing, the drug must be released from the delivery system and enter the bloodstream (absorption) so it can reach the site of action. Another common but less convenient administration route is injection, which is usually reserved for drugs that have poor absorption characteristics.

How Do Drugs Travel in the Body?

The term drug disposition refers to distribution, metabolism, and elimination of drugs after absorption into the bloodstream. After absorption, circulating blood carries drug throughout the body in a process called distribution. How much drug reaches each tissue, and how long it remains in the tissue, depends on the properties of the drug and of the tissue.

After the drug has carried out its intended action, the body should be able to eliminate it by normal physiological processes, such as transformation by enzymes into inactive products (metabolism, biotransformation), or by removal from the body in waste fluids such as urine (excretion). The acronym ADME

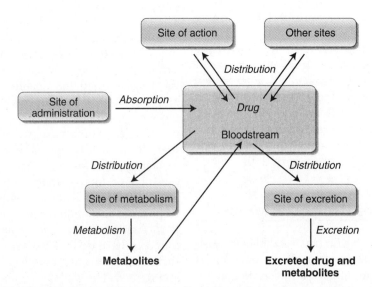

Figure 1.2. A schematic representation of drug absorption and drug disposition processes that follow drug administration.

(using the first letters from the words absorption, distribution, metabolism, and excretion) describes the absorption and disposition behavior of a drug in the body. Figure 1.2 shows a simple representation of these processes.

How Are Drugs Used Clinically in Patients?

The study of the therapeutic uses and effects of drugs in patients is called pharmacotherapeutics. The focus in pharmacotherapy is on the patient being treated, not on the drug or the disorder. Drugs do not behave the same way in all individuals, and variability in drug response is very common. Therapeutic variability seen in clinical practice may be caused by differences in patient body size and composition, age and disease, environmental factors, and genetic influences. It may

also be attributable to unexpected drug interactions that result from two drugs competing for the same mechanisms during a pharmacodynamic or an ADME process. A thorough understanding of pharmaceutical sciences is essential in providing appropriate pharmacotherapy, and in anticipating and avoiding drug interactions.

How Do Genetic Factors Affect Drug Therapy?

An important challenge for pharmaceutical sciences is to understand why individuals respond differently to drug therapy, and then to design drugs considering this variability. The field of pharmacogenomics promises to illuminate many difficult questions about the nature of disease and drug therapy that have been unanswerable so far. It is the study of how

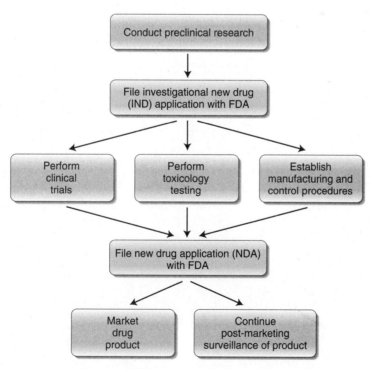

Figure 1.3. A schematic representation of the new drug development, approval, and marketing process.

genetic inheritance affects an individual's response to drugs. Greater knowledge of genes and their proteins will help pharmaceutical scientists to understand the cause of disease and design better drugs. Many pharmaceutical companies are now taking a pharmacogenomic approach in drug research to come up with drugs with consistent and predictable behavior in defined patient populations. Knowledge of genes and proteins and of their functions will also allow scientists to "fix" a genetic defect and cure diseases as an alternative to drug treatment.

How Are New Drugs Developed and Approved for Marketing?

The U.S. Food and Drug Administration (FDA) is the government agency that regulates marketed drug products and approves marketing of new drug products. The FDA defines a drug product as a finished dosage form (e.g., tablet, capsule, or solution) that contains the drug (called the drug substance or active ingredient) in a particular strength, generally in association with one or more other ingredients. The FDA considers the different strengths and dosage forms of a drug separate and distinct drug products.

The process of drug development and discovery is long, complex, and risky. Typically, it takes an average of 10 years for a drug product to make it to pharmacy shelves after its first discovery. The major steps in this discovery, development, and approval process are summarized in Figure 1.3.

CONCLUDING REMARKS

The pharmaceutical sciences comprise a broad range of overlapping disciplines, whose main goal is to design safe and effective drug products based on an understanding of drug action and disposition.

In this book, we will gain an understanding of the fundamental concepts of the pharmaceutical sciences. The first few chapters will lay out the first principles, derived from the basic sciences, on which the pharmaceutical sciences are founded. A thorough knowledge of these principles will set the groundwork for the remainder of the book. The subsequent chapters will examine the application of these first principles to drug delivery, drug disposition, and drug action, and finally to pharmacotherapy and new drug development, using an interdisciplinary and integrated approach.

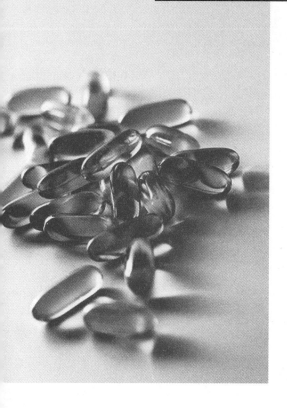

Section I • Basic Principles

Ionization of Drugs

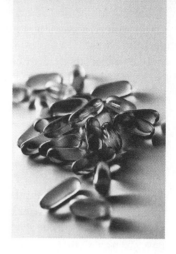

As discussed in Chapter 1, a drug's properties and subsequent behavior are determined by its structure. In particular, physicochemical properties depend on the drug's molecular structure and influence its physical, chemical, and biological performance. One critical physicochemical property is ionization: the process by which an inorganic or organic compound dissociates into two or more ions when dissolved in an aqueous solvent.

Electrolytes and Nonelectrolytes

One way of classifying compounds, including drugs, is based on whether and how much they ionize. If a compound ionizes in solution, the ions formed can conduct an electrical current. A nonelectrolyte is a compound that does not ionize when dissolved in water, but remains entirely as the neutral uncharged species. Examples of such compounds are ethanol, dextrose, and some steroids. A strong electrolyte ionizes completely and exists *solely* as positive and negative ions in solution. An example is NaCl, which exists as Na^+ and Cl^- in aqueous solution. A weak electrolyte is ionizable, but dissociates only *partially*; a fraction of dissolved molecules remain un-ionized, while others dissociate into positive or negative ions. Examples of weak electrolytes are acetic acid and ammonia.

Importance of Ionization

Whereas some drugs are nonelectrolytes and a very few are strong electrolytes, most are weak electrolytes that ionize to some extent in body fluids. Structurally, these ionizable drugs are either weak acids or weak bases, or salts of weak acids and bases. The extent of their ionization depends on strength of the ionizable functional groups and pH of the environment.

The properties of ionized (charged) and un-ionized (uncharged) forms of a drug are dramatically different from each other, even though the only change in structure is the gain or loss of a proton and the presence or absence of a charge. The two forms will be absorbed and distributed differently, will bind to receptors differently, and may be metabolized and eliminated differently. Thus, the proportion of drug ionized or un-ionized in various tissues is a critical factor in determining its overall behavior. Ionization of drugs in the drug product is also important, influencing route of administration and shelf life of the drug product.

The pH of body fluids ranges between 1 and about 8. The stomach is the most acidic region of the body with a pH ranging between 1 and 3. The pH of intestinal fluids is normally about 6 to 7, and the pH of blood is 7.4. Local pH in various tissues depends on composition and function of each tissue, and rarely exceeds 8. Thus, a drug can be expected to encounter physiological environments that vary between pH 1 and pH 8, which makes ionization in this pH range of greatest interest. If a drug does not have a functional group that ionizes in this pH region, it behaves as a nonelectrolyte and remains un-ionized over the entire physiological pH range.

Indomethacin, a weak acid anti-inflammatory drug taken orally, provides a good example of the importance of ionization in drug design. On administration, indomethacin needs to first dissolve in aqueous contents of the gastrointestinal tract. The ionized form of the drug dissolves more rapidly and to a greater extent than the un-ionized form, so that the drug dissolves faster in the small intestines than in the stomach. To enter the bloodstream, however, the drug needs to cross lipophilic cell barriers, which requires at least some of it to be in its un-ionized form in the intestines. Once indomethacin has reached its site of action, interaction with its receptor occurs with the ionized form only. Thus, both ionized and un-ionized forms are important for different aspects of the absorption, distribution, metabolism, and excretion (ADME) and pharmacodynamics of indomethacin.

From a pharmaceutical formulation perspective, it is often important to control pH of a product to minimize drug degradation, to improve patient comfort and compliance, or to improve delivery. Dosage forms, particularly liquids (such as solutions, suspensions, and emulsions), may have pH values outside the pH 1 to 8 range. Higher pH values of pharmaceutical liquids are often required to make the drug more soluble, or to maintain good stability and an adequate shelf life. Thus, in these situations, ionization behavior over a wider pH range has to be considered.

Water as a Solvent

According to the *Bronsted-Lowry* theory of acids and bases, an acid is a compound that can donate a proton and a base is one that can accept a proton. Therefore, there has to be another compound present to receive the proton from the acid, or to provide a proton to the base. In almost all situations we will deal with, this other compound is water, the solvent and medium for all living organisms. Water is also a reactant in many pharmaceutical reactions of interest to us. In addition, water is critical in determining the configuration of proteins and other biological macromolecules that play an important role in drug action.

Water is a remarkable solvent because it can behave as both an acid and a base. Compounds with this dual property are said to be amphoteric and are often called ampholytes. The water molecule possesses a dipole (two electric charges of equal magnitude but of opposite sign or polarity, separated by a small distance), giving it the ability to accept or donate a positively charged proton. Water accepts a proton in the following equilibrium:

$$H^+ + H_2O \rightleftharpoons H_3O^+ \text{ (Eq. 2.1)}$$

The species H_3O^+ is called the hydronium ion. Water can also donate a proton as follows:

$$H_2O \rightleftharpoons H^+ + OH \text{ (Eq. 2.2)}$$

The ionization product constant of water is K_w, given by:

$$K_w = [H^+][OH^-] \qquad \text{(Eq. 2.3)}$$

This relationship says that the product of protons and hydroxide ions in a solution is always constant. The value of K_w at 25°C is 10^{-14}.

Strong Acids and Bases

Let us first examine the behavior of strong acids and bases, so we can distinguish them from weak acids and bases. Strong acids such as HCl and H_2SO_4 dissociate completely in water and exist entirely in their ionized form, making them strong electrolytes.

$$HCl \longrightarrow H^+ + Cl^- \text{ (Eq. 2.4)}$$

$$H_2SO_4 \longrightarrow 2H^+ + SO_4^{-2} \quad \text{(Eq. 2.5)}$$

The H^+ ion formed will react with a water molecule to produce the hydronium ion (see Eq. 2.1), although for convenience we usually do not write the complete reaction. Thus, when a strong acid is added to water, hydrogen ion (actually hydronium ion) concentration in solution increases and pH (defined as pH = $-\log [H^+]$) decreases.

Because a strong acid dissociates completely, the molar concentration of H^+ is equal to the molar concentration of acid added for a monoprotic acid (HCl), and twice the molar acid concentration for a diprotic acid (H_2SO_4).

Similarly, a strong base like NaOH dissociates completely in water and exists entirely in its ionized form:

$$NaOH \longrightarrow Na^+ + OH^- \text{ (Eq. 2.6)}$$

The actual base here is hydroxide ion, OH^-, which will react with H^+ in water (in the reverse reaction shown in Eq. 2.2). Consequently, the concentration of H^+ will decrease and the solution pH will increase. The molar decrease in H^+ concentration will be equal to the molar concentration of NaOH added.

Weak Acids and Bases

Weak acids and bases can also dissociate in water and donate or accept protons. The main difference is that weak acids and bases are only *partially* dissociated in water because of their diminished ability to donate or accept protons.

When a weak acid is added to water, solution pH decreases, but only a fraction of acid molecules dissociate to donate protons to water. The rest of the weak acid molecules remain un-ionized. These compounds exist in solution in two forms—the uncharged, un-ionized species and negatively charged ions. Similarly, when a weak base is dissolved in water, only a fraction of molecules accept protons. Weak bases also exist in solution in two forms—the uncharged, un-ionized species and positively charged ions.

Typical weak acids have the following functionalities:

- Carboxylic acids
- Sulfonic acids
- Phenols
- Thiols
- Imides

Figure 2.1 shows the structures of weak acid functional groups.

Most weak bases fall into the following categories:

- Aliphatic amines (primary, secondary or tertiary)
- Aromatic amines (primary, secondary or tertiary)
- N-heterocycles (pyridine, imidazole)

A few drug compounds are quaternary ammonium salts that look like amines, but do not behave like weak bases. Quaternary ammonium compounds are strong electrolytes, neither acidic nor basic, and dissociate completely in water. Figure 2.2 shows the structures of weak base functional groups and of quaternary ammonium salts.

Many drug compounds are nonelectrolytes and do not behave as acids or

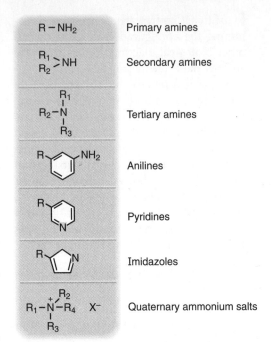

Figure 2.2. Structures of some common weak base functional groups found in drug molecules. Note that quaternary ammonium salts do not behave as weak acids or weak bases, but are strong electrolytes.

bases in aqueous solution. The following functional groups usually do not ionize in the physiological pH range:

- Alcohols and sugars
- Ethers
- Esters
- Ketones
- Aldehydes
- Most amides

Figure 2.3 shows the structures of nonelectrolyte functional groups.

Ionization of Weak Acids and Bases

Weak Acids

Consider the ionization of a weak acid such as acetylsalicylic acid, or aspirin, which has one carboxylic acid group. Its dissociation can be represented by the following:

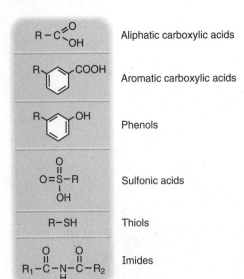

Figure 2.1. Structures of some common weak acid functional groups found in drug molecules.

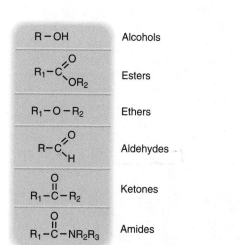

(Eq. 2.7)

In this equilibrium, acetylsalicylic acid is a weak acid because it donates a proton, and the acetylsalicylate ion is a weak base because it accepts a proton. An acid and base that can be represented by an equilibrium in which the two species differ only by a proton is called a conjugate acid–base pair.

K_a is called the acid dissociation constant. A simplified way of representing dissociation of any weak acid, denoted as HA for convenience, is:

$$HA \underset{}{\overset{K_a}{\rightleftharpoons}} A^- + H^+ \quad \text{(Eq. 2.8)}$$

where A^- is the conjugate base of the acid HA.

Weak Bases

Let us examine the conjugate acid–base pair of the weak base benzocaine, for example, with one amine group.

(Eq. 2.9)

A simplified way of representing ionization equilibrium for any base B is:

$$B + H^+ \rightleftharpoons BH^+ \quad \text{(Eq. 2.10)}$$

Here, BH^+ is the conjugate acid of the base B. By convention, we write Equation 2.10 in the reverse form:

$$BH^+ \overset{K_a}{\rightleftharpoons} B + H^+ \quad \text{(Eq. 2.11)}$$

The equilibrium is now expressed as the dissociation of the conjugate acid of the weak base, with K_a as the corresponding acid dissociation constant.

Generalizations

In summary, the dissociation equilibria for acidic forms of conjugate acid–base pairs of a weak acid or base are written as:

$$HA \overset{K_a}{\rightleftharpoons} A^- + H^+ \quad \text{(Eq. 2.12)}$$

$$BH^+ \overset{K_a}{\rightleftharpoons} B + H^+ \quad \text{(Eq. 2.13)}$$

Note that the charge is on the conjugate base form (A^-) of an un-ionized weak acid HA, and on the conjugate acid form (BH^+) of a weak un-ionized base B. Because ions behave differently from uncharged molecules, we are interested in what proportion of a weak acid or weak

R−OH	Alcohols
R₁−C(=O)OR₂	Esters
R₁−O−R₂	Ethers
R−C(=O)H	Aldehydes
R₁−C(=O)−R₂	Ketones
R₁−C(=O)−NR₂R₃	Amides

Figure 2.3. Structures of some common non-electrolyte functional groups.

base is un-ionized or ionized in a given situation; this will help us understand and predict its behavior.

Strength of Weak Acids and Bases

The **law of mass action** describes the dissociation of a weak acid and of the conjugate acid of a weak base. It states that at equilibrium the product of the concentrations on one side of an equation, when divided by the product of concentrations on the other side of the equation, is a constant regardless of the individual concentrations. Therefore, for a weak acid:

$$\frac{[H^+][A^-]}{[HA]} = K_a \qquad (Eq.\ 2.14)$$

A large value of K_a means that the acid favors giving up protons and dissociates extensively. Consequently, the reverse reaction is not favored; the conjugate base A^- is stable and does not have a high propensity to accept protons. The larger the K_a, the stronger the acid HA, and the weaker its conjugate base A^-. Therefore, K_a is a property of the conju-

Polyprotic Acids and Bases

Many drugs and natural substances contain several ionizable groups, as well as many different types of these groups, in the same molecule. These are called **polyprotic** compounds. In particular, compounds with one acidic and one basic group are called amphoteric compounds or ampholytes. Examples are amino acids such as glycine that are the building blocks of proteins.

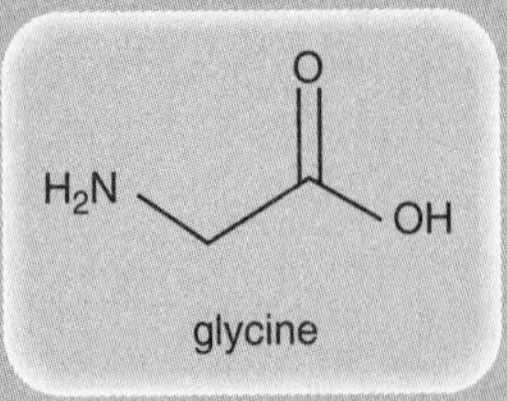

Glycine is amphoteric because it has one acidic carboxylic acid group and one basic amine group. Thus, the ionization of glycine is described by the two equilibria shown below.

K_{a1} is the acid dissociation constant for the carboxylic acid, and K_{a2} is the acid dissociation constant for the protonated amine. The pK$_a$ of the acid is 2.34 and that of the protonated amine is 9.34. Notice that a species with both positive and negative charge, called a **zwitterion**, is formed as a result of these two equilibria. Zwitterions behave like nonelectrolytes because the two charges neutralize each other. An example of an amphoteric drug is piroxicam, which has an acidic pK$_a$ of 4.5 and a basic pK$_a$ of 3.8.

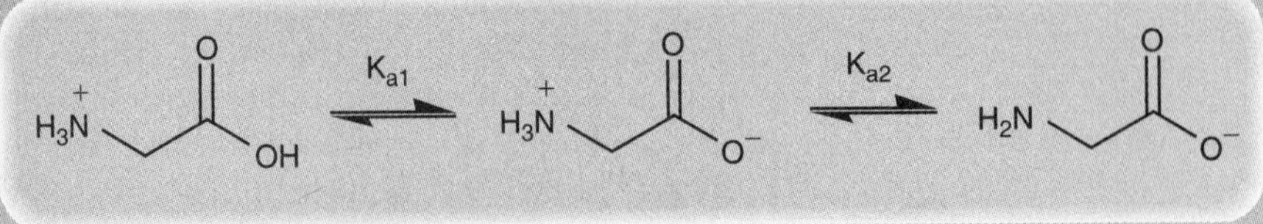

glycine

gate acid–base pair and gives us information about the strengths of both forms.

Similarly, we can define K_a for the conjugate acid of a weak base as: ·

$$\frac{[H^+][B]}{[BH^+]} = K_a \qquad (Eq.\ 2.15)$$

The larger the value of K_a, the more BH^+ dissociates to donate protons. Therefore, the larger the K_a, the stronger the conjugate acid BH^+ is, and the weaker the base B.

The pK$_a$ Value

The negative logarithm of K_a is referred to as the pK_a, giving the following relationship:

$$pK_a = -\log K_a \qquad (Eq.\ 2.16)$$

The symbol p is an operator that converts a number into its negative logarithm. This manipulation makes pK_a smaller as K_a gets larger. In other words, weak acids (or conjugate acids of weak bases) with a large K_a have a small pK_a, and weak acids with a small K_a have a large pK_a.

The pK_a value itself does not tell us whether a drug is a weak acid or base. For example, if a drug has a pK_a value of 5, it could be either a weak acid or a weak base. One way to tell is to examine the structure of the molecule and identify functional groups that are known to be acidic or basic. Another way is to see the types of salts that the compound forms; we shall discuss this below.

The pK_a is a convenient parameter for comparing the strengths of acids or bases. The lower the pK_a of a compound, the stronger the acidic form of the conjugate acid–base pair. As an example, a weak acid with a pK_a of 3 is a stronger acid than a weak acid with a pK_a of 4. Conversely, the higher the pK_a of a compound, the stronger the basic form of the conjugate acid–base pair. A weak base of pK_a 8 is a stronger base than a weak base of pK_a 7.

Each ionizable group on a drug molecule has a pK_a value that conveys its relative strength as a conjugate acid–base pair. Remember that pK_a is always defined for the conjugate acid donating a proton. Therefore, for weak acids, pK_a is defined for the *un-ionized* acid donating a proton to form the *negatively charged* conjugate base. However, the pK_a of a weak base is defined for its *positively charged* conjugate acid donating a proton to give the *un-ionized* base. Table 2.1 shows the relative strengths of some conjugate acid–base pairs. Table 2.2 lists the pK_a ranges for various types of weak acids and bases, and Table 2.3 shows the pK_a values of some common weak acid (HA) and weak base (BH^+) drugs.

TABLE 2.1. The Relative Strengths of Some Conjugate Acid–Base Pairs		
Conjugate Acid	*Conjugate Base*	*pK$_a$*
C_6H_5COOH (benzoic acid)	$C_6H_5COO^-$ (benzoate ion)	4.20
CH_3COOH (acetic acid)	CH_3COO^- (acetate ion)	4.76
$C_6H_5NH_3^+$ (anilinium ion)	$C_6H_5NH_2$ (aniline)	4.70
NH_4^+ (ammonium ion)	NH_3 (ammonia)	9.25
$CH_3NH_3^+$ (methylammonium ion)	CH_3NH_2 (methylamine)	10.6

Acetic acid and benzoic acid are weak acids. Ammonia, methylamine, and aniline are weak bases. Benzoic acid, with a lower pK$_a$, is a stronger acid than acetic acid. Conversely, acetate ion, with a higher pK$_a$, is a stronger base than benzoate ion. Methylamine, with the highest pK$_a$, is a stronger base than ammonia, which is in turn much stronger than aniline. Conversely, anilinium ion is a much stronger acid than ammonium ion, which is stronger than methylammonium ion. Acetic acid and anilinium ion have about the same strength as weak acids, with anilinium ion being a slightly stronger acid because its pK$_a$ is lower.

Salts of Weak Acids and Bases

Weak acid and base drugs are frequently available as their salts. For example, the weak acid drug naproxen is also available as its sodium salt, sodium naproxen. The weak base drug clonidine is also available in its salt form, clonidine hydrochloride. The salt of a weak acid is usually obtained by reacting it with a strong base such as NaOH, which gives the sodium salt. The salt of a weak base is obtained by reacting it with a strong acid such as HCl, which gives the hydrochloride salt. Some drug salts are also made by combining weak acids with weak bases. An example is chlorpheniramine maleate, a salt of the weak base drug chlorpheniramine with a weak acid, maleic acid.

Salt formation can give us information about whether a drug in its un-ionized form is a weak acid or base. Weak un-ionized acids form salts with strong bases, such as NaOH, KOH, and $Ca(OH)_2$, to give sodium, potassium, or calcium salts of the weak acid. Conversely, weak un-ionized bases form salts with strong acids such as HCl, H_2SO_4, and HNO_3, to give hydrochloride, sulfate, or nitrate salts.

TABLE 2.3. pK_a Values of Some Weak Acid, Weak Base, and Polyprotic Drugs[a]

| Drug | pK_a Values | |
	HA	BH+
Penicillin G	2.8	
Aspirin	3.5	
Warfarin	5.1	
Phenytoin	8.3	
Phenothiazine		2.5
Oxycodone		7.0
Scopolamine		7.6
Morphine		8.0
Captopril	3.7, 9.8	
Baclofen	5.4	9.5
Ampicillin	2.5	7.2
Doxycycline		8.2, 10.2

[a]Note that for bases, the pK_a value reflects that of the conjugate acid (BH+) form.

TABLE 2.2. pK_a Ranges of Weak Acids and Weak Bases

Weak Acids	
Type of Compound	pK_a Range
Carboxylic acids (RCOOH)	2 to 6
Sulfonic acids (RSO_3H)	−1 to 1
Phenols (ArOH)	7 to 11
Thiols (RSH)	7 to 10
Imides (—CONHCO—)	8 to 11
Sulfonamides ($RNHSO_2R$)	6 to 8
Weak Bases	
Type of Compound	pK_a Range
Aliphatic amines	8 to 11
Anilines	3 to 5
Pyridines	4 to 6
Saturated nitrogen heterocycles	9 to 11

Ionization and pH

We defined weak electrolytes, such as weak acids and weak bases and their salts, as compounds that ionize only *partially* when dissolved in water. The degree of ionization depends not only on the pK_a of the acid or base, but also on the pH of the aqueous solution in which it is dissolved.

The Henderson–Hasselbalch Equation

Equation 2.14 or 2.15 can be used to find the relationship between pK_a, pH, and concentration of drug in its acid and base forms. Taking logarithms of both sides of the equations, and rearranging appropriately, gives the Henderson–Hasselbalch equation. Whether we start with Equation 2.14 or 2.15, we get:

$$pH = pK_a + \log \frac{[base]}{[acid]} \quad \text{(Eq. 2.17)}$$

where [*base*] is the concentration of the basic form of the drug, and [*acid*] is the concentration of the acidic form

Pharmaceutical Salts

Pharmaceutical companies often prefer to develop the salt form of a drug rather than the weak acid or base form for several reasons. Salts are usually easier to crystallize into stable, manufacturable crystals, salts dissolve faster in aqueous solutions, salts are more stable on storage, and salts are easier to handle and manipulate during manufacturing. In particular, salts of amine drugs are preferred over the weak base form. Many amines are volatile and unstable, and have a short shelf life as solids. Stability and shelf life improve dramatically if an amine is converted to the hydrochloride salt, for example. The pK_a of the drug does not change when a salt is made; salts have to obey the same acid–base equilibria as the weak acids and bases they originate from.

Selecting an *appropriate* salt for a drug is an important factor in early stages of new drug development. Different salts of the same active drug are distinct products, with individual chemical and biological profiles that underlie differences in their clinical efficacy and safety. Thus, changing a drug's salt form is a common way of modifying its chemical and biological properties without modifying its fundamental structure.

Calcium supplements are a good example of potential variation in therapeutic efficacy with salt form. Various products are available, each containing a different calcium salt (such as carbonate, citrate, gluconate, and lactate). The salts have different rates of absorption and are reported to vary in their effectiveness as calcium supplements in osteoporosis.

of the drug. It is very important to remember that for a weak acid drug, [*acid*] is the concentration of the unionized HA and [*base*] is the concentration of the ion A$^-$, while, for a weak base, [*acid*] is the concentration of the ion BH$^+$ and [*base*] is the concentration of the un-ionized B.

You may find the Henderson–Hasselbalch equation written in various forms that all result from rearranging Equation 2.17 in different ways.

$$pH = pK_a - \log \frac{[acid]}{[base]} \quad \text{(Eq. 2.18)}$$

$$pK_a = pH + \log \frac{[acid]}{[base]} \quad \text{(Eq. 2.19)}$$

$$pK_a = pH - \log \frac{[base]}{[acid]} \quad \text{(Eq. 2.20)}$$

All of these equations give the same information.

The Henderson–Hasselbalch equation allows us to calculate the *ratio* between acidic and basic forms of a drug if pK_a of the drug and pH of the solvent are known. From this ratio we can determine the *fraction* or *percentage* of drug that is in its acidic or basic form in various pH environments.

Ionization in Buffered Solutions

Buffers

A buffered solution is one that resists changes in its pH when small amounts of acid or base are added, or when the solution is diluted. Buffers need an acid to react with added OH$^-$ and a base to react with added H^+. These can be any pair of a weak acid and a weak base, but are usually a conjugate acid–conjugate base pair. The pH of the buffer depends on the pK_a of the buffering substance and on the relative concentrations of conjugate acid and base, and can be calculated using the Henderson–Hasselbalch equation.

Acidic buffer solutions (with pH values less than 7) are commonly made from a weak acid and one of its salts—often a sodium salt. An example is a mixture of acetic acid ($pK_a = 4.75$) and sodium acetate in solution. If the solution contains equimolar concentrations of the acid and the salt, it has a pH of 4.75. The ions are involved in the following equilibrium:

$$CH_3COOH \underset{}{\overset{K_a}{\rightleftharpoons}} CH_3COO^- + H^+$$

(Eq. 2.21)

If additional hydrogen ions are added, they are consumed in the reaction with CH_3COO^-, and the equilibrium shifts to the left. If additional hydroxide ions enter, they react with CH_3COOH, producing CH_3COO^-, and shift the equilibrium to the right. Thus, the pH of the solution remains constant.

An alkaline buffer solution (pH greater than 7) is commonly made from a weak base and one of its salts. An example is a mixture of ammonia ($pK_a = 9.25$) and ammonium chloride solutions. If these are mixed in equimolar proportions, the solution has a pH of 9.25.

Buffer capacity is the amount of added acid or base the buffer can neutralize before the solution pH begins to change to an appreciable degree. A buffer system is most useful at a solution pH at or close to its pK_a, because there is an adequate concentration of both the conjugate acid and base forms of the buffer to neutralize added acid or base. Thus, the most effective buffers (with a large buffer capacity) contain the acid and base in large and equal amounts.

Pharmaceutical formulations are often buffered to control pH so as to minimize drug degradation, to improve patient comfort and compliance, or to improve the efficacy of delivery.

Biological Buffers

The pH of body fluids can vary from pH 8 in pancreatic fluid to pH 1 in the stomach. The average pH of blood is 7.4, and of cells is 7.0 to 7.3. Although there is great variation in pH between fluids in the body, there is little variation within each system. For example, blood pH only varies between 7.35 and 7.45 in a healthy individual. Proteins are the most important buffers in the body, because their amino and carboxylic acid groups act as proton acceptors or donors as hydrogen ions are added or removed from the environment. Other nonprotein buffer systems are also important.

The phosphate buffer system is important in maintaining pH of intracellular fluid. This buffer system consists of dihydrogen phosphate ions ($H_2PO_4^-$) as proton donor (acid) and hydrogen phosphate ions (HPO_4^{2-}) as proton acceptor (base). These two ions are in equilibrium with each other as indicated by the equation below:

$$H_2PO_4^- \rightleftharpoons HPO_4^{2-} + H^+ \quad \text{(Eq. 2.22)}$$

If additional hydrogen ions enter, they are consumed in the reaction with HPO_4^{2-}, and if additional hydroxide ions enter, they react with $H_2PO_4^-$, producing HPO_4^{2-}. Thus, the pH of cellular fluid is kept constant.

Consequences of Ionization

Many pharmaceutical systems are buffered and maintain a constant pH. When an acidic or basic drug or its salt is added to a properly buffered solution, the pH of the solution does not change. Rather, the concentrations of un-ionized and ionized drug adjust appropriately to obey the Henderson–Hasselbalch equation. The percentage of drug ionized and un-ionized is of interest because charged and uncharged drug molecules behave and react differently in drug products as well as in the body. Remember that for weak acids (and their salts), the *conjugate base* carries a negative charge, whereas for weak bases (and their salts), it is the *conjugate acid* that carries a positive charge. Thus, we also need to know whether the drug (in its uncharged form) is a weak acid or a weak base.

Once we know how much of the drug is ionized and un-ionized at any location, e.g., in a drug product, blood, urine, a tissue, or in the cell, we can explain or anticipate some of the drug's behavior, as we will learn in the following chapters.

Ionization in Unbuffered Solutions

Ionization of weak electrolyte drugs in unbuffered solutions is more complex, because pH does not remain constant as the drug dissolves. Consider a weak acid drug, such as RCOOH, and its basic sodium salt, $RCOO^-Na^+$. When RCOOH is dissolved in water, we are adding an *acid* to water and the pH will decrease. If RCOONa is dissolved in water, we are adding the *conjugate base* $RCOO^-$ to water and the pH will increase. In both cases, equilibrium will be established between the acid and conjugate base forms in accordance with the Henderson–Hasselbalch equation. The proportion of ionized or un-ionized drug in each case will depend on pK_a of the weak acid, and the final solution pH. The pK_a of the two forms is the same, because pK_a defines the equilibrium between these two forms. Thus, the fraction ionized or un-ionized in these two cases will be different because the final pH of the two solutions will be different.

pH of Unbuffered Solutions

The pH of an unbuffered solution containing a weak acid or base depends on the pK_a of the weak acid or base and its concentration in solution. Consider the example of a weak acid added to water. An approximate expression relating the $[H^+]$ concentration with the pK_a and concentration is obtained under the assumption that the concentration of $[H^+]$ is much less than the total concentration of the acid $[HA]_t$ (i.e., the acid is "very weak"). It can be used, however, to estimate the hydrogen ion concentration in the solution of the weak acid.

$$[H^+] \approx \sqrt{K_a[HA]_t}$$

where $[HA]_t$ is the total concentration of weak acid added to the solution.

The pH of the solution can be calculated from $[H^+]$.

This equation shows that a large K_a (small pK_a) and a large concentration result in a more acidic solution. When a salt of a weak *base* is added to water, it is similar to adding a weak acid to water, and the pH will be given by the equation above.

Similarly, the $[H^+]$ of a solution after a base is added to water is given by:

$$[H^+] = \frac{K_w}{[OH]} \approx \sqrt{\frac{K_w \cdot K_a}{[B]_t}}$$

where $[B]_t$ is the total concentration of base added. This expression also gives the acidity of a solution made with the salt of a weak acid.

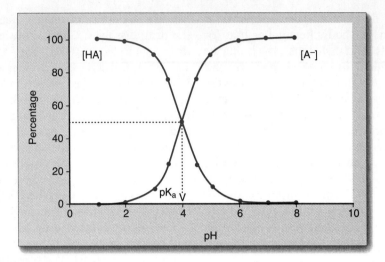

Figure 2.4. Percentage of un-ionized [HA] and ionized [A$^-$] forms as a function of pH for a weak acid with pK$_a$ = 4. At pH = pK$_a$, the weak acid is 50% ionized and 50% un-ionized.

Similarly, if we add a weak base (RNH$_2$) to water the pH will increase, and if we dissolve the acidic salt of the weak base (e.g., a salt such as RNH$_3^+$Cl$^-$, also written as RNH$_2$.HCl) in water, the pH will decrease. In both cases, there will be equilibrium between RNH$_3^+$ and RNH$_2$ in solution, but the relative amounts of ionized and un-ionized drug will be different in the two solutions, because the final pH of the two solutions will be different.

pH–Ionization Profiles

Figure 2.4 shows the percentage of [*acid*] and [*base*] forms as a function of pH for a weak acid of pK$_a$ = 4. Figure 2.5 shows a similar profile for a weak base of pK$_a$ = 8. These graphs were constructed using the Henderson–Hasselbalch equation, which allows us to calculate the ratio of [*acid*]/[*base*] at any pH value if we know the pK$_a$. From this ratio, the percentage (or fraction) of each form can be

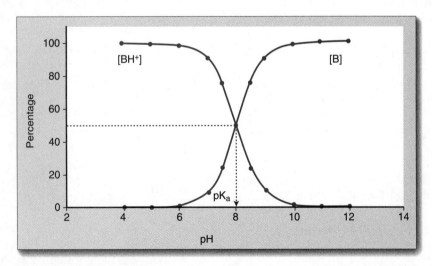

Figure 2.5. Percentage of un-ionized [B] and ionized [BH$^+$] forms as a function of pH for a weak base with pK$_a$ = 8. At pH = pK$_a$, the weak base is 50% ionized and 50% un-ionized.

TABLE 2.4. Dependence of Fraction or Percent Ionization on the pH and the pK_a of a Weak Acid or Weak Base		
$pH–pK_a$	Percent (Conjugate Acid Form)	Percent (Conjugate Base Form)
−4	99.99	0.01
−3	99.9	0.10
−2	99.0	1.00
−1	90.9	9.10
−0.8	86.3	13.7
−0.6	79.9	20.1
−0.4	71.5	28.5
−0.2	61.3	38.7
0	50.0	50.0
0.2	38.7	61.3
0.4	28.5	71.5
0.6	20.1	79.9
0.8	13.7	86.3
1	9.10	90.9
2	1.00	99.0
3	0.10	99.9
4	0.01	99.99

determined. For example, if [acid]/[base] = 0.1, then the fraction of the acid form = 0.1/(1 + 0.1) = 0.0909 (or 9.09%).

Table 2.4 shows how the degree of ionization of a weak acid or weak base changes with the relative values of pH and pK_a. Overall, the following generalizations can be made:

- A weak acid will be more ionized (negatively charged) when the pH is above its pK_a, whereas a weak base will be more ionized (positively charged) when the pH is below its pK_a.
- Small changes in pH (within 2 pH units) near the pK_a of the compound result in large changes in the percentage ionized and un-ionized.
- Changes in pH away (more than 2 pH units) from the pK_a of the compound result in small changes in the degree of ionization.
- A weak acid is almost completely un-ionized when the pH is 4 units below its pK_a, and completely ionized when the pH is 4 units above its pK_a.
- A weak base is almost completely un-ionized when the pH is 4 units above its pK_a, and completely ionized when the pH is 4 units below its pK_a.

KEY CONCEPTS

In this chapter, we have considered one important physicochemical property of a drug, ionization.

- When dissolved in water, a strong electrolyte dissociates completely, a weak electrolyte dissociates only partially, and a nonelectrolyte does not dissociate.
- Many drugs are weak electrolytes and are classified as weak acids and weak bases.
- The pK_a value of a weak acid or base is a measure of its strength.
- The extent of ionization of a weak electrolyte depends on its pK_a and the pH of the medium.
- The Henderson–Hasselbalch equation can be used to calculate the relative proportions of ionized and unionized forms of weak electrolytes.
- Drugs are present in very different proportions of uncharged and charged forms in various physiological fluids.
- The chemical, ADME, and pharmacological properties of the charged and uncharged forms can be dramatically different.

ADDITIONAL READING

1. Amiji M, Sandmann BJ. Applied Physical Pharmacy, 1st ed. McGraw-Hill/Appleton & Lange, 2003.

2. Connors KA. Thermodynamics of Pharmaceutical Systems—An Introduction for Students of Pharmacy. Wiley Interscience, 2002.

3. Florence AT, Attwood D. Physicochemical Principles of Pharmacy, 3rd ed. MacMillan Education, Ltd, 1998.

4. Martin AN, Bustamante P. Physical Pharmacy—Physical Chemical Principles in the Pharmaceutical Sciences, 4th ed. Lippincott Williams & Wilkins, 1993.

REVIEW QUESTIONS

1. Compare and contrast the ionization behavior of nonelectrolytes, weak electrolytes, and strong electrolytes when they are dissolved in water.
2. Describe what is meant by weak acid, weak base, strong acid, and strong base.
3. List the functional groups that have weak acid, weak base, and non-electrolyte properties in the physiological pH range.
4. Explain what is meant by conjugate acid–base pair. Which form of the pair, the conjugate acid or conjugate base, is charged for a weak acid? A weak base? Is this charge positive or negative?
5. How do the equilibrium acid dissociation constant, K_a, and the pK_a give you information about the strength of a weak acid or base?
6. Explain the difference between a buffered and an unbuffered solution. How does the pH of an unbuffered solution change when an acid or base is added to it? When a salt of a weak acid or weak base is added to it?
7. Discuss the use of the Henderson–Hasselbalch equation in making buffers and in determining percentage of drugs ionized at different pH values.

PRACTICE PROBLEMS

1. The K_a for the dissociation of acetic acid is 1.74×10^{-5}. What is its pK_a? ($pK_a = -\log K_a = 4.76$)
2. The pK_a of propranolol is 9.5. What is its K_a?
3. Glyburide is a weak acid drug used in the treatment of diabetes. It has a $pK_a = 6.8$.
   a) What is the K_a of glyburide?
   b) Which form of the conjugate acid– base pair is charged, and what charge (positive or negative) does it bear?
   c) What percentage of glyburide is ionized in the small intestines (pH = 6)? In the blood (pH = 7.4)?
4. Naproxen (Aleve) is an anti-inflammatory drug with a molecular weight of 230 and a $pK_a = 4.2$. It has the following structure:0

   a) Is naproxen a weak acid or weak base?
   b) At what buffer pH will the concentration of the conjugate acid

and conjugate base be equal?
   c) When naproxen is added to an unbuffered solution, will the pH of the solution go up or down? Why?
   d) What fraction of naproxen is ionized in a buffer at pH 3 and a buffer at pH 6?
   e) In a 25 mg/mL solution of naproxen in a pH 6 buffer, what will be the molar concentration of the drug in its ionized and un-ionized forms?
   f) Naproxen is also available as its sodium salt. When naproxen sodium is added to an unbuffered solution, will the pH of the solution go up or down? Why?
5. Cimetidine (Tagamet) is a drug used to treat duodenal ulcers to reduce excessive secretion of gastric acid. The drug has a $pK_a = 6.8$ and is also available as its hydrochloride salt.

   a) Is cimetidine a weak acid or a weak base?
   b) What fraction of cimetidine is un-ionized in the stomach (pH = 1), small intestines (pH = 6), and blood (pH = 7.4)?
   c) When cimetidine hydrochloride is added to an unbuffered solution, will the pH of the solution go up or down? Why?

Solubility and Lipophilicity

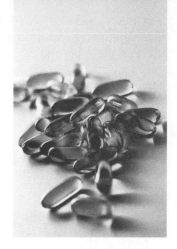

To be a successful drug, a compound has to be somewhat soluble in polar environments such as water and aqueous solutions, and in nonpolar environments such as lipids. Aqueous solubility is necessary because most of the body is made up of water; thus a drug must dissolve in these aqueous environments to enter and travel through the body. Lipid solubility is needed because cells and tissues have lipids that act as barriers, and the drug needs to dissolve in these barriers to cross them and reach the site of action. Thus, a drug needs to have a combination of hydrophilic (water-loving) and lipophilic (lipid-loving) properties.

Water Solubility

The aqueous solubility of a compound is a measure of its hydrophilicity or polarity. When a drug product is administered to the body it usually encounters an aqueous environment in which the drug must dissolve. For example, an orally administered drug must dissolve in gastric fluids. If a drug is not sufficiently water soluble and has trouble dissolving, all of it may not be available to the body. Thus, adequate aqueous solubility is an important property for a drug.

Water as a Solvent

Water is a good solvent for molecules that can interact with it in some way. Recall that the water molecule has a dipole that can form certain kinds of bonds with compatible molecules. The primary interactions that allow a drug molecule to dissolve in water are:

- *Ion–Dipole Interaction:* Ion–dipole bonds are formed between an ion and an uncharged polar molecule with a permanent dipole moment, like water. This interaction represents the strongest force for water solubility of drugs. Thus, ionized molecules (i.e., those with a charge) are generally very soluble in water.
- *Van der Waals Forces:* The attractive forces between electrically neutral molecules are collectively called van der Waals forces. These intermolecular forces are much weaker than covalent bonds, and operate when molecules are at a close or moderate distance from each other.
- *Dipole–Dipole Interaction:* Polar molecules with permanent dipole moments but no charge can interact with each other at close distances. Permanent dipoles usually exist in molecules that have an electronegative atom (such as O, N, S, or a halogen) attached to a carbon. Thus, water can interact with drug molecules with dipoles, even if they are not charged. This interaction is usually weaker than the ion–dipole bond.
- *Dipole-Induced Dipole Interaction:* A polar molecule with a permanent dipole can temporarily induce a dipole in a nonpolar molecule, resulting in an attractive force that brings the two molecules together. Thus, water can induce a dipole in a nonpolar drug molecule. Obviously, this interaction is very weak and results in low water solubility.
- *Hydrogen Bonds:* Hydrogen bonds are abnormally strong dipole–dipole attractions that involve molecules with –OH, –NH, or FH groups. When a bonded electronegative atom (such as oxygen, nitrogen, or fluorine) pulls electrons away from the hydrogen atom, the result is a concentrated positive charge on the hydrogen (called the *hydrogen bond donor*). This hydrogen is strongly attracted to small, electron-rich O, N, and F atoms (called the *hydrogen bond acceptor*) on other molecules. Larger electron-rich groups and atoms like Cl will also attract the hydrogen, but because their electrons are not as tightly concentrated, the resulting dipole–dipole attraction is too weak to be considered a "real" hydrogen bond.

Hydrogen bonds contribute significantly to aqueous solubility of drugs because water can function as both a donor and acceptor of hydrogen bonds. Once one hydrogen bond forms, the probability of a second one forming may be increased, leading to an increased probability of a third forming, and so on. This can lead to a very strong and stable structure, even though it is made up of individually weak hydrogen bonds. This phenomenon is very important in the chemical and biological properties of water.

Intrinsic Aqueous Solubility

For simplicity, first consider a nonelectrolyte drug dissolved in water. The solubility of a compound is the concentration of a saturated solution of the compound in a given solvent (in our case, water) at a given temperature. In a saturated solution, the solid form of the drug is in equilibrium with drug in solution, as follows:

$$\text{Drug}_{\text{solid}} \rightleftharpoons \text{Drug}_{\text{solution}} \quad \text{(Eq. 3.1)}$$

This means further addition of solid drug will not change the solution concentration because no more drug can dissolve. The equilibrium constant K is given by:

$$K = \frac{[\text{Drug}]_{\text{solution}}}{[\text{Drug}]_{\text{solid}}} \qquad \text{(Eq. 3.2)}$$

The numerator of Equation 3.2 is the concentration of drug dissolved in the saturated solution. The denominator is, by convention, equal to 1. The constant K is called the intrinsic solubility (S_0) of the nonelectrolyte drug in water at the temperature of the experiment; in other words S_0 is the concentration of the saturated solution of drug, as shown below:

$$S_0 = K = [\text{Drug}]_{\text{solution}} \qquad \text{(Eq. 3.3)}$$

Intrinsic water solubility depends on the drug's chemical structure and solid-state structure as well as the temperature of the solution. The intrinsic solubility of most compounds increases as temperature increases, so solubility is always stated along with the temperature of measurement. The temperatures of most interest for pharmaceutical application are normal body temperature (37°C) and controlled room temperature (15° to 30°C).

Polar solvents like water are able to solvate molecules and ions through dipole interactions, particularly hydrogen bonding, allowing the compound to dissolve in water. If the drug has many polar functional groups capable of interacting with water, its intrinsic aqueous solubility will be high.

Nonpolar solvents, such as hydrocarbons and lipids, cannot reduce attraction between the ions of electrolytes and are said to have a low dielectric constant. These solvents also cannot break covalent bonds and cause weak electrolytes to ionize, resulting in poor solubility for ionic and polar solutes. However, nonpolar solutes dissolve in nonpolar solvents quite well because of induced dipole interactions. Thus, nonpolar drugs dissolve poorly in water, but dissolve well in lipids; this leads to the simple maxim of *like dissolves like*.

Crystalline and Amorphous Solids

Intrinsic solubility also depends on the solid-state structure of the drug, because solubility is an equilibrium condition between the drug in the solid and solution phases. Many drug substances can exist in more than one solid form with different spatial arrangement of molecules. There are two main classes of solids, crystalline and amorphous, based on the arrangement of atoms or molecules in the solid-state structure.

Crystalline solids possess a regular, repetitive internal arrangement of atoms, molecules, or ions in a structure called a crystal lattice. The concept of symmetry describes the repetition of structural features; crystals therefore possess symmetry. The unit cell is the simplest repeating unit in a crystal; it consists of a specific group of atoms or molecules bonded to one another in a set geometric arrangement. This unit and its constituent atoms or molecules are then repeated over and over to construct the crystal lattice.

Crystalline solids show a definite melting point, converting rather sharply from solid to liquid state over a narrow temperature range. The melting point is an indication of the strength of the crystal lattice; the stronger the lattice, the higher the melting point.

There are four types of crystalline solids:

1. Ionic: these have ions occupying crystal lattice points in the crystal. Ionic solids have high melting and boiling points because of the strong ion–ion forces holding these ions in the structure.
2. Molecular: these have neutral molecules occupying crystal lattice points. Forces holding these molecules in the crystal are weaker intermolecular forces. Because these forces are not as strong as the ion–ion forces in ionic solids, molecular solids tend to have lower melting points compared with ionic solids.

3. Macromolecular: these have very strong covalent bonding in the crystal and therefore have extremely high melting points.
4. Metallic: these are elemental crystals whose atoms are held in position in the crystal lattice by metallic bonding forces.

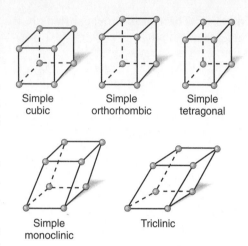

Most drugs are either molecular or ionic solids. Crystalline solids are categorized as members of 32 possible crystal classes on the basis of types of symmetry. Each crystal class is then placed into one of six different crystal systems so that several different classes are members of each system; five of these systems are shown in Figure 3.1.

Crystalline drugs occur as single molecular crystals as stated above or as molecular adducts containing a second component in addition to the drug. Solvates are crystalline adducts containing molecules of a solvent incorporated within the crystal lattice. If the incorporated solvent is water, solvates are commonly known as hydrates.

Amorphous solids consist of disordered arrangements of molecules and do not possess a distinguishable crystal lattice. These materials do not have a characteristic melting temperature but soften over a very wide temperature range, generally lower than the melting points of the crystalline forms of the same compound. A

Figure 3.1. Types of crystal lattice structures in which drugs can crystallize. The molecules in a crystalline solid are designated as points, forming an array called a lattice. The lines between adjacent molecules help to show the particular three-dimensional grid with a repeating structure.

given drug may exist in several crystalline forms as well as in an amorphous form. For example, chloramphenicol-3-palmitate, a broad-spectrum antibiotic, is known to exist in one amorphous form and at least three different crystalline forms.

The crystal lattice of a drug has to be disrupted by the solvent before the drug can dissolve. If the molecules of a drug are held together tightly in the crystal lattice, the driving force for the drug to dissolve is

Forms of Insulin

Insulin is available in both the amorphous and crystalline forms. The intermediate-acting insulin suspension for injection contains the amorphous form of the drug, whereas the longer-acting product contains crystalline insulin. The differing rates of dissolution of these two solid forms after injection are responsible for the differing response rates. The amorphous form has a higher intrinsic solubility, dissolves faster, and enters the bloodstream more rapidly after injection. The crystalline form has a crystal lattice, a lower intrinsic solubility, and a slower dissolution rate. It therefore reaches the bloodstream more slowly.

lower. Hence, crystalline drugs have lower intrinsic solubility compared with the same drug in its amorphous form.

Polymorphs

Each of the crystal classes mentioned above can be further characterized as various crystal forms with a unique symmetry. Many drug substances can exist in more than one crystal form; this property is known as polymorphism, and the individual crystal forms are called polymorphs. Different polymorphs arise from differences in the crystallization process, particularly the solvent used, the rate of cooling during crystallization, and the pressure on crystallization. Polymorphs have the same molecular structure but different crystal forms. A large number of pharmaceuticals, such as the barbiturates, sulfonamides, and steroids, exhibit extensive polymorphism.

Polymorphs, although chemically identical, generally have different crystal lattice energies, melting points, and intrinsic solubilities. The different solubilities of polymorphic forms of a given drug may lead to differences in the rate at which the drug is absorbed into the body after administration. The objective of achieving faster drug dissolution in the body may suggest the use of the amorphous or the lower melting point polymorph in the drug product. These forms, however, might crystallize into the stable form at any stage of the "life cycle" of a pharmaceutical product, i.e., during manufacturing, packaging, distribution, and storage, leading to unexpected changes in behavior. The polymorphic behavior of drugs is a major concern of the pharmaceutical industry because it has considerable formulation, therapeutic, legal, and commercial implications.

Ritonavir Polymorphism

Ritonavir (Norvir; Abbott) is a protease inhibitor drug used in the treatment of patients infected with the HIV-1 virus. During early development, ritonavir was thought to exist in only one monoclinic form during development and early manufacturing. This form, now called Form I, was poorly absorbed into the bloodstream after oral administration, requiring Norvir to be formulated as a soft-gelatin capsule filled with an ethanol–water solution containing dissolved drug. Two years after marketing, several batches of Norvir capsules showed that the drug was dissolving much slower than the desired rate. Evaluation of the failed batches revealed that a second polymorphic crystal form of ritonavir (Form II) had precipitated from the formulation during storage. This polymorph had a 50% lower intrinsic solubility compared with Form I, resulting in the lower rate of dissolution observed. To ensure continuous supply of this life-saving drug, an oral liquid formulation had to be introduced to the market until the issue of polymorphic forms was resolved. Precipitation of Form II was also observed in the oral solution of Norvir when the solution was refrigerated, and patients were advised to store this solution at room temperature to avoid precipitation.

Substantial time and effort went into identifying and correcting the problem, and a new oral soft-gelatin capsule formulation was subsequently developed and introduced onto the market.

Solubility of Weak Acids and Bases

The ionization of weak acids and bases in water complicates the solubility equation. For drugs that ionize in water, observed solubility depends not only on the intrinsic solubility of the un-ionized drug but on the extent of ionization as well. In general, aqueous solubility of ions is much greater than solubility of the corresponding un-ionized form.

When a solid weak electrolyte drug is added to an aqueous medium, it will dissolve to the extent of the intrinsic solubility of the un-ionized form. The dissolved drug will then ionize in accordance with the Henderson–Hasselbalch equation and the pH of the aqueous medium. As the drug ionizes, more solid drug will dissolve to maintain a saturated solution of the un-ionized form of drug. This process will continue until both the solubility equilibrium and ionization equilibrium are satisfied.

We can write the following equations for the solubility and subsequent ionization of a weak acid and a weak base in a buffered solution:

$$HA_{solid} \rightleftharpoons HA_{solution} \rightleftharpoons H^+ + A^-$$

(Eq. 3.4)

$$B_{solid} \rightleftharpoons B_{solution} + H^+ \rightleftharpoons BH^+$$

(Eq. 3.5)

The saturated solutions of both HA and B will contain some ionized and some un-ionized forms of the drug, depending on the pH of the buffer. The total observed solubility, S_t, therefore, is the total concentration of drug (ionized and un-ionized) in solution, as shown by the following equations:

$$\text{Weak acid: } S_t = [HA]_{solution} + [A^-]$$

(Eq. 3.6)

$$\text{Weak base: } S_t = [B]_{solution} + [BH^+]$$

(Eq. 3.7)

The concentration of un-ionized drug in this saturated solution is actually the intrinsic solubility of the drug, as defined earlier for nonelectrolytes. Therefore, we can rewrite Equations 3.6 and 3.7 as follows:

$$\text{Weak acid: } S_t = S_{0(HA)} + [A^-]$$

(Eq. 3.8)

$$\text{Weak base: } S_t = S_{0(B)} + [BH^+]$$

(Eq. 3.9)

Knowing the concentration of the un-ionized form, the pK_a of the drug, and the pH of the medium allows us to calculate the concentration of the ionized form using the Henderson–Hasselbalch equation. After incorporating these relationships into Equations 3.8 and 3.9, we get the following general equations:

Weak acid:

$$S_t = S_0 + \frac{K_a \bullet S_0}{[H^+]} = S_0 \left[1 + \frac{K_a}{[H^+]} \right]$$

(Eq. 3.10)

Weak base:

$$S_t = S_0 + \frac{[H^+] \bullet S_0}{K_a} = S_0 \left[1 + \frac{[H^+]}{K_a} \right]$$

(Eq. 3.11)

pH–Solubility Profiles

Figure 3.2 shows a graphical representation of the pH–solubility profiles for a weak acid and a weak base. The graphs show that if the pH of the solution allows ionization of a weak electrolyte drug, total solubility will be greater than intrinsic solubility. As the degree of ionization increases, total solubility of the drug also increases. If the pH of the solution keeps the drug essentially un-ionized, total solubility is equal to intrinsic solubility of the drug. A weak base will show higher solubility at a low pH and a lower

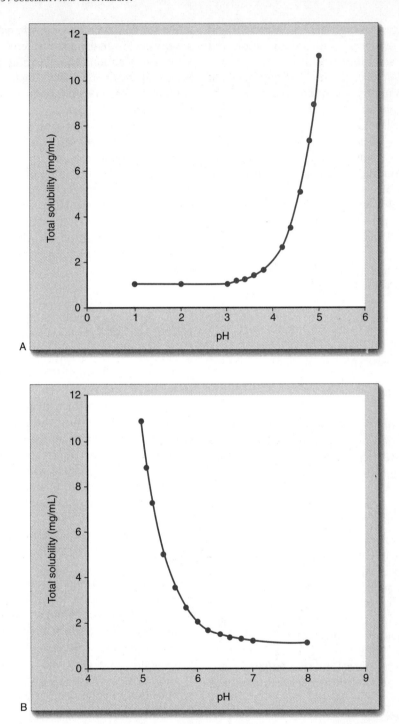

Figure 3.2. The pH–solubility profiles for a weak acid and a weak base. Graph A shows the total solubility as a function of pH for a weak acid of $pK_a = 4$. Graph B shows the total solubility as a function of pH for a weak base of $pK_a = 6$. Both compounds have an intrinsic solubility of 1 mg/mL.

solubility at a high pH. A weak acid will show a higher solubility at a high pH and a lower solubility at a low pH.

Equations 3.8 and 3.9 predict that total solubility will increase infinitely as ionization increases. However, the solubility of the ionized drug is actually limited by a parameter called the *solubility product*, which depends on the type and concentration of the counter-ions present in solution.

A useful way to write the relationship between pH, pK_a, and solubility of weak acids and bases is as follows:

$$\text{Weak acid: } pK_a = pH - \log \frac{S_t - S_0}{S_0}$$

(Eq. 3.12)

$$\text{Weak base: } pK_a = pH - \log \frac{S_0}{S_t - S_0}$$

(Eq. 3.13)

Equations 3.12 and 3.13 can be used to calculate the total solubility of a drug at any pH if the pK_a and intrinsic solubility are known.

Solubility of Salts

Many weak acid and weak base drugs are available as their salts. The physical properties of salts (crystal structure, melting point, and so forth) are usually very different from those of their parent weak acid or weak base. However, salt formation does not change the pK_a and intrinsic solubility of a weak acid or weak base. Therefore, in a *buffered* solution, total solubility of a weak acid and its salt (or a weak base and its salt) is the same.

Nevertheless, we have seen that when weak acids, bases, or their salts are dissolved in an *unbuffered* solution, the pH of the solution changes. When a weak acid is dissolved in water to make a saturated solution, the pH of the solution becomes lower than the pK_a of the acid, resulting in

a low solubility. Conversely, when a *salt* of a weak acid is dissolved in water to make a saturated solution, the solution pH increases above the pK_a, resulting in a higher solubility. Analogous behavior is seen with weak bases and their salts.

One may generalize and say that saturated solutions of salts in unbuffered solutions promote a pH that is on the ionized side of the pK_a of the drug. Therefore, salts appear to have a higher solubility in water than their parent weak acid or base. This is entirely related to a change in solution pH; the intrinsic solubility does not change when a salt is made.

Lipophilicity

A compound has to have a balance of hydrophilic and lipophilic properties for it to be a successful drug. Thus, the chemical structure of a drug has to be designed to make sure the molecule is compatible with both aqueous and lipid environments. The ability of a drug to dissolve in a lipid phase when an aqueous phase is present is important because it mimics typical situations found in the body.

Lipophilicity is a key factor in determining the *in vivo* behavior of drugs such as:

*   Permeation through biological membranes (absorption and distribution)
*   Transport of drug throughout the body
*   Binding of drug to plasma proteins
*   Accumulation of drug in tissues
*   Recognition of drug by receptor
*   Affinity of drug for receptor
*   Specificity of the drug–receptor interaction

The Partition Coefficient

The balance between lipophilicity and hydrophilicity of a compound in its unionized, nonelectrolyte form is characterized by a parameter called the partition coefficient, P. Because partition coefficients are difficult to determine in living systems, laboratory experiments measure the partition coefficient as the relative affinity of a compound for water and a model lipid solvent. The choice of lipid solvent has been subject to much debate. The most commonly used solvent is n-octanol, and extensive data are available for partitioning of thousands of drugs between octanol and water. Other model lipophilic solvents used more recently include chloroform and isopropyl myristate.

Water and octanol are immiscible with each other. Determination of P involves placing these solvents in contact with each other and adding the compound of interest to this system. Molecules of the compound will distribute between the two solvents, or phases, until equilibrium is reached, as illustrated in Figure 3.3. After the system is at equilibrium, concentrations of the compound in each phase are measured.

If the compound is more hydrophilic than lipophilic, its concentration in water will be higher, whereas if it is more lipophilic than hydrophilic, its concentration in octanol will be higher. Denoting C_o as the concentration in octanol and C_w as the concentration in water, the partition coefficient (P) is defined as:

$$P = \frac{C_o}{C_w} \qquad \text{(Eq. 3.14)}$$

Thus, P provides a measure of the relative affinity of a compound for lipid and aqueous phases. A compound with $P = 1$ has equal affinities for lipid and water. A P value greater than one implies the compound is lipophilic; the larger the value of P, the greater its lipophilicity. A P value less than one implies a compound is hydrophilic; the smaller the value, the lower its lipophilicity.

Remember that partition coefficient is defined only for the *un-ionized* form of a drug. For a weak electrolyte, this means that P is measured at a pH at which the compound is entirely un-ionized. In this respect, partition coefficient is analogous to the intrinsic solubility of a compound; both are dependent on the chemical structure of the drug, but without the complication of ionization. We will consider the effect of ionization on partition coefficient below.

The Log P Value

Partition coefficient is often stated as a logarithmic ($\log P$) value for convenience. The $\log P$ of thousands of drugs and potential drugs has been measured over the years. We can make some generalizations about the viability of a compound as a drug based on this large data set.

A compound with $\log P < 0$ (or $P < 1$) is usually considered too hydrophilic to be a suitable drug candidate, particularly if it needs to cross lipophilic biological membranes for its activity. At the other

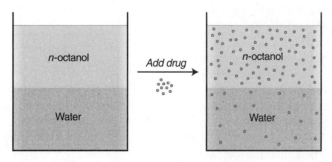

Figure 3.3. Partitioning of a drug compound between octanol and water. In this example, more drug is in the octanol phase than in the aqueous phase at equilibrium.

extreme, compounds with log $P>3.5$ (or $P>3,000$) are usually too lipophilic to be good drugs because they tend to be poorly water soluble. Nevertheless, some successful drugs have log P values that lie outside this desirable range, which shows that the body is more complex than simple physicochemical approximations make it out to be. However, measurement of partition coefficient provides a simple *in vitro* method to make some prediction about the behavior of a compound in the body and to select the most promising drug candidates from a large pool of compounds.

Effect of Structure on Partition Coefficient

The effect of various chemical substituents on partitioning behavior of organic compounds has been extensively studied and documented. If a potential drug compound has a log P value that is too high or too low, scientists often attempt to modify its chemical structure by adding or removing appropriate substituents to change partition coefficient in a predictable manner. Table 3.1 shows examples of substituents that influence the partition coefficient of compounds.

Apparent Partition Coefficient

The definition of partition coefficient applies to only the un-ionized form of the compound. Ionization of an electrolyte in the aqueous phase complicates its partitioning behavior. Weak acids and bases ionize to some extent in water, depending on their pK_a and the pH of the aqueous phase. Electrolytes cannot ionize in lipids or octanol because these nonpolar solvents cannot stabilize ionic charge. In other words, the ionized form of a drug can be present in the aqueous phase, but cannot partition into octanol.

When the influence of pH on partitioning is studied, a buffer is used to maintain the pH of the aqueous phase at the desired value. Two equilibrium

TABLE 3.1. Substituents That Influence the Partition Coefficient of Compounds	
Substituent	*Structure*
Substituents That Increase Partition Coefficient	
Alkyl	$-CH_3$, $-CH_2-$, and so on
Aryl	$-C_6H_5$
Sulfur-containing groups	$-S-$, $-SCH_3$
Halogens	$-Cl$, $-Br$, $-I$
Substituents That Decrease Partition Coefficient	
Hydroxyl	$-OH$
Carboxyl	$-COOH$
Carbonyl	$-C=O$
Amino	$-NH_2$, $-NH-R$
Ether	$-O-$

conditions have to be satisfied in these situations:

1. The ratio of ionized to un-ionized drug in the aqueous phase must obey the Henderson–Hasselbalch equation.
2. The un-ionized form has to partition between the two phases as governed by its partition coefficient.

Consequently, ionization in the aqueous phase decreases the amount of un-ionized form available to distribute into octanol.

The apparent partition coefficient (P_{app}) is defined as the ratio of the concentration in octanol to the *total* concentration, i.e., ionized (C_i) plus un-ionized (C_u), in the aqueous phase:

$$P_{app} = \frac{C_o}{(C_i + C_u)_w} \qquad \text{(Eq. 3.15)}$$

If the buffered aqueous phase pH causes practically all the drug to be in its un-ionized form, then $C_i = 0$ and Equation 3.15 can be written as:

$$P_{app} = \frac{C_o}{(C_u)_w} = P \qquad \text{(Eq. 3.16)}$$

Therefore, the apparent partition coefficient P_{app} is equal to the partition coefficient P when the drug is completely un-ionized. Performing a partition coefficient measurement at an aqueous pH at which ionization is negligible is one way of determining the P of weak acid and base drugs. Figures 3.4 and 3.5 illustrate partitioning equilibria of a weak acid and weak base between octanol and a buffer.

If the aqueous phase pH allows some drug molecules to ionize, measured $P_{app}<P$. In such cases, P_{app} can be related to P if the fraction (α) of drug ionized in the aqueous phase is known. The value of α is easily determined using the Henderson–Hasselbalch equation if pK_a of the drug and pH of the aqueous phase are known. Inasmuch as only un-ionized drug can partition into octanol:

$$P = \frac{P_{app}}{(1-a)} \qquad \text{(Eq. 3.17)}$$

This equation applies if $\alpha<1$. If pH is such that the entire drug is ionized and $\alpha = 1$, then there is no un-ionized drug in the aqueous phase to distribute into octanol, and $P_{app} = 0$.

Therefore, a drug with a large partition coefficient may be so extensively ionized in aqueous body fluids that very little drug is able to cross into the lipid phase. The apparent partition coefficient of this drug will be close to zero. This concept is important because biological membranes contain lipids, and the ability of drugs to penetrate into these membranes will depend not only on the P and pK_a of the drug but also on the pH of surrounding fluids.

Amphiphilicity

Some molecules have their hydrophilic functional groups located at one end of the molecule and their hydrophobic functional groups at the other end. Such molecules, which have distinct hydrophilic and lipophilic regions, are called **amphiphiles**. Examples of amphiphilic compounds include soaps and detergents, fatty acids, and phospholipids.

Amphiphiles form unique, organized structures when exposed to water, as illustrated in Figure 3.6. This spontaneous behavior occurs because the polar groups (often called *head groups*) are attracted to water, forming hydrogen bonds with water molecules, whereas the hydrophobic groups (often called *tails*) are repelled and try to remove themselves from water. This type of interaction, driven by the exclusion of nonpolar sections or residues of a molecule from water, is called a **hydrophobic bond** or hydrophobic interactions.

The hydrophobic bond does not imply bonding between the nonpolar parts of amphiphilic molecules. Rather, it is the result of the repulsive interaction between water and nonpolar groups. For a hydrophobic molecule to dissolve in water,

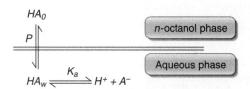

Figure 3.4. Equilibrium distribution of a weak acid between octanol and water. The extent of ionization in the aqueous phase depends on the pK_a of the acid and the pH of the aqueous phase. Only the un-ionized form HA (partition coefficient = P) can distribute into n-octanol. This system must obey the following relationships at equilibrium:

$$\log \frac{[HA]_w}{[A^-]_w} = pK_a - pH$$

$$\frac{[HA]_o}{[HA]_w} = P$$

The apparent partition coefficient P_{app} of the weak acid between octanol and aqueous phases is given by:

$$P_{app} = \frac{[HA]_o}{[HA]_w + [A^-]_w}$$

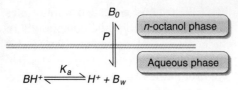

Figure 3.5. Equilibrium distribution of a weak base between octanol and water. The extent of ionization in the aqueous phase depends on the pK$_a$ of the base and the pH of the aqueous solution. Only the un-ionized form B (partition coefficient = P) can distribute into n-octanol. The following relationships must be obeyed by this system at equilibrium:

$$\log \frac{[BH^+]_w}{[B]_w} = pK_a - pH$$

$$\frac{[B]_o}{[B]_w} = P$$

The apparent partition coefficient P_{app} of the weak base between octanol and aqueous phases is given by:

$$P_{app} = \frac{[B]_o}{[B]_w + [BH^+]_w}$$

it must disrupt the existing hydrogen-bonded network of water molecules to create a cavity. However, hydrophobic molecules cannot form new interactions with water molecules to compensate for loss of hydrogen bonds, so that dissolving a hydrophobic molecule in water is unfavorable. If multiple hydrophobic residues of molecules cluster together, fewer hydrogen bonds are disrupted; in effect, water forces out hydrophobic residues.

One consequence of hydrophobic-bonding forces is that amphiphiles migrate to the air–water interface, forming a single layer of molecules called a monolayer, with polar *head groups* in water and nonpolar *tails* in the air. Orientation of amphiphiles at the surface results in a reduction of the surface tension of water. Similar monolayers can also form at the solid–liquid oil–water interface.

At higher concentrations, hydrophobic bonding causes amphiphiles to aggregate into structures known as micelles, in which nonpolar tails are in

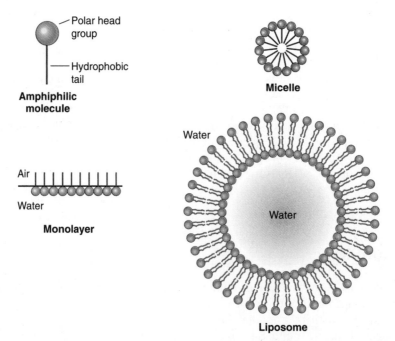

Figure 3.6. Organization of amphiphilic molecules into monolayers, bilayers, micelles, and liposomes.

the interior, away from water, whereas polar heads form the outer surface of the sphere. By gathering hydrophobic chains together in the center of the micelle, disruption of the hydrogen-bonded structure of liquid water is minimized. Polar head groups extend into the surrounding water where they can participate in hydrogen bonding. Micelles, which can be made up of 50 or more amphiphile molecules, are often spherical in shape, but may also assume cylindrical or other similar shapes.

Hydrophobic bonding is a very important aspect of cell membrane structure and of molecular folding and shaping of proteins. Certain amphiphilic molecules form stable sheetlike structures called bilayers more readily than they form spherical micelles. Examples include phospholipids that organize into bilayers, an important component of cell membranes. Bilayers can be made to form small saclike structures termed vesicles or liposomes, which have been used as unique drug delivery systems.

KEY CONCEPTS

- Aqueous solubility is a measure of hydrophilicity, and partition coefficient is a measure of lipophilicity of a drug.
- A high partition coefficient often goes hand-in-hand with poor intrinsic solubility; i.e., functional groups that enhance water solubility make a drug less lipid soluble, and vice versa.
- Ionization behavior of a drug molecule has a strong impact on total water solubility and apparent partition coefficient.

General Principles of Aqueous Drug Solubility

- The intrinsic solubility depends on the polarity of the drug molecule and the structure of the solid state.
- Intrinsic solubility does not depend on pH of the aqueous medium.

Solubility of Weak Acid Drugs

- Total solubility increases as pH increases (and the drug ionizes).
- The lowest solubility will be observed at pH values about 3 units below the pK_a; this will be the intrinsic solubility of the weak acid.

Solubility of Weak Base Drugs

- Total solubility increases as pH decreases (and the drug ionizes).

- The lowest solubility will be observed at pH values 3 units above the pK_a; this will be the intrinsic solubility of the weak base.

Solubility of Salts of Weak Acids and Bases

- Solubility of salts in buffered solutions is the same as the solubility of the parent weak acid or base.
- Solubility of salts in unbuffered solutions is higher than the corresponding weak acid or base because the pH changes to favor ionization of the drug.

General Principles for Partitioning of Drugs

- The partition coefficient of a drug depends on its chemical structure.
- The partition coefficient is defined for the un-ionized drug and does not vary with pH.
- The *apparent* partition coefficient of weak acids and bases changes with pH of the aqueous phase.
- The apparent partition coefficient of a weak acid decreases as pH increases.
- The apparent partition coefficient of a weak base decreases as pH decreases.

ADDITIONAL READING

1. Yalkowsky SH. Solubility and Solubilization in Aqueous Media (ACS Professional Reference Books). American Chemical Society, 1999.

2. Amiji M, Sandmann BJ. Applied Physical Pharmacy, 1st ed. McGraw-Hill/Appleton & Lange, 2003.

3. Florence AT, Attwood D. Physicochemical Principles of Pharmacy, 3rd ed. MacMillan Education, Ltd., 1998.

4. Martin AN, Bustamante P. Physical Pharmacy—Physical Chemical Principles in the Pharmaceutical Sciences, 4th ed. Lippincott Williams & Wilkins, 1993.

REVIEW QUESTIONS

1. Why does a drug need to have both hydrophilic and lipophilic properties?
2. What determines the intrinsic solubility of a weak acid or weak base?
3. What is polymorphism? How does it affect intrinsic solubility?
4. Describe the change in total solubility of a weak acid and weak base as the pH *decreases* below the pK_a.
5. Describe the change in total solubility of a weak acid and weak base as the pH *increases* above the pK_a.
6. Why do salts of weak acids and bases appear to have a higher water solubility than the parent acid or base?
7. What is meant by the partition coefficient of a compound? How is it measured?
8. What is meant by log *P*? What is the approximate range of desirable log *P* values for a drug? What is the problem if the log *P* value is outside this range?
9. Describe the change in apparent partition coefficient of a weak acid and weak base as the pH *decreases* below the pK_a.
10. Describe the change in apparent partition coefficient of a weak acid and weak base as the pH *increases* above the pK_a.

PRACTICE PROBLEMS

1. Consult the information about naproxen given in Problem 4 of Chapter 2.
   a) A saturated solution of naproxen is made in a buffer at pH 3, and a buffer at pH 6. Which solution will have a higher concentration, and why?
   b) If the intrinsic solubility of naproxen is 0.0001 M, calculate the total solubility when naproxen is dissolved in a buffer of pH 4.2. Express the solubility in units of mg/mL.

2. Consult the information about cimetidine given in Problem 5 of Chapter 2.
   a) Is cimetidine more soluble in stomach fluids or in small intestinal fluids?
   b) Cimetidine and cimetidine hydrochloride are allowed to dissolve in water (unbuffered) until the solutions are saturated. Which solution will have a higher concentration? Why?
   c) Cimetidine and cimetidine hydrochloride are allowed to dissolve in a pH 7 buffer until the solutions are saturated. Which solution will have a higher concentration? Why?

3. A new drug is a sodium salt of a carboxylic acid. It has a molecular weight = 150, a $pK_a = 5$, and an intrinsic solubility = 0.002 M. What is the maximum concentration of drug that can be dissolved in a buffer at pH 6? Give the concentration in both molar and mg/mL units.

4. A partition coefficient experiment was carried out with a nonelectrolyte drug. Drug was added to an *n*-octanol–water system that contained 100 mL of each solvent and allowed to equilibrate. At equilibrium, the concentration of drug in the octanol phase was 0.52 M and in the aqueous phase was 0.33 M.
   a) What is the partition coefficient of the drug?
   b) What is the log *P*?
   c) Will the partition coefficient change if the pH of the aqueous phase is changed?

5. Diphenhydramine (Benadryl) is an antihistamine and has the following structure:

The *n*-octanol–water partition coefficient of diphenhydramine is 3,500, and its $pK_a = 9.0$.

a) What is the log *P* value of diphenhydramine? Would you call this drug more hydrophilic or lipophilic?

b) Will the apparent partition coefficient of diphenhydramine be greater at pH 7 or at pH 9? Calculate the apparent partition coefficient at pH 7 and at pH 9.

c) Will the aqueous solubility of diphenhydramine be greater in a buffer of pH 7 or a buffer of pH 9?

d) If you wanted to make a salt of diphenhydramine, would you react it with an acid or a base?

6. Warfarin (Coumadin) is an anticoagulant drug. It is a weak acid with a $pK_a = 5.1$ and a log *P* = 0.9.

a) Calculate the partition coefficient of warfarin.

b) Will warfarin be more ionized at pH 2 or pH 7? Calculate the fraction ionized at each of these pH values.

c) Will the apparent partition coefficient be higher at pH 2 or at pH 7? Calculate these apparent partition coefficient values.

d) If 100 mg of warfarin is added to an *n*-octanol–buffer experiment, calculate the total milligrams in the octanol phase and in the buffer phase at pH 2 and at pH 7.

e) Will warfarin be more water soluble at pH 2 or pH 7?

Rates of Pharmaceutical Processes

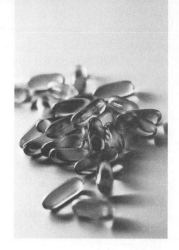

In previous chapters our focus has been on properties of drug systems at equilibrium. Ionization, partitioning, and aqueous solubility are measurements made when the process has reached equilibrium; no further change occurs unless the system is perturbed in some way. Equilibrium constants such as the acid dissociation constant, partition coefficient, and solubility give an indication of *how far* or *to what extent* a process or reaction can proceed. Equilibrium constants, however, do not reveal *how quickly* the process or reaction will occur.

The *rate* or speed of pharmaceutical processes or reactions is of great importance to pharmaceutical scientists. Drug therapy is a dynamic process, and time is a critical parameter in design of drug products and behavior of drugs in the body. A drug product must remain intact on the shelf for a specified length of time. When administered, the drug needs to dissolve at the appropriate rate to be absorbed. The drug then needs to reach its site of action and act in a timely manner. Finally, the drug needs to be removed from the body in an appropriate time frame.

The mathematical study of the rate of appearance or disappearance of a substance in a reaction or process is called kinetics. In this chapter, we will learn mathematical principles that apply to the kinetics of common pharmaceutical processes. In chapters to follow, these concepts will be applied to drug stability, dissolution, disposition, and receptor binding.

Rate

The rate of a reaction or process is the speed or velocity at which the process occurs. Consider the following process:

$$\text{Drug} \longrightarrow \text{Product or Outcome} \quad \text{(Eq. 4.1)}$$

The process shown in Equation 4.1 could represent any of the following situations:

- Drug decomposing to give a decomposition product
- Solid drug dissolving in water to give a solution
- Drug being absorbed from the small intestines into the blood
- Drug being metabolized in the liver to give inactive products

A common feature in all these examples is that the amount, A, of drug in its original form decreases with respect to time, t. The rate of this process can be expressed as a differential expression describing change of A with time:

$$\text{rate} = -\frac{dA}{dt} \quad \text{(Eq. 4.2)}$$

The negative sign indicates that the amount, A, of drug is decreasing as the process proceeds.

In most cases, we follow change in concentration of drug rather than amount of drug. The rate of a process in which concentration, C, of drug decreases with respect to time, t, is given by:

$$\text{rate} = -\frac{dC}{dt} \quad \text{(Eq. 4.3)}$$

The rate of a process or reaction is experimentally determined by measuring disappearance of drug or appearance of products during defined time intervals.

First-Order Processes

Reactions in which the rate depends on concentration of only one reactant are called **first-order reactions**. Most applications we will deal with in this text can be treated as first-order processes. More complex processes might involve two, three, or more reactants, all of which change in concentration as a function of time; these are called second-order, third-order, or multiple-order reactions, respectively. Such processes are outside the scope of our discussion.

The rate of most pharmaceutical processes depends on concentration of drug available to participate in the process. In other words, rate is *directly proportional* to drug concentration:

$$-\frac{dC}{dt} \propto C \quad \text{(Eq. 4.4)}$$

The rate of the process is initially fast when C is large and slows as the reaction proceeds and C decreases. The higher the concentration of drug, the faster the rate of the process is.

Therefore, in a first-order process, the *amount* of drug removed in a certain time interval decreases as the reaction proceeds, whereas the *fraction* or *percentage* of drug removed in each time interval remains constant.

Most pharmaceutical processes include the drug as a reactant, but other compounds or substances may also be involved. For example, drug decomposition often involves hydrolysis of the drug by water. Concentration of the drug decreases with time, but concentration of the second reactant, water in the case of a hydrolysis reaction, remains essentially unchanged because water is present in a great excess compared with the drug.

Thus, although water is involved in the reaction, its concentration can be treated as a constant to simplify the reaction kinetics. These types of processes can be approximated by first-order kinetics and are called *pseudo*first-order reactions.

First-Order Rate Constant

Equation 4.4 can be rewritten as:

$$-\frac{dC}{dt} = k_1 C \text{ or } \frac{dC}{dt} = -k_1 C \qquad \text{(Eq. 4.5)}$$

The proportionality constant, k_1, is called the first-order rate constant, which has units of time^{-1} (e.g., yr^{-1}, day^{-1}, hr^{-1}, min^{-1}, s^{-1}). The magnitude of k_1 is a reflection of the speed or rate of the process. A large k_1 indicates a fast process or reaction. The value of k_1 can be considered the fraction of the concentration that is removed during a unit length of time.

Integrated Rate Expression

Equation 4.5 can be integrated to give a more useful expression:

$$C = C_0 e^{-k_1 t} \qquad \text{(Eq. 4.6)}$$

where C is the concentration remaining after time t, C_0 is the initial concentration (at $t = 0$), and k_1 is the first-order rate constant of the process. Taking natural logarithms of both sides of Equation 4.6 allows it to be written in its logarithmic form:

$$\ln C = \ln C_0 - k_1 t \qquad \text{(Eq. 4.7)}$$

Equation 4.7 may also be written using common logarithms:

$$\log C = \log C_0 - \frac{k_1 t}{2.3} \qquad \text{(Eq. 4.8)}$$

Equations 4.6, 4.7, or 4.8 allow the calculation of the first-order rate constant if two concentrations and the time

Example of a First-Order Process

Consider the decomposition reaction of a drug with $k_1 = 0.12$ yr^{-1}. This means that 12% of available drug is removed in the first year, so that 88% of the drug remains after 1 year. In the second year, 12% of the *drug remaining after the first year* is removed, and so on.

If the initial concentration of the drug were 100 mg/tablet, 12 mg (100 mg $\times$ 0.12) are lost in 1 year, leaving behind 88 mg. The amount lost in the second year will be 10.6 mg (88 mg $\times$ 0.12), leaving behind 77.4 mg/tablet after 2 years. The amount lost in the third year will be 9.3 mg (77.4 mg $\times$ 0.12) leaving behind 68.1 mg/tablet after 3 years. And so on. The actual *amount* of drug removed each year decreases with time, but the *percentage* or *fraction* removed each year remains constant.

If the initial concentration of the drug had been 200 mg/tablet, the remaining concentrations would be 176 mg/tablet after 1 year, 154.9 mg/tablet after 2 years, and so on. Thus, the *amount* of drug removed in a time interval increases as the initial concentration increases, but the *percentage* or *fraction* removed does not depend on concentration.

Calculation of k_1

The initial concentration of drug in blood after an intravenous injection is 12 mg/L. The first-order rate constant for elimination of drug from the blood is 0.032 hr^{-1}. What is the estimated concentration in blood after 3 hours?

We know C_0 (12 mg/L) and k_1 (0.032 hr^{-1}) and want to calculate C at $t = 3$ hours. We can use Equation 4.6, 4.7, or 4.8 to do this. Using Equation 4.6:

$$C = C_0 e^{-k_1 t} = 12 \, \text{mg} / \text{L} \cdot e^{-0.032 \times 3} =$$

$$10.9 \, \text{mg} / \text{L}$$

Alternatively, we may be told that the initial concentration after an intravenous injection is 12 mg/L, and 3 hours later it is 10.9 mg/L. Calculate the first-order rate constant for the process. Again, we can use Equation 4.6, 4.7, or 4.8 to solve this. Rearranging Equation 4.7:

$$k_1 = -\frac{\ln C_0 - \ln C}{t} = \frac{\ln 12 - \ln 10.9}{3 \, \text{hr}} =$$

$$\frac{2.4849 - 2.3888}{3 \, \text{hr}} = 0.032 \, \text{hr}^{-1}$$

interval between them are known. Alternatively, if k_1 and C_0 are known, the concentration at any time in the process can be determined.

Graphical Representation

The kinetics of a pharmaceutical process is generally followed by measuring drug concentration as a function of time. A graphical representation of the process can be obtained by plotting concentration, C, on the y axis and time, t, on the x axis. When a first-order process is graphed in this manner we get the exponential curve shown in Figure 4.1, as described by Equation 4.6.

Although Figure 4.1 provides a graphical view of a first-order reaction, such a plot is not very useful for calculating the rate constant, or concentration of drug remaining at any given time. A more effective graph is obtained by plotting the same data according to either Equation 4.7 or 4.8, both of which are equations of straight lines. Figure 4.2 shows data from Figure 4.1 plotted according to Equation

4.7. The x axis represents time, t, and the y axis represents $\ln C$. The y intercept is, therefore, $\ln C_0$, and the slope gives the first-order rate constant, k_1.

Semilogarithmic (semilog) graph paper allows us to conveniently plot first-order data without having to calculate $\ln C$. Semilog paper uses common logarithms, so that C versus t may be plotted directly according to Equation 4.8, giving a linear relationship between $\log C$ and t. Figure 4.3 shows a graph of data from Figure 4.1 on semilog paper.

The linearity of Figures 4.2 and 4.3 proves that the process follows first-order kinetics and obeys Equation 4.6.

Half-Life

The half-life of a pharmaceutical process is the time taken for amount or concentration of drug to decrease by one half. In other words, it is the time needed for drug concentration to decline to half of the initial concentration.

The expression for half-life of a first-order process can be derived from

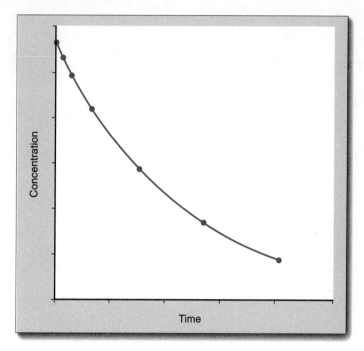

Figure 4.1. Plot of concentration, C, against time, t, for a first-order process. The concentration declines in an exponential manner, as given by the equation $C = C_0 e^{-kt}$, where C_0 is the concentration at $t = 0$, and k is the first-order rate constant.

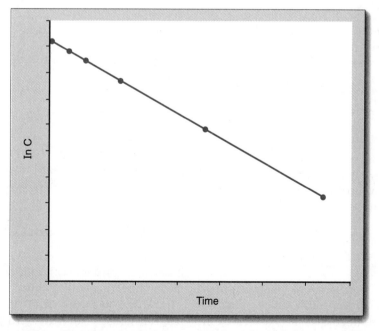

Figure 4.2. Plot of the natural logarithm of concentration, C, against time, t, for a first-order process, according to the equation $\ln C = \ln C_0 - kt$, where C_0 is the concentration at $t = 0$ and k ($-$slope) is the first-order rate constant. Note that the data fall on a straight line; $C_0 =$ the y intercept and $k = -$slope.

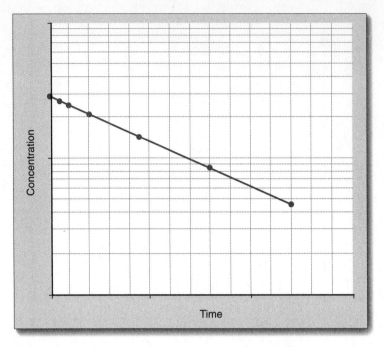

Figure 4.3. Plot of concentration, C, against time, t, on semilogarithmic paper for a first-order process, according to the equation $\log C = \log C_0 - kt/2.303$, where C_0 is the concentration at $t = 0$ and k ($-2.303 \times$ slope) is the first-order rate constant. Note that the y axis is the log axis and the data fall on a straight line; $C_0 = $ the y intercept and $k = $ negative slope.

Equation 4.6, 4.7, or 4.8, and by further setting $C = 0.5\ C_0$. This manipulation gives an expression for half-life, denoted by $t_{1/2}$:

$$t_{1/2} = \frac{0.693}{k_1} \qquad \text{(Eq. 4.9)}$$

For first-order processes, half-life depends only on the rate constant k_1. Thus, for a given process, half-life is a constant and does not change with concentration.

Zero-Order Processes

Although a majority of pharmaceutical processes follow first-order kinetics, zero-order kinetics is also observed in some circumstances. Zero-order reactions are those in which the rate is a constant and does *not* change with time. Remember that rate decreases with time in

first-order reactions as drug concentration declines.

A zero-order process is defined by the following equation:

$$-\frac{dC}{dt} = k_0 \quad \text{or} \quad \frac{dC}{dt} = -k_0 \qquad \text{(Eq. 4.10)}$$

Equation 4.10 indicates that rate of change of concentration remains constant as the reaction proceeds.

Zero-Order Rate Constant

The term k_0 in Equation 4.10 is the zero-order rate constant with units of concentration/time ($\text{mg} \cdot \text{mL}^{-1} \cdot \text{min}^{-1}$, $\text{mg} \cdot \text{L}^{-1} \cdot \text{hr}^{-1}$, and so forth). Note that the rate and rate constant of a zero-order process are the same; both directly indicate how concentration declines with time. Therefore, in a zero-order process, the *fraction* or *percentage* of drug removed in each

Calculation of Half-Life

A 10-mg/mL drug solution degrades by first-order kinetics with a $k_1 = 0.0433$ month^{-1}. How long will it take for the drug concentration to drop to 5 mg/mL?

$$t_{1/2} = \frac{0.693}{k_1} = \frac{0.693}{0.0433} = 16 \text{ months}$$

This question is asking for the half-life of a first-order process. So, if this were a 20-mg/mL solution, half-life would still be 16 months, at the end of which the drug concentration would be 10 mg/mL. Thus, half-life does not depend on initial concentration.

---

time interval decreases as the reaction proceeds, whereas the *amount* of drug removed in a certain time interval remains constant.

Equation 4.10 is often written in terms of amount rather than concentration:

$$\frac{dA}{dt} = -k_0 \qquad \text{(Eq. 4.11)}$$

For the equation in this form, units of k_0 are mass per time (mg/hr, mg/day, and so on).

Integrated Rate Expression

Equation 4.10 can be integrated to give a more useful expression:

$$C = C_0 - k_0 t \qquad \text{(Eq. 4.12)}$$

where C is the concentration remaining after time t, C_0 is the initial concentration (at $t = 0$), and k_0 is the zero-order rate constant. This equation is used to calculate any one parameter if other terms in the equation are known.

Example of a Zero-Order Calculation

A drug suspension with an initial concentration of 100 mg/mL degrades over time. The concentration after 7 days is 95 mg/mL, after 14 days is 90 mg/mL, and after 21 days is 85 mg/mL. Does the degradation reaction follow zero-order kinetics? What is the zero-order rate constant?

The data show that the rate of reaction is constant; 5 mg/mL are lost every 7 days, so the reaction is zero-

order. The zero-order rate constant is given by using Equation 4.12 and any two data points:

$$k_0 = \frac{C_0 - C}{t} = \frac{100 - 95}{7} = \frac{95 - 90}{7} = \text{?}$$

$$\frac{90 - 85}{7} = 0.71 \text{ mg} \cdot \text{mL}^{-1} \cdot \text{day}^{-1}$$

This, in fact, is also the rate of the reaction.

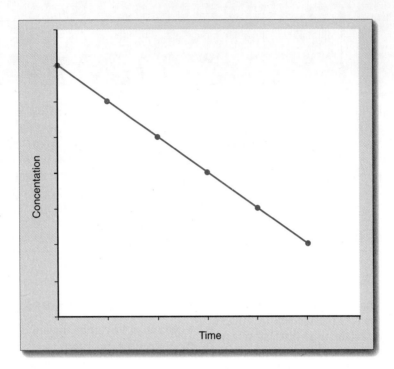

Figure 4.4. Plot of concentration, *C*, against time, *t*, for a zero-order process. Note that the data fall on a straight line.

Graphical Representation

The decrease in drug concentration for a zero-order process can be graphed according to Equation 4.12. Note that this is a linear, not exponential, expression. Consequently, a plot of *C* against *t* gives a straight line with a slope of k_0 and an intercept of C_0, as shown in Figure 4.4. A linear plot here confirms that the process follows zero-order kinetics.

Half-Life

Earlier in this chapter we learned that the half-life of a given first-order reaction is a constant. In contrast, the half-life of zero-order reactions is not a constant, but changes with initial concentration or amount. Recall that half-life is the time needed for drug concentration to decline to half of the initial concentration. For zero-order reactions, half-life is given by:

$$t_{1/2} = \frac{0.5 C_0}{k_0} \qquad \text{(Eq. 4.13)}$$

Equation 4.13 shows that half-life of zero-order processes depends on both k_0 and C_0. Therefore, at a higher C_0, half-life will be longer. Also, half-life will decrease as concentration declines. This changing value of $t_{1/2}$ of zero-order reactions makes the calculation of half-life meaningless for such processes.

Mixed-Order Processes

In pharmaceutical systems, we often encounter processes that show first-order behavior at low reactant concentrations and zero-order behavior at high reactant concentrations. In the intermediate concentration range, the reaction follows neither first-order nor zero-order kinetics. A process whose order changes as some condition of the reaction changes is said to follow mixed-order kinetics. Examples of mixed-order processes are reactions involving enzymes. The dependence of rate on reactant concentration for zero-order,

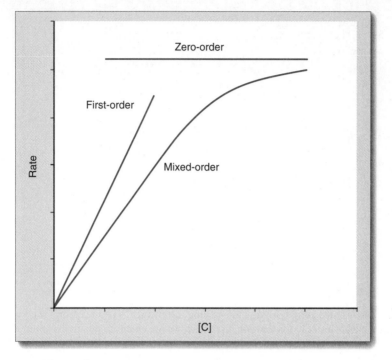

Figure 4.5. Dependence of reaction rate on reactant concentration, C, for zero-order, first-order, and mixed-order processes.

first-order, and mixed-order processes is illustrated in Figure 4.5.

Transition State Theory

The rate laws discussed so far have been simple: a reactant is consumed and a product is formed. However, all reactions are theoretically reversible so that the forward reaction is matched by a corresponding reverse reaction. The reaction progresses to equilibrium, with an equilibrium constant given by the ratio of rate constants of the forward and reverse reactions.

Reaction Progress Diagram

As a reaction progresses, reactants are converted to products or are changed in some other manner. All reversible reactions tend to proceed in the direction that decreases the energy of reactants. However, the reaction may not proceed very quickly even in this direction. Before re-actants can be transformed into products, they must pass through an intermediate state called the transition state or activated complex, a state with higher energy than either reactants or products. This "barrier" prevents the reactants from instantly turning into products.

The transition state is an unstable transitory combination of reactant molecules that can either go on to form products or fall apart to return to unchanged reactants. The energy difference between reactants and transition state is referred to as the activation energy of the process. The activation energy is, therefore, a measure of the energy barrier that reactant molecules must surmount if the reaction is to proceed. A reaction may occur very slowly or not at all if very few molecules overcome the energy barrier and make the transition toward the lower energy state.

A reaction progress diagram, as shown in Figure 4.6, is useful to visualize the reaction process. Here, compounds A and B

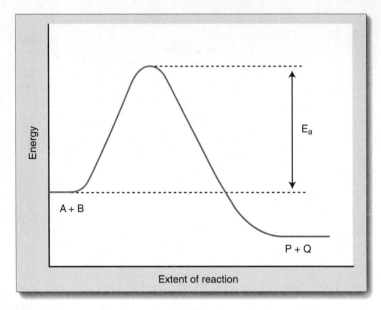

Figure 4.6. The reaction progress diagram showing the energetics of a reaction. The y axis is energy and the x axis is the reaction coordinate that shows the extent to which the reaction has proceeded. Note that the transition state has a higher energy (E_a) than either the reactants ($A + B$) or products ($P + Q$).

react to form products P and Q. Reactant molecules approach each other and progress along the reaction coordinate to the transition state. The original bonds in reactant molecules weaken and new bonds are partially formed. Some of the transition state species progress to products, and others fall back to reactants.

The rate of reaction is proportional to the number or concentration of molecules in the transition state. The higher the activation energy barrier, the fewer reactant molecules are able to reach the transition state, resulting in a slower reaction. Reaction rate is not affected by what happens after the transition state is reached.

Effect of Temperature on Rate

Chemical intuition suggests that the higher the temperature, the faster a given chemical reaction will proceed. This can be readily deduced from the transition state theory. As temperature increases, there are more collisions between reactant molecules, causing original bonds to

weaken and new bonds to be formed more readily. The proportion of reactant species that reach the transition state increases. The result is a faster rate of reaction and a larger rate constant.

The Arrhenius equation describes this relationship between rate constant and temperature:

$$k = A e^{-E_a/RT} \qquad \text{(Eq. 4.14)}$$

In this equation, k is a rate constant of any order, T is the temperature of reaction *in Kelvin,* E_a is the activation energy of the reaction, R is the universal gas constant, and A is the Arrhenius constant, also called the preexponential factor. The activation energy can be looked on as a measure of the sensitivity of a reaction to temperature. A is constant for a given reaction and can be viewed as the rate constant when E_a is zero.

Equation 4.14 can be written in its logarithmic form for convenience:

$$\ln k = \ln A - \frac{E_a}{RT} \qquad \text{(Eq. 4.15)}$$

Equation 4.15 states that the higher the activation energy E_a, the smaller the rate constant k, and the slower the reaction. It also shows that for a reaction with a given activation energy, the higher the temperature, the larger the k and the faster the reaction.

The activation energies of most drug decomposition reactions fall in the range of 12 to 24 kcal/mol, with a typical value of about 19 to 20 kcal/mol. Thus, we can make an estimate about the effect of temperature on drug decomposition in pharmaceutical products when the exact activation energy is unknown. The general rule of thumb is that for every 10°C rise in temperature, the first-order rate constant increases by a factor of two, or doubles. This helps us to establish the proper storage conditions (freezer, refrigerator, or room temperature) for pharmaceutical products.

Catalysis

Increasing temperature is one way of speeding up a chemical reaction. Another approach is to lower the activation energy barrier for the reaction. A catalyst may be broadly defined as a substance that alters the rate of a chemical reaction without shifting the equilibrium of the reaction and without being itself consumed. Catalysts usually work by providing an alternative reaction route with lower activation energy. Decrease in E_a increases the number of molecules that reach the transition state and the number of collisions that will result in reaction. Even quite modest reductions in the activation energy can produce large increases in reaction rate.

Although the catalyst undoubtedly enters into the reaction mechanism at some point, it does so in a cyclic manner and does not itself undergo a permanent change. Therefore, a relatively small amount of catalyst can produce significant changes in reaction rate and may be reused during the reaction. The rate of the catalyzed reaction is usually directly proportional to the concentration of the catalyst.

A catalyst does not change the beginning or end point of a reaction, just the *path* taken to go from beginning to end. In other words, a catalyst does not change the equilibrium constant of a reaction, but changes the rate at which equilibrium is achieved. Figure 4.7 illustrates the change in the reaction energetics when a catalyst is involved.

Chemical Catalysis

Catalysis is observed in many different types of pharmaceutical processes and may be desirable or undesirable. Catalysts are used successfully in many types of synthetic reactions for the manufacture of new drug substances. The reaction is speeded up, and the new drug is synthesized faster and in higher yields. In other systems, catalysis is undesirable; for example, many components of drug products (buffers, preservatives, stabilizers, and so forth) may act as catalysts for drug decomposition reactions, and reduce the shelf life of the product.

Chemical catalysis may be homogeneous or heterogeneous. In homogeneous catalysis, reactants, products, and catalyst are all present in one phase, usually liquid. For example, a number of drugs undergo decomposition in aqueous solution. Hydrolysis of drugs in aqueous solutions is a common mechanism for their degradation. These hydrolysis reactions are often catalyzed by acids and bases, requiring that the pH of the solution be adjusted to provide maximum stability and shelf life for the drug.

In heterogeneous catalysis, catalyst and reactants are in separate phases; most commonly, reactants and products are in the gas or liquid phase whereas the catalyst is a solid. These types of catalytic reactions are used in manufacture of drug substances. The catalyst may be a finely

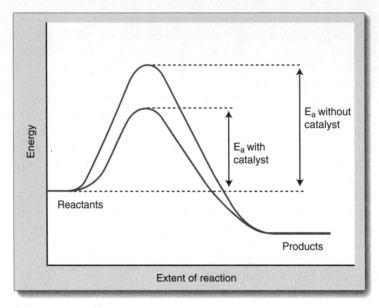

Figure 4.7. The effect of a catalyst on reaction energetics. The catalyst lowers the activation energy (E_a), allowing the reaction to proceed more rapidly.

divided solid such as platinum, or it may be the walls of the reaction vessel. Many chemical reactions that occur in the presence of such solid surfaces do not proceed at all in the absence of the solid catalyst.

Enzyme Catalysis

Enzymes are proteins that act as catalysts in various biochemical reactions in our body and are able to dramatically increase the rates at which these reactions occur. Enzyme-catalyzed reactions typically proceed 100 to 1,000 times faster than they would if they were not catalyzed. Enzyme activity enables cells to carry out complex chemical reactions rapidly at the relatively low temperatures of the body. In the absence of enzymes, our cells would not be able to carry out these reactions at a significant rate.

In typical enzyme-catalyzed reactions, reactant and product concentrations are usually hundreds or thousands of times greater than the enzyme concentration. Consequently, one enzyme molecule is able to catalyze the reaction of many reactant molecules.

In this context, the reactant is called a substrate. The substrate usually binds reversibly to a specific part of the enzyme called the active site or catalytic site. Binding is possible only if the shapes of the substrate and active site are complementary, and if the substrate can form attractive intermolecular bonds with the functional groups exposed at the enzyme's active site. Thus, enzymes are very specific in the substrates to which they bind.

Binding of substrate at the active site provides an environment favoring catalytic events. Enzyme–substrate interaction causes covalent bonds in the substrate to stretch or become distorted. The bonds weaken, causing them to break more readily to form products. Product molecules do not have the appropriate shape or structure to be attracted to the active site and are, therefore, released. The active site is now available to catalyze breakdown of another substrate molecule. This sequence of events is illustrated in Figure 4.8.

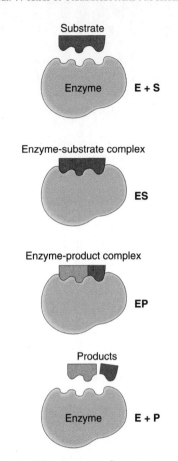

Figure 4.8. The sequence of events in an enzyme-catalyzed reaction. The enzyme, *E*, catalyzes the reaction of substrate, *S*, forming products, *P*. The enzyme remains unchanged after the reaction, and is available to catalyze the reaction of another molecule of substrate.

In Chapter 6, Drugs and Their Targets, we will elaborate on the mechanism and forces involved in the binding of substrates to proteins such as enzymes. This chapter considers only the kinetics of enzyme catalysis.

Michaelis–Menten Kinetics

The reaction rate of an enzyme-catalyzed reaction is proportional to concentration of the enzyme–substrate complex, ES, formed by a specific combination of enzyme, E, with its substrate, S. This complex reacts further, yielding product, P,

and regenerating free enzyme. These reactions can be represented by:

enzyme + substrate ⇌

    ⇌ enzyme - substrate complex -

    ⟶ product + enzyme   (Eq. 4.16)

Equation 4.16 can be written simply as:

$$E + S \underset{}{\overset{K}{\rightleftharpoons}} ES \rightarrow E + P \qquad \text{(Eq. 4.17)}$$

Consider this process in two successive steps: formation of the complex, and formation of product from the complex.

Formation of the complex is *reversible*. The law of mass action gives K, the association constant for the first equilibrium reaction:

$$K = \frac{[ES]}{[E][S]} \qquad \text{(Eq. 4.18)}$$

where [E], [S], and [ES] represent the concentrations of enzyme, substrate, and complex, respectively, at equilibrium. The magnitude of K gives information about the extent of substrate–enzyme binding, i.e., how much substrate is bound by enzyme in the complex. A substrate that is extensively bound to an enzyme has a large K, showing that there is a high affinity between enzyme and substrate; affinity is a measure of the strength of the enzyme–substrate interaction.

Formation of product from the complex is *irreversible* and its rate depends on the concentration of the enzyme–substrate complex. Therefore, rate of formation of ES controls the rate and extent of the overall reaction. The higher the affinity of drug for enzyme, the larger the concentration of the complex, and the faster the reaction.

For mathematical convenience, we define a *dissociation constant* K_m for the enzyme–substrate complex (inverse of

Equation 4.18), rather than the association constant K we saw above:

$$K_m = \frac{1}{K} = \frac{[E][S]}{[ES]} \quad \text{(Eq. 4.19)}$$

K_m is called the Michaelis constant.

The rate of reaction shown in Equation 4.17 depends on concentration of only one species, the ES complex. This makes it a *first-order* reaction with rate or velocity V given by:

$$\text{rate} = V = k[ES] \quad \text{(Eq. 4.20)}$$

where k is the *first-order rate constant* of the reaction.

Steady-State Approximation. In practice, there is no simple way of determining the value of [ES]. Therefore, it must be expressed in terms of other easily measured quantities. This is accomplished by making an assumption called the **steady-state approximation**. For enzymatic catalysis, this approximation states that at steady state the value of [ES] is constant throughout the reac-

tion, and is very small compared with [E] or [S].

Without going into the details of the derivations, let us examine the final outcome of this approximation. Combining and manipulating Equations 4.19 and 4.20 gives the **Michaelis–Menten equation** for the rate of an enzyme-catalyzed reaction at steady state:

$$V = \frac{V_{max}[S]}{K_m + [S]} \quad \text{(Eq. 4.21)}$$

where V_{max} is the maximum rate of reaction. A graphical representation of the Michaelis–Menten equation is shown in Figure 4.9.

Equation 4.21 can be rearranged as follows:

$$\frac{V}{V_{max}} = \frac{[S]}{K_m + [S]} \quad \text{(Eq. 4.22)}$$

When $K_m = [S]$, $V/V_{max} = 1/2$. In other words, the reaction proceeds at half its maximum rate when the substrate concentration is equal to the Michaelis

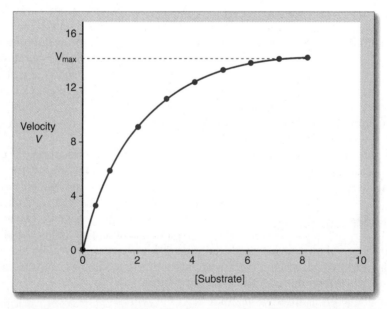

Figure 4.9. Graphical representation of the rate of an enzyme-catalyzed reaction as a function of substrate concentration. The maximum velocity or rate of the reaction is V_{max}.

constant. Put another way, K_m represents the substrate concentration at which half the enzyme molecules are occupied by substrate molecules. This relationship is shown graphically in Figure 4.10.

Significance of V_{max} and K_m. V_{max} and K_m define the kinetic behavior of an enzyme as a function of [S]. V_{max}, a measure of how fast the given amount of enzyme can go at full speed, is the maximum rate of the reaction and has units of concentration per time or amount per time.

K_m is an approximate measure of the amount of substrate required to reach full speed. K_m has units of either concentration or amount.

When [S] is small compared with K_m, Equation 4.21 reduces to:

$$V = \frac{V_{max}}{K_m}[S] = k_1[S] \qquad \text{(Eq. 4.23)}$$

Consequently, a plot of V versus [S] is linear at low substrate concentrations, with slope $= V_{max}/K_m$. This means that an increase in substrate concentration in this region will give a proportionate increase in rate of product formation. Because rate is directly proportional to substrate concentration, this represents a first-order reaction with a first-order rate constant of V_{max}/K_m.

At high substrate concentrations, [S] is large compared with K_m, and Equation 4.21 reduces to:

$$V = V_{max} = k_0 \qquad \text{(Eq. 4.24)}$$

Thus, the rate of reaction reaches its maximum value at high substrate concentrations. Because rate no longer depends on substrate concentration, this is a zero-order reaction with a zero-order rate constant of V_{max}.

At intermediate substrate concentrations (not very low or very high), enzyme-catalyzed reactions show mixed-order kinetics. We can see that although some reactions exhibit simple first-order or zero-order behavior under certain conditions, their true mechanisms may be quite complex.

The change of kinetic order of enzyme-catalyzed reactions as substrate concentration increases can be explained in the following manner. The concentration of

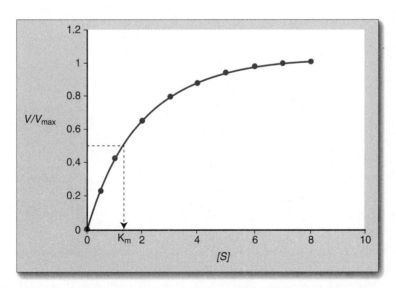

Figure 4.10. Graphical representation of Equation 4.22. When $V/V_{max} = 0.5$, [S] $= K_m$. K_m, Michaelis–Menten coefficient; [S], concentration of substrate; V, velocity of reaction; V_{max}, maximum velocity of reaction.

enzyme available is usually quite small. At low substrate concentrations ($<<K_m$), there is sufficient enzyme to bind with all the substrate molecules, and the rate of reaction depends directly on substrate concentration. At intermediate substrate concentrations, there is not sufficient enzyme available to bind with all the substrate; the reaction rate still increases with substrate concentration, but not proportionately. At very high substrate concentration, all enzyme molecules are occupied by substrate, and the enzyme is said to be saturated. An increase in substrate concentration beyond this saturation point will give no further increase in reaction rate.

Temperature Dependence of Enzymatic Reactions

As a consequence of the transition state theory, chemical reactions are usually accelerated by an increase in temperature because a greater proportion of molecules possess the required activation energy at the higher temperature. For enzymatic reactions, the rate increases with temperature up to a certain point and then abruptly decreases. This phenomenon occurs because most enzymes are stable only in a narrow temperature range—around a body temperature of 37°C (99°F) for enzymes of interest to us. At temperatures substantially different from this ideal temperature, enzymes are unstable and lose their activity.

pH Dependence of Enzymatic Reactions

Enzyme activity is also influenced by the pH of the reaction medium. An enzyme may exist in several different ionic forms depending on the pH of the medium. In some instances only one of these ionic forms may be catalytically active; in other cases one form may be more active than the others. The optimum pH for different enzymes varies over a broad range, from about pH 2 for pepsin to about pH 10 for arginase. Some enzymes exhibit a broad optimal range extending over several pH units, whereas others have a very sharp pH optimum.

KEY CONCEPTS

Because drug therapy is dynamic, the rate at which a pharmaceutical process proceeds is very important. Some important concepts discussed in this chapter are:

- The rate of a reaction or process is the speed at which the process occurs, and is characterized by following the concentration as a function of time.
- In a first-order process, the *amount* of drug lost in a certain time interval decreases as the reaction proceeds, whereas the *fraction* or *percentage* of drug removed in the time interval remains constant.
- In a zero-order process, the *fraction* or *percentage* of drug removed in each time interval decreases as the reaction proceeds, whereas the *amount* of drug removed in the time interval remains constant.

- The half-life is the time taken for the amount or concentration of the drug to decrease by one half.
- The activation energy of a reaction is an energy barrier that reactant molecules must surmount if the reaction is to proceed. The Arrhenius equation describes the dependence of the reaction rate constant on activation energy and temperature.
- Catalysts, chemical and biochemical, accelerate reactions by lowering the activation energy.
- Enzyme-catalyzed reactions are mixed-order processes described by the Michaelis–Menten equation. The reaction is first-order at low substrate concentrations, mixed-order at intermediate substrate concentrations, and zero-order at high substrate concentrations.

REVIEW QUESTIONS

1. What is the difference between the rate and the rate constant of a reaction?
2. How do the rates of first-order and zero-order reactions change with time?
3. How is the graph of *reactant concentration versus time* different for first-order and zero-order reactions?
4. What type of graph will give a straight line for a zero-order reaction? First-order reaction?
5. What are the units of zero-order and first-order rate constants?
6. What is meant by the half-life of a reaction or process? How is the half-life of a first-order reaction related to the rate constant?
7. What is the transition state of a reaction process? How does the rate of reaction depend on the characteristics of the transition state?

8. Why is the activation energy of a reaction important in determining its rate?
9. How do rates of chemical reactions change with temperature?
10. How do catalysts speed up reactions?
11. What are the differences between homogeneous and heterogeneous catalysis?
12. What are enzymes, and how do they catalyze reactions?
13. What do the values of V_{max} and K_m mean? What are their units?
14. Under what conditions does an enzyme-catalyzed reaction approach first-order kinetics? Zero-order kinetics?

PRACTICE PROBLEMS

1. The first-order rate constant for the hydrolysis of aspirin at pH 7 and 25°C is 0.013 hr^{-1}.

a) Express this rate constant in units of min^{-1} and s^{-1}.
b) What is the half-life of aspirin in hours?
c) If you make a 1 mg/mL solution of aspirin at pH 7 and 25°C, what will its concentration be after 24 hours?
d) For the aspirin solution in c), how many hours will it take for the solution concentration to decrease to 90% of its initial 1 mg/mL concentration?

2. The half-life for a solution of acetaminophen at pH 2 and 25°C is 0.8 years, and the activation energy of the reaction is 16.7 kcal/mol. Assume that the reaction follows first-order kinetics.
a) What is the first-order rate constant of the reaction?
b) How long will it take for the concentration of a 10-mg/mL solution of acetaminophen at pH 2 and 25°C to drop to 80% of its initial concentration?
c) If the concentration of the solution in b) had been 6 mg/mL, what would be the time to reach 80% of the initial concentration?

3. A dose of drug is administered by intravenous injection to an individual, and the concentration of the drug in the plasma is measured as a function of time. The plasma concentration declines with time, and the values obtained at different times are as follows:

Time after injection (hr):	2	4	6
Plasma concentration (mg/L):	100	67	45

a) Does the loss of drug from plasma follow first-order kinetics? How can you tell?
b) What is the first-order rate constant for the process?
c) What will the plasma concentration be after 8 hours?

4. A 200 mg/mL drug suspension degrades by zero-order kinetics. The concentration after 6 months is 195 mg/mL.
a) What is the zero-order rate constant?
b) What will be the concentration of the suspension after 2 years?
c) How long will it take for the concentration to decrease to 150 mg/mL?

5. Calculate the rate of an enzyme catalysis reaction, when the substrate concentration is 10 µM, if the maximum velocity of the reaction is 20 µM/min and the K_m is 5 µM.

6. Calculate the K_m of an enzymatic reaction if V_{max} of the reaction is 30 µM/min and the velocity is 5 µM/min at a substrate concentration of 10 µM.

7. What is the velocity of an enzymatic reaction in terms of V_{max} when the substrate concentration is 3 times the K_m?

Membranes and Tissues

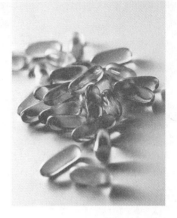

A chemical compound is not a drug unless it affects the human body in some way. In earlier chapters, we examined important physicochemical properties of drugs and the kinetics of processes in which a drug might participate. This chapter reviews the structure and function of biological membranes and tissues that are involved in determining drug pharmacokinetics and pharmacodynamics. In subsequent chapters, we will integrate this biological information with the drug's physicochemical and kinetic properties to gain insight into drug action and behavior.

The cell is the smallest fundamental structural and functional unit in our body. The major components of a cell are the cell membrane, nucleus, and cytoplasm, as illustrated in Figure 5.1. Everything between the cell membrane and the nucleus is the cytoplasm. It is composed of the *cytosol* (primarily water with dissolved salts, nutrients, gases, enzymes, and proteins), components of the *cytoskeleton*, and various *organelles* (such as ribosomes, endoplasmic reticulum, and Golgi apparatus). The cytosol is often called the intracellular fluid, separated from the extracellular fluid (the aqueous region outside the cell) by the cell membrane. We will focus on only one component of the

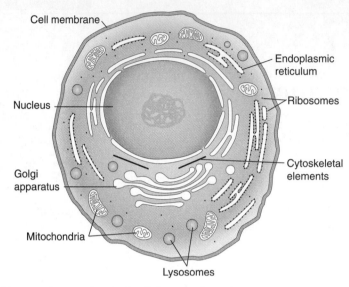

Figure 5.1. Diagram of a typical animal cell showing the major components.

The Cell Membrane

cell—the cell membrane—in this chapter. Other cell components will be reviewed in subsequent chapters as their functions are discussed.

The Cell Membrane

The cell membrane or plasma membrane is the outermost layer of a cell. Its major functions are to:

- hold together the aqueous cell contents (*structure*)
- separate cellular contents from the aqueous external fluid (*barrier*)
- control transport of substances in and out of the cell (*regulation*)
- respond to the environment (*sensitivity*)

Components of Cell Membranes

The primary constituents of the cell membrane are lipids and proteins, and carbohydrates attached to lipids and proteins. A brief review of these biomolecules is presented here. More complete discussions of the structure and proper-

ties of lipids, proteins, and carbohydrates can be found in introductory biochemistry textbooks; suggestions are included at the end of this chapter.

Lipids are a wide variety of structurally diverse biomolecules primarily made up of nonpolar groups. As a result of their nonpolar character, lipids typically dissolve more readily in nonpolar solvents than in water. This solubility characteristic is of critical importance because lipids tend to associate into nonpolar structures and barriers like the cell membrane. Besides their important role in membranes, some lipids are stored and used in cells as an energy source, whereas others are involved in cellular regulatory mechanisms. Lipids can link covalently with carbohydrates to form glycolipids and with proteins to form lipoproteins.

Proteins are macromolecular chains built from amino acids, which coil or fold to adopt a characteristic three-dimensional structure. There are four levels of structure for a protein: primary, secondary, tertiary, and quaternary (Fig. 5.2). This overall structural organization gives each protein its unique three-dimensional configuration and determines its properties. The tertiary and quaternary

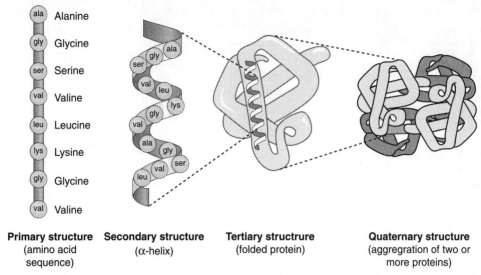

| Primary structure | Secondary structure | Tertiary structrure | Quaternary structure |
| (amino acid sequence) | (α-helix) | (folded protein) | (aggregation of two or more proteins) |

Figure 5.2. Level of structure of proteins. Amino acids linked by peptide bonds form the chain of the primary structure. Secondary structure results from interactions (mainly hydrogen bonding) between the side chains of the amino acid residues in the chain. The side chains of the amino acids interact further via hydrogen bonds or disulfide bonds to fold the protein into its three-dimensional tertiary structure that is compatible with the environment. The quaternary structure arises as a result of association of two or more protein molecules to form a complex.

folded structure of a protein depends on the surrounding environment. A protein will fold spontaneously to adopt and preserve a conformation most compatible with its surroundings. The folded protein is stabilized by a variety of intermolecular forces, including hydrogen bonds, van der Waals forces, and hydrophobic bonds.

Carbohydrates are compounds named for their characteristic content of carbon, hydrogen, and oxygen, which occur in the ratio of 1:2:1. They are very important as our body's fuel and energy stores, and form the structural framework of DNA and RNA. Short chains containing three to seven carbons are called monosaccharides or sugars, the individual building blocks of carbohydrates. Monosaccharides in the ring form can link together through a glycoside bond to form oligosaccharides or, in greater numbers, polysaccharides.

A glycoconjugate is a complex hybrid molecule made up of a carbohydrate and a noncarbohydrate portion. The two major types of glycoconjugates of interest in cell membranes are glycoproteins and glycolipids. The carbohydrate confers specific biological functions on the proteins and lipids carrying them. When embedded in the cell membrane they cover the cell surface with specific oligosaccharide structures that are often crucial to cell function.

The Lipid Bilayer

The well-known *fluid–mosaic model* provides a good, simple description of cell membrane structure. It proposes that the basic structural unit of almost all cell membranes is the lipid bilayer in which a variety of proteins are embedded. It also depicts the cell membrane as a fluid structure in which many of the constituent molecules are free to diffuse in the plane of the membrane.

Phospholipids

The primary lipids of biological membranes are phospholipids, a group of phosphate-containing molecules. Glycerol

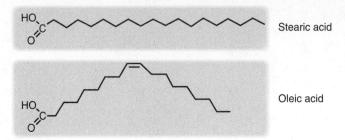

Figure 5.3. Structures of two typical fatty acids that make up phospholipids. Stearic acid is a saturated acid, whereas oleic acid is unsaturated. In a phospholipid, the carboxylic group of the fatty acid is esterified with one of the hydroxyl groups of glycerol. Note that stearic acid with no double bonds is a linear molecule, whereas the *cis* double bond in oleic acid gives the molecule a kink.

forms the backbone of most common phospholipids, with one hydroxyl linked to a phosphate group. The two other hydroxyl groups are esterified with carboxyl groups of two fatty acids, which can be either saturated or unsaturated. Fatty acids of phospholipids usually contain an even number of carbons, e.g., myristic acid (14 carbons), palmitic acid (16 carbons), and arachidonic acid (20 carbons). Structures of two typical fatty acids, stearic acid (a saturated C-18 acid) and oleic acid (an unsaturated C-18 acid) are shown in Figure 5.3.

The other end of the phosphate bridge links to an alcohol, most commonly a nitrogen-containing alcohol like *choline*. Other alcohols that may link at this position include ethanolamine, serine, threonine, and inositol. Structures of these alcohols are shown in Figure 5.4.

The alcohol gives the phospholipid its name, e.g., *phosphatidylcholine, phosphatidylserine*. Phosphatidylcholine is a major component of most cellular membranes. This phospholipid is actually a family of closely related molecules because different fatty acids may bind at the 1- and 2-carbons of the glycerol residue. Figure 5.5 illustrates the structure of a typical phospholipid molecule.

The attached alcohol gives the phospholipid its unique properties. The alcohol also plays other important roles; it can break off from the phospholipid and serve as a molecule for transmitting messages in and out of the cell, as we shall see in Chapter 15, Ligands and Receptors. The phosphate group on the phospholipid molecule carries a negative charge, whereas the alcohol may be positively charged because of ionization of the amine group. Thus, the phospholipid may be negatively charged or may bear no net charge (zwitterionic) at physiological pH.

Phospholipids are amphiphilic lipids; recall from Chapter 2, Solubility and

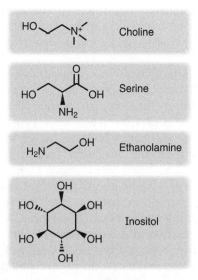

Figure 5.4. Structures of some common alcohols that make up phospholipids. Note that choline, serine, and ethanolamine are amines and can be ionized at physiological pH. Inositol is a nonelectrolyte and does not ionize.

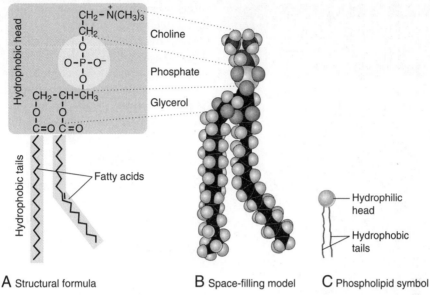

A Structural formula   **B** Space-filling model   **C** Phospholipid symbol

Figure 5.5. Structure of a typical phospholipid, phosphatidylcholine. A and B. Structural formula and space-filling model of phosphatidylcholine. Note that the fatty acids (one of which is unsaturated) make up the hydrophobic portion, whereas the hydrophilic portion includes glycerol, phosphate, and the alcohol (choline in this case). Note further that the hydrophilic head is zwitterionic because phosphate is negatively charged and choline is ionized and positively charged at physiological pH. C. Cartoon of phospholipid molecules as shown in diagrams of cell membranes.

Lipophilicity, that amphiphilic molecules have a hydrophobic part and a hydrophilic part, enabling them to organize into various structures such as micelles and bilayers as a result of hydrophobic bonding. In the phospholipid molecule, fatty acids make up the hydrophobic "tail" whereas the polar alcohol end makes up the polar "head group." Thus, phospholipids can spontaneously assemble to form a *lipid bilayer,* as illustrated in Figure 5.6.

Characteristics of the Bilayer

The bilayer is a sheetlike structure composed of two layers of phospholipid molecules whose polar alcohol head groups face the surrounding water and whose fatty acid chains form a continuous hydrophobic interior, approximately 3 nm thick. The bilayer is closed, separating intracellular and extracellular aqueous compartments of the cell. It is stabilized

and held together by a variety of forces such as:

- hydrophobic interactions between fatty acid chains of phospholipid molecules
- van der Waals interactions among fatty acid chains, causing close packing of these hydrophobic tails
- hydrogen bonding between polar head groups and water molecules
- electrostatic interactions between charged head groups

The presence of unsaturated fatty acids influences how the phospholipids pack in the bilayer. Double bonds form "kinks" in the fatty acid chain, decreasing efficiency of packing and "loosening" the bilayer. Conversely, saturated fatty acids form more rigid membranes.

Other amphiphilic or lipophilic molecules such as steroids (e.g., cholesterol), fatty acids, and so forth are interspersed

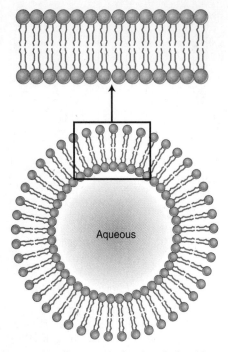

Aqueous

Figure 5.6. Illustration of a phospholipid bilayer. Note that the bilayer is composed of two layers of phospholipid molecules with their polar head groups facing outward. The bilayer forms closed structures with aqueous inner and outer compartments.

in the bilayer. These compounds are present in different amounts in different types of cells in our body. The unique lipid composition of each membrane contributes to the fluidity or rigidity of the membrane. The melting temperature of this complex lipid mixture is below normal body temperature, making the bilayer mobile, like a viscous fluid. Thermal motion allows phospholipids and other molecules to rotate freely around their long axes and to diffuse sideways within the membrane.

Many cell membrane lipids are covalently bonded with carbohydrates to form glycolipids. These are often located on the exterior surface of cell membranes where they function as receptors or are involved in cell–cell interactions. Glycolipids are essential for the development and growth of organisms and have been implicated in a number of serious

illnesses such as cancer or viral or microbial infections.

The hydrophobic interior of the lipid bilayer restricts movement of molecules; ions and other polar compounds pass very slowly or not at all through the bilayer, whereas small lipophilic compounds can cross the bilayer readily.

Cellular Proteins

Although the lipid bilayer provides the framework of the cell membrane, other types of molecules, such as proteins, are also present. The presence of these proteins modifies the properties of the bilayer considerably.

Soluble Proteins

Soluble proteins, such as plasma proteins and enzymes, are found in aqueous environments in the body and adopt specific confirmations compatible with water. The interior of the folded protein molecule contains a high proportion of hydrophobic amino acids, which tend to cluster and exclude water. This core is stabilized by van der Waals forces and by hydrophobic interactions. The exterior of the folded protein is primarily composed of hydrophilic amino acids that are charged or able to hydrogen-bond with water, making the protein water soluble. Soluble proteins are usually globular and tightly packed.

Membrane Proteins

Membrane proteins are located in or near the hydrophobic region of the lipid bilayer of cell membranes. Proteins that sit on the inner or outer surface of the cell membrane (extrinsic or *peripheral* proteins) are folded such that a large percentage of their hydrophobic amino acids are close to or anchored within the membrane lipids. Amino acids facing aqueous environments of the cytoplasm or extracellular fluid are mostly hydrophilic, allowing the protein to be compatible with water. Proteins

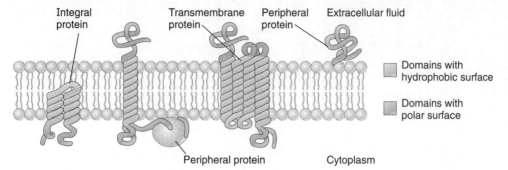

Figure 5.7. The phospholipid bilayer with membrane proteins. Note that the proteins are oriented so that their hydrophobic domains reside in the lipid bilayer, whereas their hydrophilic regions are exposed to the aqueous cytoplasm or extracellular fluid.

embedded in the lipid bilayer are called intrinsic or *integral* proteins; most of these have a portion that is exposed to the aqueous environment on the outer or inner surface of the bilayer. The portion that resides in the bilayer is composed of hydrophobic amino acid residues, whereas the portion exposed to water is largely hydrophilic. Many integral membrane proteins extend through the bilayer (*transmembrane proteins)* and have portions extending onto both the inner and outer bilayer surfaces. Figure 5.7 shows the cell membrane with its lipid bilayer and the location of peripheral and integral proteins. Although proteins are mobile within the bilayer, their large size makes them diffuse much more slowly than the membrane lipids.

Membrane proteins play a variety of roles and are often named on the basis of their function.

- Marker proteins identify cells to each other. The immune system uses these proteins to identify foreign invaders.
- Receptor proteins are involved with the passage of information between the extracellular and intracellular regions of cells.
- Transport proteins regulate transport of materials in and out of cells. Transport proteins can be classified into two types: channel proteins and carrier proteins.

○ Channel proteins are usually transmembrane proteins that create a water-filled channel through which ions and some small hydrophilic molecules can pass. In general, channels are quite specific for the type of solute or ion they will allow to pass. Many channels are gated, meaning that they can be opened or closed according to the needs of the cell. The channel transports when the gate is open and does not transport when the gate is closed.

○ Carrier proteins are transmembrane proteins that have one or more sites at which a substrate (e.g., an ion or molecule) can bind. The carrier protein then transports the substrate into or out of the cell.

Like lipids, many proteins are covalently bonded to carbohydrates to form glycoproteins. The carbohydrates attached to proteins allow for a more comprehensive system of cellular communication; glycoproteins are widely present in the cell membrane (see Fig. 5.8). Most glycoproteins and glycolipids in cell membranes have their carbohydrate chains almost exclusively on the external surface of the cell. The negative charge on the external surface of most cell membranes is ascribed to the negatively charged sialic acid, a carbohydrate attached to many glycoproteins and glycolipids.

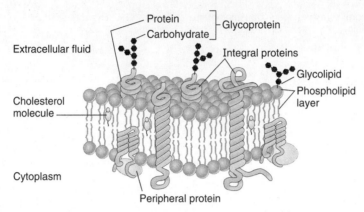

Figure 5.8. Diagram of a cell membrane, showing the phospholipid bilayer and the various types of membrane proteins, glycoproteins, and glycolipids.

Tissues

Cells are often arranged into groups called tissues, representing the next level of organization in the body. Cells in a tissue have similar structural and functional characteristics and, together, can impart additional properties. The four main types of tissues are muscle tissue, nervous tissue, connective tissue, and epithelial tissue. The latter is of particular interest to us, because it is the barrier that controls the movement of drugs into, within, and out of the body. Such multicellular barriers are often called *functional membranes.*

Epithelial Tissue

The internal cavities and external surfaces of the body are lined with a tissue called the epithelium or epithelial tissue. The specialized junctions between epithelial cells enable this tissue to act as a barrier to the movement of water, solutes, and cells from one body compartment to another. All materials that enter or leave the body do so through some type of epithelial barrier. Epithelial tissue serves both as a protective barrier for the body and as an active interface with the environment. It may also carry out other specialized functions, such as secretion of mucus, absorption of nutrients, and excretion of waste. Examples of epithelial tissue are the outer layers of skin, linings of body cavities exposed to the environment (e.g., the mouth, gastrointestinal tract, and respiratory tract), and the tissues that cover all internal organs.

Epithelial tissue provides the interface between masses of cells on one side and a cavity or space (lumen) on the other. The surface of the cell exposed to the lumen is called its apical or *lumenal* surface; the sides and base of the cell are the basolateral or *basal* surface.

Structure of Epithelial Tissues

Epithelial tissue is composed of epithelial cells often arranged in sheets. These sheets rest on a connective tissue called the *basement membrane,* anchoring the cells and attaching them to other tissues. In certain organs, the basement membrane assumes major significance; for example, the basement membrane in the kidney serves as a filter for plasma on its way to becoming urine. In other locations, the absence of a basement membrane is functionally important; the absence of a basement membrane in the liver permits plasma to come into direct contact with liver cells.

There are various types of epithelia depending on the shape of cells and number of cell layers. When classified by number, epithelial tissue is distinguished as *simple* (one layer) or *stratified* (more than one layer). When classified by shape, epithelial tissue may be *squamous* (flat, scalelike), *cuboidal* (cube-shaped), or *columnar* (tall and column-shaped). *Transitional* epithelium is found in organs that must stretch and contract such as the bladder. It is composed of several layers of cells that alter their shape with change in physiological state, i.e., variation in internal pressure and capacity. In the contracted condition the cells have a cuboidal or columnar shape; in the stretched condition some of the cells flatten out and assume a squamous shape. Some of the different types of epithelia are illustrated in Figure 5.9.

A stratified epithelium provides more protection to the organ against external assaults such as friction. Also, the outer layers of the cells can be sloughed off as the epithelium encounters friction. For example, the oral mucosa is composed of stratified squamous cells. Simple epithelia provide minimal protection, but make it easier for substances to cross the tissue; thus, they are found in tissues that are involved in movement of molecules from one side of the epithelium to the other. For example, capillary walls and lung epithelia are composed of simple squamous cells and the intestinal epithelium of simple columnar cells.

Epithelial cells often display surface specializations such as cilia (seen in cells lining the trachea) or microvilli (present in the epithelium of the small intestines). Cilia are motile, hairlike surface projections found on specialized cells and play a role in moving fluid or mucus

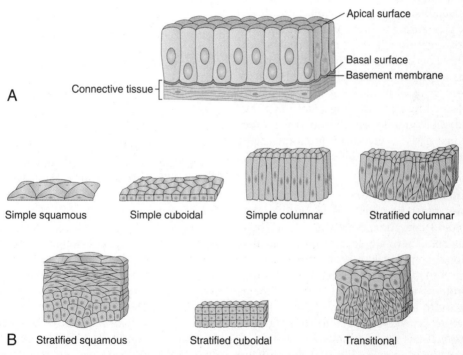

Figure 5.9. **A.** Structure of a typical epithelial tissue. The epithelial cells are separated from the underlying connective tissue by a basement membrane. The apical surface of cells is exposed to the environment, whereas the basal surface rests on the basement membrane. **B.** Types of epithelia based on number of layers and the shape of the cells. Simple epithelia consist of one cell layer, whereas stratified epithelia have multiple layers. Epithelial tissue is classified on the basis of cell shape as squamous (flat, scalelike), cuboidal (cube-shaped), columnar (tall and column-shaped), or transitional (columnar and squamous).

over the surface of the epithelium. Microvilli are nonmotile, fingerlike projections of the cell surface, commonly found in epithelial cells involved in absorption of materials from the lumenal side. Epithelial tissue can also exhibit down-growths, called glands, into the underlying connective tissue; glands are responsible for the secretion and excretion of a variety of substances.

Cell Junctions

If groups of cells are to come together to form a tissue or part of an organ, it is imperative that each cell be held in its proper place and be able to communicate with its neighbors. Cells are held together by contacts and adhesive forces between cell membrane molecules acting as weak "cellular glue." Several specialized *cell junctions* are responsible for cellular adhesion, cellular communication, or cell sealing to prevent substances from flowing through the intracellular space. These specialized cell junctions occur at many points of cell–cell and cell–matrix contact in all tissues, but they are particularly important and abundant in epithelia. Cell junctions fall into three functional classes: anchoring junctions, tight junctions, and gap junctions.

Anchoring Junctions.   Cells within tissues must be anchored to one another and to components of the extracellular matrix. There are several types of junctional complexes to serve this mechanical function. In each case, anchoring proteins extend through the cell membrane to link cytoskeletal proteins in one cell to cytoskeletal proteins in neighboring cells, as well as to proteins in the extracellular matrix (Fig. 5.10B). All are built from specific membrane proteins and filaments of the cytoskeleton. Anchoring junctions not only hold cells together, but also provide tissues with structural cohesion. These junctions are most abundant in tissues that are subject

to constant mechanical stress such as skin and heart.

Tight Junctions. One important characteristic of epithelial tissues is that the cells are closely packed, with specialized contacts between cells. **Tight junctions** are formed when specific proteins on the cell membranes of adjacent epithelial cells make direct contact across the intercellular space, forming a complex, impenetrable network (Fig. 5.10A).

The cells are thus sealed in a narrow band just beneath their apical surface. This seal creates a continuous sheet of cells that restricts the movement of most molecules through spaces between cells. Tight junctions are essential for the barrier function of epithelial tissue; their presence prevents potentially harmful molecules, especially macromolecules, from crossing the epithelium from the lumenal side to the basolateral side, and vice versa.

Tight junctions also restrict the movement of membrane proteins along the lipid bilayer, from the lumenal side of the membrane to the basolateral side. This means that most epithelial membranes have a distinctive apical and a basolateral side, with different proteins on each side. Each of these sides has not only different structure and composition but also different functions. This phenomenon is known as *membrane polarity,* and the epithelial membrane is said to be *polarized.*

The diameter of a typical tight junction is approximately 0.2 nm, so molecules with molecular weights greater than approximately 200 cannot pass between cells. The more the contacts between membrane proteins of adjacent cells, the tighter the junction becomes. However, this seal between cells is not absolute or uniform. The tight junction is almost always impermeable to macromolecules, but its permeability to small molecules varies greatly in different epithelia. Chapter 8, Transport Across Biological Barriers, will address the role of tight junctions in the transport of drug molecules across tissues.

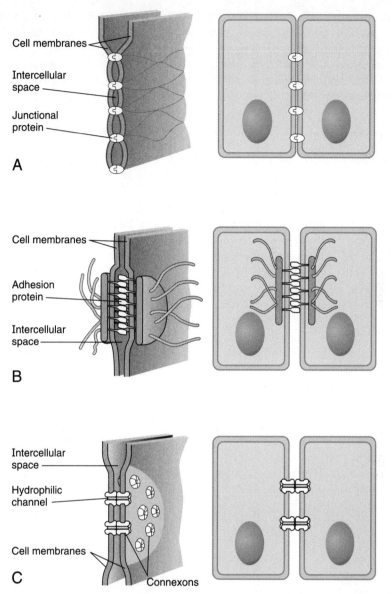

Figure 5.10. A diagram showing the different types of junctions between cells. **A.** Tight junctions seal neighboring cells together and prevent movement of materials through the intercellular space. **B.** Anchoring junctions link neighboring cells but permit materials to move around them through the intercellular space. **C.** Gap junctions allow neighboring cells to exchange materials and to communicate with each other.

Gap Junctions. Gap junctions are communicating junctions that allow cells in a tissue to respond as an integrated unit. Gap junctions are composed of clusters of channel proteins or *connexons*; one protein resides in the membrane of one cell and aligns and joins a channel protein of a neighboring cell, forming a continuous aqueous pathway. These channels permit substances and chemical information to be transmitted between cells, and allow the coordinated behavior of a group of cells. Molecules and ions with molecular weights below approximately 1,000 are able to pass directly from the cytoplasm of one cell to another through these structures (Fig. 5.10C). In contrast to tight and anchoring junctions, gap junctions do not seal membranes together, nor do they restrict passage of material through the intercellular space between cells.

The Endothelium

A special type of epithelial tissue, called the endothelium or endothelial membrane, makes up the walls of blood and lymph vessels and the internal surfaces of body cavities. A single layer of endothelial cells forms the walls of most capillaries. Endothelial cells are usually simple squamous cells, more loosely packed than epithelial cells. They do not have tight junctions, allowing freer movement of many small dissolved molecules through spaces between cells. The junctions between cells in the endothelium are often called *leaky* because they allow the passage of most small molecules (including drugs) and some larger molecules from the apical to the basolateral side and vice versa.

Specialized endothelial membranes line the capillaries in some parts of the body. Capillaries in the kidney and liver are very leaky, and may allow large molecules and even red blood cells to move between cell junctions. In contrast, the endothelium of capillaries in the brain has tight junctions like most epithelial membranes, allowing almost no movement of small molecules through these junctions.

KEY CONCEPTS

- Cell membranes are made up of lipids, proteins, and carbohydrates.
- The cell membrane is composed of a lipid bilayer with embedded membrane proteins.
- Many membrane lipids and proteins are glycosylated, giving them unique properties.
- Membrane proteins are responsible for controlling transport, communication, and recognition between cells.
- Cells with similar structure and function are arranged in tissues.

- Epithelial tissue lines the internal cavities and external surfaces of the body.
- Specialized junctions between cells control structure, communication, and transport through the intercellular space.
- Tight junctions prevent movement of substances through the intercellular space between epithelial cells.
- Endothelial tissue is a special type of epithelium; it does not have tight junctions.

ADDITIONAL READING

1. Berg JM, Stryer L, Tymoczko JL. Biochemistry, 5th ed. WH Freeman, 2002.
2. Nelson DL, Cox MM. Lehninger Principles of Biochemistry, 4th ed. WH Freeman, 2004.
3. Alberts B, Johnson A, Lewis J, Raff M, Roberts K, Walter P. Molecular Biology of the Cell, 4th ed. Garland Science, 2002.
4. Scott MP, Matsudaira P, Lodish H, et al. Molecular Cell Biology, 5th ed. WH Freeman, 2003.

REVIEW QUESTIONS

1. What are the biomolecules that make up the cell membrane? Briefly describe their structure.
2. What are the functions of a cell membrane?
3. What is the structure of phospholipids? Why do these molecules spontaneously form a bilayer?
4. Discuss the fluid–mosaic model of cell membrane structure. What makes the membrane "fluid"?
5. Describe the types and functions of membrane proteins.
6. What role do carbohydrates play in the cell membrane?
7. What are the types and functions of epithelial tissue?
8. Describe the three major types of cell junctions. What are their functions?
9. How is the endothelial membrane different from most epithelial tissues?

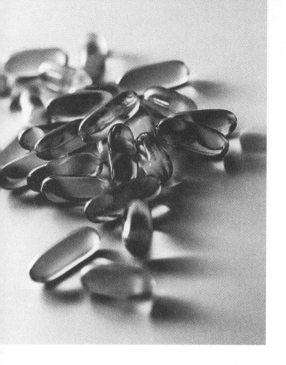

Section II • Drug Structure and Design

Drugs and Their Targets

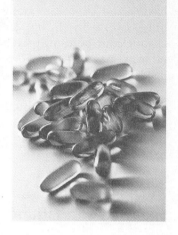

Cellular processes are detected, modulated, and directed by complex systems made up of diverse biomolecules such as DNA, RNA, proteins, lipids, and carbohydrates. These molecules regulate the internal environment of living organisms and are essential to survival. Many diseases and illnesses are linked to problems in the synthesis or properties of a particular biomolecule. A drug target is a biomolecule that plays a role in a disease process and is the intended site of action of a drug. Proteins, particularly enzymes and cell membrane receptors, are the most common targets of existing drugs and of drug discovery research. Other less common targets are hormones, ion channels, DNA, and nuclear receptors.

Proteins are the engines of the cell, regulating activation of genes, relaying signals within and between cells, and driving metabolic processes. Proteins are required for the structure, function, and regulation of the body's cells, tissues, and organs. For cells and tissues to remain healthy they must be able to make proteins, and the proteins they make must be able to function correctly. Changes in the composition or abundance of critical proteins can lead to disease.

Drug–protein interactions play a vital role in almost all aspects of a drug's behavior and function. Many of today's drugs work by fitting into pockets, channels, or pores in proteins. Furthermore, drugs are transported, metabolized, and excreted with the help of proteins. This chapter discusses the role of proteins as important drug targets, and the nature of drug–protein interactions responsible for drug pharmacokinetics and action.

Proteins and Ligands

Proteins are folded into a highly organized tertiary structure, a three-dimensional shape with a distinct inside and outside. Many proteins self-associate into assemblies composed of two to six or more individual polypeptide chains; this represents the quaternary structure of proteins. For example, the acetylcholine receptor, a membrane protein of critical importance in neuromuscular communication, is a five-chain molecule. Only one final folded structure of the protein is functional.

Proteins are linked in networks of physical interactions and functional relationships to each other. Interactions between different proteins play pivotal roles in various aspects of the structural and functional organization of cells. The complexity of life requires proteins to be able to transfer specific signals, build tissues, control the function of enzymes, and regulate production and activities of many substances.

In general, drugs act by interaction with four kinds of regulatory protein targets:

- Receptor proteins: Receptors receive and process extracellular signals. An example of a drug that targets receptors is the antiallergy drug Zyrtec, which interacts with and blocks the histamine H_1 receptor.
- Ion channel proteins: Channel proteins control passage of solutes and

ions in and out of cells. Local anesthetics bind to and inhibit sodium ion channel proteins.
- Enzymes: Enzymes catalyze biochemical and metabolic reactions. The drug celecoxib binds to and inhibits the COX2 (cyclooxygenase 2) enzyme.
- Transporters: Transporters help to transport materials in and out of a cell. Prozac inhibits the serotonin transporter in the brain.

The term receptor is reserved mainly for those proteins that play an important role in intercellular communication via chemical messengers. As such, enzymes, ion channels, and transporters are usually not classified as receptors. The ways that these proteins interact with other molecules are similar, however, as we shall see shortly.

Receptors perform their cellular functions by binding to chemical messenger molecules called ligands. A ligand is an ion or a molecule that binds to the receptor to form a complex and consequently participate in a biological action. Ligands may be endogenous (already present in the body), or introduced into the body as drugs; examples of endogenous ligands are signaling compounds such as neurotransmitters and hormones. Most drugs take the place of endogenous ligands in exerting their action. For example, morphine and related pain-relieving drugs use the same receptors in the brain used by endorphins, compounds produced by the body to control pain. Ligands may be small molecules or macromolecules; the term small molecule generally refers to molecular weights less than 1,000. Most small molecule drugs have molecular weights in the range between 300 and 700.

The three-dimensional shape of a protein creates several pockets or active sites (also called *binding sites*) where molecules of appropriate structure may bind (see Figure 6.1). These molecules are said to have an affinity (attraction) for the protein. Protein misfolding can

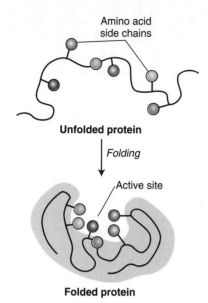

Figure 6.1. An illustration of the active site formed by the folding of a protein. Note that the unfolded protein does not have a unique binding site; such a site is created when the protein folds in a specific way.

change the active site configuration and interfere with binding of ligands, causing Alzheimer's, mad cow disease (in humans, variant Creutzfeldt-Jakob disease), cystic fibrosis, amyotrophic lateral sclerosis, and Parkinson's. Many cancers are also believed to result from protein misfolding.

Protein–Ligand Interactions

Most protein function is controlled by ligands that bind reversibly to proteins and either stimulate or inhibit their activity. The rate and extent of binding of a particular protein to a particular ligand are influenced by many factors, such as:

- structure, physicochemical properties, and concentration of the ligand
- structure and concentration of the protein
- affinity between the ligand and the protein

- competition by other substances that also bind to the protein active site

Different branches of pharmaceutical sciences use different nomenclature for ligand molecules, depending on whether the protein is a receptor or an enzyme.

Receptor Agonists and Antagonists

If the protein is a receptor, the endogenous ligand is called an agonist, a compound that binds to the receptor and then stimulates a cellular effect. *Drugs* that bind to receptors are classified as either agonists or antagonists. Agonist drugs activate their receptors, triggering a response that increases or decreases the cell's activity in a manner similar to the endogenous ligand. Antagonist drugs block the access or binding of the body's natural agonists to their receptors, and thereby prevent or reduce cell responses to natural agonists. Both the agonist and antagonist are released unchanged at the end of the process. Drugs are *receptor modulators* in that they can only influence some preexisting function of the receptor, but cannot impart any new property to it. We will explore these concepts further in Chapter 16, Mechanisms of Drug Action.

An example of an agonist drug is albuterol, which binds to *adrenergic* receptors on cells in the respiratory tract, causing relaxation of smooth muscle cells and thus opening airways in asthmatic patients. Using an appropriate antagonist may also widen constricted airways. For example, the drug ipratropium bromide binds to *cholinergic* receptors in the respiratory tract, preventing binding of the endogenous ligand acetylcholine, a neurotransmitter that causes contraction of smooth muscle cells and narrows the airways. Blocking acetylcholine binding to its cholinergic receptor prevents bronchoconstriction and makes breathing easier. Thus, a given disease or condition may be treated in different ways.

Enzyme Inhibitors

If the protein is a soluble protein like an enzyme, the molecule that binds to it is called a substrate rather than a ligand. Enzymes catalyze chemical reactions involving substrates and turn them into products; the substrate is consumed in the reaction. Enzyme catalysis is important for most cellular metabolic processes. At any given moment, enzymes are facilitating most of the activities inside a cell and endogenous substrates are being converted into products. Many drugs have been designed to target enzymes, and most of these are enzyme inhibitors. The action of an inhibitor is to take the place of the natural substrate and prevent it from being converted into product. For example, the cholesterol-lowering drug lovastatin inhibits an enzyme called HMG-CoA reductase, critical for production of cholesterol in the body. We will discuss enzyme inhibitors further in Chapter 16, Mechanisms of Drug Action.

Enzymes are also important in drug biotransformation reactions, in which the drug (substrate) undergoes a reaction while bound to the enzyme (protein) and the reaction products (metabolites) are released in a subsequent step. A side effect of many drugs is that they are enzyme *inducers*; for example, one side effect of the antibiotic rifampin is that it activates enzymes involved in metabolizing oral contraceptives. When women taking an oral contraceptive also take rifampin, the contraceptive may be ineffective because it is metabolized and removed from the body more quickly than usual.

The Binding Equilibrium

Whether the protein is a receptor or enzyme, most ligands bind by a *reversible* process, in which bonds formed between ligand and protein are noncovalent and weak, and can be readily broken to give back the starting materials. *Irreversible* protein–ligand binding can occur when a ligand attaches to a protein by a covalent bond; such binding cannot be easily reversed to give the original protein. Irreversible binding is rare and accounts for a few types of drug toxicity (such as chemical carcinogenesis) and the action of certain antibiotics on microorganisms. Many poisons and toxins also act by forming covalent bonds with enzyme or receptor proteins. An example is the nerve gas sarin, which forms an irreversible covalent bond with the enzyme acetylcholinesterase. The enzyme's active site is blocked and it becomes nonfunctional. New acetylcholinesterase molecules have to be synthesized by cells to carry out the enzyme's function.

Figure 6.2 illustrates the reversible binding of a ligand (or drug) to a protein. For simplicity, assume that the protein has only one type of binding site where the ligand can bind. In reality, proteins are quite large compared with most ligands and may contain more than one binding site, but this requires a complex analysis beyond our scope.

Consider the reversible binding between a receptor and its ligand or an enzyme and its substrate. This analysis is very similar to the discussion of enzyme catalysis and Michaelis–Menten kinetics in Chapter 4, Rates of Pharmaceutical Processes. In the present context, the

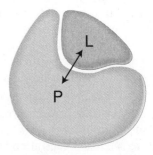

Figure 6.2. Binding of protein, P, to a ligand, L, at an active site. The arrow indicates that the binding is reversible.

receptor is denoted as R and the ligand as L. The same treatment applies to an enzyme, E, binding to its substrate, S. The equilibrium can be written as:

$$\text{receptor} + \text{ligand} \rightleftharpoons \text{complex}$$

$$\text{(Eq. 6.1a)}$$

$$\text{enzyme} + \text{substrate} \rightleftharpoons \text{complex}$$

$$\text{(Eq. 6.1b)}$$

Equation 6.1a and 6.1b can be rewritten simply as:

$$R + L \rightleftharpoons RL \quad \text{(Eq. 6.2a)}$$

$$E + S \rightleftharpoons ES \quad \text{(Eq. 6.2b)}$$

RL represents the receptor–ligand complex, while ES is the enzyme–substrate complex.

The law of mass action defines K, the association constant for these equilibria:

$$K = \frac{[RL]}{[E][L]} \quad \text{(Eq. 6.3a)}$$

$$K = \frac{ES}{[E][S]} \quad \text{(Eq. 6.3b)}$$

The square brackets denote concentrations of the corresponding molecule at equilibrium.

Affinity

The magnitude of K gives information about the extent of ligand–receptor (or enzyme–substrate) binding, i.e., how much ligand (or substrate) is bound by the receptor (or enzyme) in the complex. A ligand that is extensively bound to a receptor has a large K, showing that there is a high affinity between receptor and ligand. The same is true for enzyme–substrate binding. Again, note the simi-

larity between this discussion and the earlier discussion of enzyme catalysis.

The strength of binding is often expressed as the inverse of the association constant K. A *dissociation constant*, K_d for the receptor–ligand complex or K_m for the enzyme–substrate complex, is defined as:

$$K_d = \frac{1}{K} = \frac{[R][L]}{[RL]} \quad \text{(Eq. 6.4a)}$$

$$K_m = \frac{1}{K} = \frac{[E][S]}{[ES]} \quad \text{(Eq. 6.4b)}$$

K_m is the Michaelis constant we have seen previously. K_m and K_d have units of concentration. These constants can be thought of as the concentration of ligand (or substrate) required to occupy 50% of the receptor (or enzyme) active sites. The lower the K_d, the higher is the affinity of receptor for ligand; the same holds true for K_m.

Consequences of Binding

In some situations, the only outcome of complex formation between a protein and another molecule is to tie up the molecule for some time, making it unavailable to perform its function. This occurs when proteins in the plasma (such as albumin) bind to drugs and prevent them from leaving the bloodstream and entering tissues. The complex eventually dissociates, according to the equilibrium shown in Equation 6.1, and releases the drug.

In other situations, however, the formation of the complex is only a first step in some important physiological process with a definite outcome, as indicated below.

$$\text{protein} + \text{binding molecule} \underset{}{\overset{K}{\rightleftharpoons}}$$

$$\text{complex} \rightarrow\rightarrow \text{outcome} \quad \text{(Eq. 6.5)}$$

Catalytic Outcomes

If the protein is an enzyme, the outcome in Equation 6.5 is usually *catalytic* in that the substrate is transformed into a new product after initial binding to the protein. The kinetics of such a catalytic process is described by Michaelis–Menten kinetics. Figure 6.3 illustrates enzymatic catalysis of substrate(s) to product(s).

Catalytic reactions can be suppressed by enzyme inhibitors that bind to the enzyme and prevent the substrate from binding. As we saw earlier, many drugs are enzyme inhibitors, preventing the endogenous ligand from binding and performing its normal function. For example, angiotensin-converting enzyme inhibitors (also called ACE inhibitors; e.g., captopril and enalapril) are drugs that block the conversion of the substrate angiotensin I to a substance that increases salt and water retention in the body. ACE inhibitors are used in the treatment of high blood pressure.

Noncatalytic Outcomes

The outcome of complex formation may be *noncatalytic*, in that the ligand is not chemically changed on binding to its receptors, but is eventually released unchanged. Instead, binding induces a conformational change in the receptor that triggers biochemical events in the cell as illustrated in Figure 6.4. The ligand eventually dissociates from the receptor–ligand complex. We will discuss binding

Protein–Protein Interactions

We have considered protein–small molecule interactions in detail, because a majority of drugs are small molecules. Most cellular processes, however, are mediated by protein–protein interactions, which are vital to the functioning of our body.

Enzymes perform transcription of DNA to RNA, whereas other proteins bind to specific regions of DNA to promote or inhibit its transcription, and thus, gene regulation. Nearly all the cellular machinery for synthesis, replication, manipulation, modification, and degradation involves proteins interacting with other proteins and macromolecules. Proteins are directed to the correct compartments of cells by binding to other proteins. Many endogenous ligands are proteins, which bind to receptors on cell membranes to send signals between cells. Proteins form structural connections between cells. Proteins are substrates and inhibitors of enzymes. Protein–protein interactions underlie large-scale movements in organisms such as muscle contraction.

Protein–protein interactions can sometimes be undesirable. Protein aggregation is associated with a number of diseases, including prion-related diseases, Alzheimer's disease, and Down's syndrome.

It is important to note that interaction forces between proteins are weak. It is through the synergism of multiple weakly interacting proteins that a cell can generate responses. If every protein had high affinity for every other protein, it would be difficult for the cell to regulate the activity of any one pathway. Thus, weak protein–protein interactions play a central role in finely tuned cellular signaling. They also provide us an opportunity to control cellular responses by using small molecule drugs to interfere with and alter protein–protein interactions.

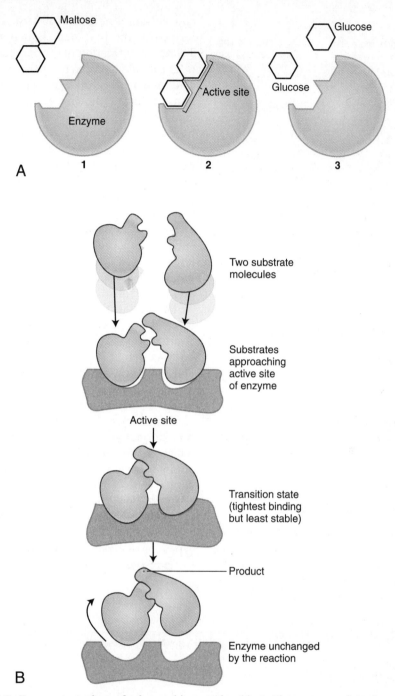

Figure 6.3. Enzymatic catalysis of substrate(s) to product(s). **A.** The enzyme maltase has an active site complementary to the structure of maltose and binds only to maltose. A reaction occurs when maltose binds to the enzyme, releasing two glucose molecules as products. A single maltase molecule can catalyze the reaction of more than 1,000 maltose molecules per second. **B.** Example of the enzyme-catalyzed synthesis of a product from two substrate molecules.

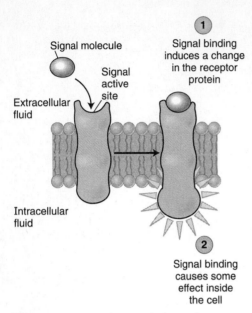

Figure 6.4. A signal molecule (an endogenous ligand or a drug) binds to a cell membrane receptor on the extracellular surface and induces a change in receptor protein that causes some effect inside the cell.

to receptors in more depth in Chapter 16, Mechanisms of Drug Action.

Similarities Between Receptors and Enzymes

Both receptor–ligand and enzyme–substrate binding are generally reversible events. The outcome depends on the concentration of ligand–protein complex formed in the first step (Equation 6.2). Therefore, formation of the complex controls the rate and extent of the outcome. The higher the affinity of ligand for protein, the larger the concentration of the complex, and the greater the outcome of ligand–protein binding will be. The formation of the complex is dependent on pH, temperature, and the presence of ions and other molecules. Binding can be saturated at high concentrations of the ligand or substrate. Molecules bound by enzymes and receptors may be small, such as a sugar or amino acid, or may be large, such as another protein. For example, insulin, a macromolecule, is the ligand for the insulin receptor.

The similarities between enzymes and receptors are easily recognized by direct comparison, as shown in Table 6.1. The body contains many different receptors and enzymes, and often the distinction between them is unclear. Sometimes a receptor has enzymatic activity. Many enzymes, such as those with allosteric regulation, also qualify as receptors when the broadest use of the term is applied. If we consider any ligand interacting with a macromolecule to be a receptor–ligand interaction, then any interaction of small molecules with protein, DNA, or RNA can be classified as types of receptor–ligand complexes if some response occurs.

TABLE 6.1. Similarities Between Enzymatic and Receptor Processes		
	Enzyme	*Receptor*
Binding molecule	Substrate	Ligand
Complex	E–S	R–L
Outcome	Product formation	Complex formation, or response
Number of binding sites	One or more	One or more
Type of binding	Specific or nonspecific	Specific or nonspecific
Measurement of binding affinity	K_m	K_d
Types of binding molecules	Inhibitors, activators	Agonists, antagonists
Regulation	Allosteric activation	Gene regulation

Molecular Recognition

Protein surfaces are irregular. This irregularity enables proteins to bind specific ligands (we will use the term ligand generally to mean a substrate as well) and to associate specifically with other proteins, and it underlies the formation of quaternary structure. The primary concept behind protein–ligand binding is that of *complementarity*, or "fit," between ligand and active site. This matching between a protein surface and another molecule depends on much more than shape. It extends to the weak bonds that hold complexes together; hydrogen bond donors line up with acceptors, nonpolar groups are opposite other nonpolar groups, and positive charges are opposite negative charges.

The two types of complementarity for us to consider are physicochemical complementarity, i.e., the presence of several physicochemical bonding interactions between the two molecules, and steric complementarity, i.e., whether the shape of the ligand fits the shape of the active site. Both determine the strength of the overall interaction.

Physicochemical Complementarity

Covalent bonds are not routinely formed between a protein and ligand during normal cellular processes. Therefore, several types of weaker noncovalent bonds are necessary to attract and keep the two molecules together as a complex. In most cases, the initial attraction between the two interacting species is provided by a long-range force such as an ionic interaction between opposite charges on the protein active site and the ligand. As the ligand approaches the protein, short-range forces such as hydrogen bonds provide additional attractive and orienting forces. Finally, van der Waals forces and hydrophobic interactions come into play to further orient and stabilize the complex. Thus, most protein–ligand interactions rely on many different molecular forces to form the final complex. Of the various physicochemical interactions involved in protein–ligand binding, ionic and hydrophobic interactions are probably the most important.

Because the initial interaction between a ligand and protein is often ionic, the ionization state of weak acid and base drugs is very important. Charged atoms (from ionized amino acids) often line the protein active site, imparting a localized charge in specific regions of the pocket. Opposite charges on the active site and ligand will attract each other, beginning the complex formation process. *Electrostatic complementarity* is important in preventing inappropriate molecules from binding to the active site, as the ligand must contain correctly placed complementary charged atoms for interaction to occur.

Another critical force for ligand–protein binding is hydrophobic interaction. Nearly two thirds of the body is water, and this aqueous environment surrounds all our cells. For a ligand and protein to interact, there must be a driving force that compels the ligand to leave water and bind to the protein; hydrophobic ligands are able to accomplish this. Thus the partition coefficient of the ligand is also an important factor in protein–ligand binding.

Steric Complementarity

Although physicochemical complementarity is important for the initial attraction between ligand and protein, the ligand must also have stereochemical complementarity to sustain the ligand–protein complex. This means that the ligand must have a defined three-dimensional shape and size that fit well into the active site. Let us briefly review the basic concepts of stereochemistry as they pertain to stereochemical complementarity in protein–ligand binding. Undergraduate textbooks in chemistry are good resources for a more thorough discussion of stereochemistry.

Stereoisomers are molecules that have the same molecular formula and sequence of bonds but different spatial arrangements; the only difference between them is the three-dimensional orientation of atoms or functional groups in space. Despite having identical chemical formulas and bonding, stereoisomers can have dramatically different chemical, physical, and biological properties. There are two main types of stereoisomers of interest in understanding stereocomplementarity: enantiomers and geometric isomers.

Enantiomers and Chirality. Chirality is the geometric property of a rigid object (like a molecule or drug) not being superimposable with its mirror image. A molecule that cannot be superimposed on its mirror image is said to be chiral (the Greek word for "handed"). This is in contrast to *achiral* molecules, which can be superimposed on their mirror images.

Chirality is analogous to our right and left hands—they are mirror images but are not superimposable. The two mirror images of a chiral molecule are termed enantiomers. Like hands, enantiomers come in pairs. Chirality usually occurs when a compound contains at least one asymmetric or chiral center in its structure. A chiral center is an atom at which the interchange of any two substituents attached to it creates a new stereoisomer. Various nomenclature systems have been used for enantiomers; the most common ones designate the two forms in the pair as L- and D-, or as R- and S-.

Chirality is a property found in many biologically important molecules such as amino acids, carbohydrates, and lipids. For example, the natural amino acids share a common stereochemistry; they are all L-amino acids. Our bodies use only D-sugars; DNA and RNA are made up of D-sugars, resulting in a right-handed DNA double helix. Consequently, most cellular targets are chiral and can recognize differences between enantiomers of a chiral ligand. Our receptors, such as the taste receptors in our tongue, can distinguish between stereoisomers of a ligand; for example, one isomer of leucine tastes sweet and the other tastes bitter. Chemicals with different enantiomeric forms can smell different also. One isomer of limonene smells of oranges, the other of lemons.

Enantiomeric pairs have identical physicochemical properties, such as boiling point, melting point, density, and solubility. Enantiomers, however, can have marked differences in their interaction with proteins such as enzymes and receptors, and can behave very differently in biological systems as a result of their different three-dimensional shape. Figure 6.5

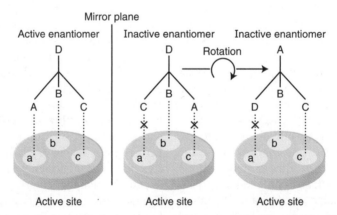

Figure 6.5. Binding of two hypothetical enantiomers of a drug to a receptor active site. The active enantiomer has a three-dimensional structure that allows drug domain A to interact with active site domain a, B to interact with b, and C to interact with c. All three binding interactions are necessary. In contrast, the inactive enantiomer cannot be aligned to have the same three interactions with the binding site simultaneously. The difference in three-dimensional structure allows the active enantiomer to bind and have a biological effect, whereas this is not possible for the inactive enantiomer.

illustrates the binding of two hypothetical enantiomers of a drug to a receptor active site. In other words, the R enantiomer of a drug will not necessarily behave the same way as the S enantiomer of the same drug when taken by a patient. In essence, the two enantiomers of a chiral drug should be considered different drugs. The ability of biomolecules to distinguish between the various steric forms of a ligand or drug is called chiral recognition or *chiral discrimination*.

For example, the two enantiomers of amphetamine (D-amphetamine and L-amphetamine) have the same melting points, solubilities, and pK$_a$ values; however, the D isomer is more potent.

Geometric Isomers. Geometric isomers (or *cis–trans* isomerism) occur because of restricted rotation around a bond such as a carbon–carbon double bond, or in a ring such as cyclohexane. The *cis* and *trans* configurations are not mirror images of each other, and the two forms show significant differences in their physicochemical properties, such as ionization and lipophilicity, and in their biological activity.

Geometric *cis* and *trans* isomers can be isolated as pure substances, and mixtures of isomers are not commonly seen. However, the two *trans* isomers in a cyclic compound can exist as an enantiomeric pair. Differences in biological activity

Racemic Mixtures

A racemic mixture or racemate is a sample of a compound that contains all its possible stereoisomers in equal proportions. Thus, for a compound with one chiral center, a racemate has the two enantiomers in a 1:1 ratio. Enantiomers in a racemic mixture are difficult to separate from each other as pure stereoisomers because they have the same physicochemical properties. For this reason, the majority of synthetic drugs were produced as racemic mixtures for many years, and the properties of the individual stereoisomers were not known. More than 500 currently useful drugs are racemic mixtures containing an active drug and its enantiomer in equal proportions.

It is now clear that stereoisomers can have significantly different biological properties, and that a single stereoisomer is often therapeutically superior to a racemic mixture. The isomer with the desired activity is called the eutomer and the one without the desired activity or with an undesired activity is the distomer. New methods to produce single isomers on a commercial scale are now available, removing a major obstacle in the use of single isomer drugs.

Chirality now plays a major role in the development of new pharmaceuticals; approximately 30% of marketed drugs are sold as a single isomeric form. The antiinflammatory drug naproxen is marketed as the S isomer, because the R form is a liver toxin. Similarly, L-dopa has anti-Parkinsonian activity, whereas D-dopa exhibits none of the desired anti-Parkinsonian activity and can cause granulocytopenia (loss of white blood cells that leaves patients prone to infections). There are other examples such as penicillamine, used to treat arthritis, in which the S enantiomer is active while the R form is extremely toxic. The (S, S) form of the antituberculosis drug ethambutol is active while the (R, R) form causes optical neuritis that can lead to blindness.

between *cis* and *trans* isomers may, therefore, be caused by either nonspecific physicochemical effects or stereoselectivity of receptor binding. Figure 6.6 illustrates geometric isomerism and how geometric isomers can bind differently to a target protein.

An example of *cis–trans* isomerism in drugs is found in *trans*-diethylstilbestrol, which has estrogenic activity, and *cis*-diethylstilbestrol, which has only 7% of the estrogenic activity of *trans*-diethylstilbestrol.

Selectivity and Specificity

These two terms are often used interchangeably and describe the same general concept. Selectivity refers to the ability of a ligand or drug to interact with a certain protein's active site without binding significantly to other proteins. Selectivity is generally a desirable prop-

erty in a drug, e.g., it is desirable that an antibacterial drug affect bacteria at concentrations too small to affect host cells.

Specificity is the ability of a *protein* to bind to a ligand with a defined structure, while having little or no interaction with other molecules of similar structure. Proteins can be specific, somewhat specific, or nonspecific in their binding to ligands. Most receptors are highly specific in their binding to other molecules.

Nonspecific or partially specific binding occurs when ligands with a variety of structures are able to bind to a given protein, and where physicochemical complementarity is most important. For example, albumin, a protein found in plasma, can bind to a variety of lipophilic drug molecules, particularly weak acids and neutral drugs. Similarly, α_1-acid glycoprotein, another plasma protein, binds with many basic drugs, regardless of their structure. Many enzymes show *group*

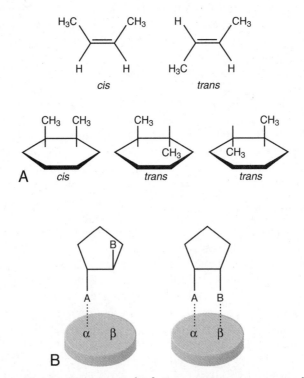

Figure 6.6. **A.** Geometric isomerism as a result of *cis–trans* orientation across a double bond or in a ring. **B.** Binding of geometric isomers to a target. On the left, the *trans* isomer does not have the B group in proper configuration for effective binding. On the right, the *cis* isomer has both the functional groups in a favorable orientation for binding to the receptor.

specificity, in which a general group of compounds can serve as substrates.

Specificity and selectivity increase when stereochemical complementarity plays a major role in protein–ligand binding, such as the binding between receptors and their ligands, or several enzymes with their substrates.

A few drugs produce their biological action without binding to a particular target. Such nonspecific activity is usually related to a physicochemical property of the drug, such as lipophilicity or pK_a. For example, antacids neutralize stomach acid because of their alkalinity, and osmotic diuretics help eliminate water by producing an osmotic gradient in the kidneys and increasing urine production. For other drugs, nonspecific activity is often manifested as a side effect or toxicity. Examples are sedation and general depression of the central nervous system by some lipophilic drugs, and bactericidal

effects of certain compounds. A wide variety of chemical structures can show the same nonspecific activity if their physicochemical properties are similar.

Models of Binding

Two simple models have been proposed to describe the binding between a ligand and a protein: the lock-and-key model and the induced-fit model. These are illustrated in Figure 6.7. Other more complex models have also been proposed but are outside the scope of this book.

Lock and Key

The lock-and-key model proposes that the surfaces of ligand (key) and protein (lock) must fit exactly or there will be no binding. The ligand and protein need to have compatible, interlocking shapes,

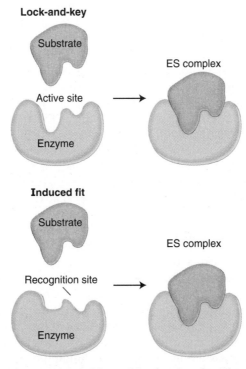

Figure 6.7. The lock-and-key and induced-fit models of protein–ligand interaction. This diagram uses an example of an enzyme binding to its substrate.

like two puzzle pieces or a lock and key. Some drugs attach to only one type of receptor and are therefore selective; others, like a master key, can bind to several types of receptors throughout the body, making them partially selective. In this simplest scenario, the protein and ligand interact with no change in their conformation on binding.

Induced Fit

Molecular interactions that involve conformational changes in one or both interacting molecules are more versatile. The induced-fit model states that when the ligand first binds, its interaction with the protein is weak. However, this initial binding causes a change in the conformation of the protein, allowing the ligand to bind more tightly. Protein conformational change is possible because proteins are flexible molecules, and because the forces that maintain secondary and tertiary protein structure are also weak. Thus, enough energy is available at body temperature to break interactions that hold the folded protein together, and allow for a different folded structure in the presence of ligand. This can be thought of as a stabilization of a particular protein conformation by ligand binding to allow for optimal binding. Induced fit also allows for binding of more than one ligand at the same active site. When the binding of a specific ligand causes a protein to change from an inactive to an active conformation, the process involves an induced fit.

Allostery and Cooperativity

Proteins often contain several active sites for different types of ligands. Until this point, we have considered ligands that bind independently to these sites, i.e., the affinity of the ligand for the protein active site remains the same regardless of ligand concentration. There are many examples, however, in which ligands do not bind independently, but a ligand bound at a site influences the ability of another ligand to bind to a second site on the same protein.

Proteins have the ability to coordinate what is going on at these different binding sites in such a way that the binding of one ligand alters the affinity for another ligand on the same protein. There need not be a direct connection between the two ligands; they may bind to opposite sides of the protein, or even to different subunits of protein. This mechanism is called allostery; the interaction is termed allosteric binding and is illustrated in Figure 6.8.

One explanation of allostery involves protein flexibility. In some ligand–protein interactions, binding to a ligand induces conformational changes in the protein, as described by the induced-fit model discussed earlier. Conformational changes may also take place in locations far removed from the first binding site. Often, the result of the first protein–ligand interaction is to change the shape of other active sites, so that subsequent ligand binding (of a similar or different ligand) is altered. These can be relatively minor adjustments of the protein chain or can be significant changes in three-dimensional conformation. An example of drug activity caused by allostery is found in the drug nevirapine, an inhibitor of the enzyme HIV reverse transcriptase (HIV-RT). Nevirapine binds to HIV-RT at an allosteric site that is not the active site of the enzyme. This binding changes the conformation of the active site, so that HIV-RT is no longer able to function normally.

For identical ligands, the allosteric mechanism is called a cooperative effect. If ligand binding were independent, each site would exhibit the same affinity for ligand. In cooperative binding, however, the apparent individual site binding affinities differ from one another and from the independent affinity of each site. Binding may exhibit either positive cooperativity or negative cooperativity, in which the apparent ligand affinity

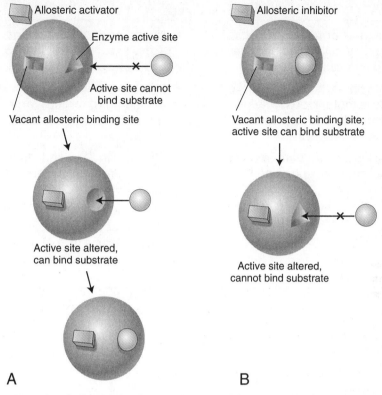

Figure 6.8. Examples of allosteric binding resulting in either an increase (**A**) or decrease (**B**) of the target's affinity for its ligand or substrate.

increases or decreases as more ligands bind, respectively. Cooperativity is evident in the binding of oxygen to hemoglobin. Hemoglobin is a protein with four subunits linked together, each subunit containing a single heme—a ringlike structure with a central iron atom that binds to an oxygen atom. Deoxyhemoglobin is relatively uninterested in oxygen, but when one oxygen attaches, the second binds more easily, and the third and fourth easier yet. The same process works in reverse: once fully oxygenated

hemoglobin lets go of an oxygen, it lets go of the next more easily, and so forth. In fact, hemoglobin is usually observed in only two states—all four subunits carrying oxygen, or completely oxygen free.

One reason that cooperative binding is widespread in biological systems is that it is an important way for cells to modulate the response to an input signal. Positive cooperativity causes the system to respond more sensitively to changes in ligand concentration. Negative cooperativity damps the response to ligand concentration.

KEY CONCEPTS

- Proteins perform their biological function by binding to endogenous compounds called ligands.

- Drugs work by binding to targets, usually receptor or enzyme proteins, and thus influencing protein–ligand binding in some way.

- Agonist drugs stimulate receptors just like the corresponding ligands. Antagonist drugs interfere with ligand binding and thus reduce its effect. Enzyme inhibitor drugs reduce the activity of enzymes.

- Ligand or drug binding to target active sites requires physicochemical and steric complementarity.

- Ligands and drugs show selectivity in binding to targets; targets show specificity in binding to ligands or drugs.

- The lock-and-key and induced-fit models are simple approaches to understanding specificity and selectivity.

- Allosteric or cooperative effects often modulate the binding of ligands or drugs to their targets.

ADDITIONAL READING

1. Bohm HJ, Schneider G (eds). Protein–Ligand Interactions: From Molecular Recognition to Drug Design. John Wiley and Sons, 2003.

2. Nelson DL, Cox MM. Lehninger Principles of Biochemistry, 4th ed. W.H. Freeman, 2004.

3. Hardman JG, Limbird LE, Gilman AG (eds). Goodman and Gilman's The Pharmacological Basis of Therapeutics, 10th ed. McGraw-Hill Professional, 2001.

4. Katzung BG (ed). Basic and Clinical Pharmacology, 8th ed. McGraw-Hill/Appleton & Lange, 2000.

REVIEW QUESTIONS

1. What is meant by the term drug target?

2. Explain the term affinity as it applies to ligand–protein interactions. How is affinity measured?

3. Discuss the difference between a receptor agonist, a receptor antagonist, and an enzyme inhibitor.

4. Differentiate between catalytic and noncatalytic outcomes of ligand–target binding.

5. What is meant by complementarity? Discuss the two types of complementarity.

6. Explain why chiral recognition is important in the binding of small molecule ligands to targets.

7. What is a racemic mixture? Discuss the advantages and disadvantages of using single isomers of drugs instead of racemic mixtures.

8. Explain the terms selectivity and specificity as they apply to ligand–protein binding.

9. Discuss the lock-and-key and induced-fit models of ligand–protein binding.

10. Explain the mechanisms of allosteric and cooperative binding.

Drug Discovery and Optimization

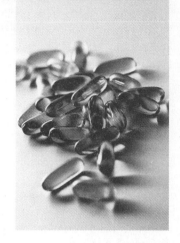

Most drugs on the market were not discovered in their final form but went through a process of experimentation and modification to make the best possible therapeutic agent. The starting point in drug discovery is identification of a lead compound, a substance that possesses the desired biological activity but that may have other undesirable characteristics. The lead compound serves as an initial prototype that is modified to retain or enhance the desired activity and to eliminate or minimize unwanted properties.

Lead Compound Versus Drug

A lead compound has the desired pharmacological activity, but may have other unfavorable properties such as high toxicity, problems with one or more absorption, distribution, metabolism, and excretion (ADME) processes, or an unusually complex or expensive manufacturing process. The lead has to be transformed into a drug by modifying its structure to impart suitable *drug-like* properties such as low toxicity and the ability to reach the site of action in appropriate concentrations. Other considerations such as ease and cost of synthesis must also be taken into

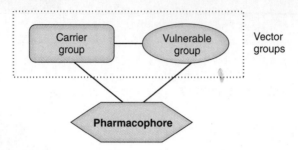

Figure 7.1. Typical components of the chemical structure of a drug molecule. The pharmacophore is needed for biological activity. The vector groups define the physicochemical properties of the molecule; carrier groups control absorption, distribution, and excretion; and vulnerable groups determine metabolism.

account. Lead-optimization is the process by which the structure of the lead compound is modified to build in these desirable properties.

We know that most drugs show a structurally specific relationship to biological activity, meaning that a definite pattern of structural features is necessary for a biological response. This is because the behavior of a majority of drugs is related to their binding to biological targets. The molecular structure of such drugs can be subdivided into various components as shown in Figure 7.1.

The pharmacophore is the part of the molecule that interacts with the target protein or receptor; a change in this portion will alter biological activity. The pharmacophore and the target must have physicochemical and stereochemical complementarity. Several parts of the molecule can together make up the pharmacophore; as an example, see Figure 7.2, which shows the pharmacophore that binds to the δ-opioid receptor.

Vector groups may not bind to the target but play a vital role in determining pharmacokinetics of the drug and may also aid in minimizing toxicity. Vector groups may be classified further as carrier groups and vulnerable groups. Carrier groups control ionization and lipophilicity of the molecule and consequently influence absorption, distribution, and excretion of the drug. Vulnerable groups are susceptible to

enzymatic action and are responsible for determining the drug's metabolism.

Identification of a Lead Compound

Several approaches are available to identify a lead compound, each one with its advantages and drawbacks. To find a lead, one generally needs a convenient laboratory test called a bioassay or a screen that can determine whether a compound has the desired biological activity.

Random Screening

Random screening is the testing of large numbers of compounds in a bioassay without regard to their chemical structure. This approach relies on luck and serendipity

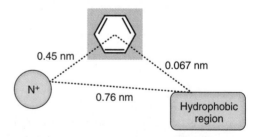

Figure 7.2. The pharmacophore recognized by the δ-opioid receptor. This pharmacophore consists of an aromatic ring, a protonated amine, and a hydrophobic region, all spatially oriented as shown.

and has been the traditional way of identifying lead compounds; in fact, many of today's important drugs were discovered this way. The use of random screening has declined as more advanced technologies have become available. However, this approach is still useful in identifying leads with unexpected or unusual structures that cannot be foreseen.

Historically, plants and other natural products were major sources of medicinal substances. For example, the foxglove plant (*Digitalis purpurea*) had been used to treat congestive heart failure. As medicinal chemistry evolved, it was found that digitalis and other related substances in foxglove are responsible for the therapeutic effect. These active compounds were isolated, synthesized, and developed into products so that dosage could be accurately controlled.

Screening in Animals

Typically, screening for new drug leads has involved *in vivo* studies in animals. This approach provides the most relevant feedback if a good animal model is available to demonstrate the desired effect. The compounds are administered to animals and screened for efficacy. A positive effect provides strong support to continue further development. However, there are several drawbacks to using animals for initial screening. The process tends to be slow and requires large quantities of the test compounds. The use of animals is also very labor intensive. Together, these disadvantages make animal screening an expensive proposition. Toxic effects of the compound may also complicate or mask the interpretation of efficacy.

Screening in Cells and Tissues

Screening in isolated tissues or cultured cells requires smaller quantities of compound than with animal screening. Such *in vitro* testing is also faster, cheaper, and less labor intensive. In addition, because the screening system is less complex than a whole animal system, the results may allow determination of the mechanism of action, i.e., whether a compound is an agonist or an antagonist.

Screening in Binding Assays

If the target protein is known, a protein-binding assay can be used to conveniently screen compounds for affinity to the target. This screening approach requires the least amount of compound. It is also rapid, and thousands of compounds can be screened per day in a given assay. Specificity is often readily determined by testing the compound in preparations of several different related target proteins.

Tissue homogenates or intact cells containing the target protein are incubated with a radiolabeled ligand known to have affinity for the protein. The compound to be screened is added, and the amount of ligand remaining bound is determined. This assay gives a comparison of the relative affinities of the known ligand and the new compound for the target protein. Compounds that inhibit ligand binding by a certain specified percentage are evaluated further. Receptor assay screening, however, gives little information about ultimate efficacy in an animal. In addition, it is often impossible to predict whether a compound will be toxic.

Compound Diversity

Medicinal chemists often synthesize new and unusual molecules in the laboratory without any predetermined goal for biological activity. The objective is to make compounds of diverse structures to find unexpected biological activity. Random screening of such compounds in a series of biological tests can often result in identification of a lead compound. Random screening of large numbers of compounds can use up a lot of time and resources, so a narrower approach is often taken. The synthesis is restricted to compounds having a vague resemblance to known weakly active compounds, to decrease cost of screening and increase probability of success. The keys to success with random screening are acquisition of diverse and large libraries of compounds, diversity being at least as important as number of compounds.

Natural Products Chemistry

The natural environment is a rich source of structurally diverse chemical compounds. Natural products are materials derived from nature for use as drugs or in pharmaceutical drug discovery and design. They may be extracted from tissues of terrestrial plants, marine organisms, or microorganism fermentation broths. A crude extract from any one of these typically contains many novel, structurally diverse chemical compounds. Chemical diversity in nature is based on biological and geographical diversity, so researchers travel the world obtaining samples to evaluate in drug discovery screens. This effort to search for natural products is known as bioprospecting.

Natural products have formed the basis of traditional medicine systems for thousands of years. Modern pharmaceutical science has improved on these natural medicinals by extracting, concentrating, and identifying the active compound from the natural product mixture. Many drugs on the market today were discovered from natural sources. The analgesic activity of the bark of the white willow tree (*Salix alba*) was known from folklore and gave us aspirin. The antibiotic activity of penicillin, obtained from molds of the genus *Penicillium,* was discovered serendipitously in the laboratory. Scientists have isolated dozens of natural antibiotics, such as streptomycin and vancomycin, mostly from soil microbes in the Actinomycete family.

An inherent problem with widespread use of natural products, however, lies with harvesting and processing products with low concentrations of the active compound. Scientists are, therefore, primarily interested in natural compounds as a template or starting point for laboratory synthesis of related drug leads.

Natural products chemicals have played, and will continue to play, a key role in drug discovery. Screening natural products extracts, however, is expensive when compared with synthetic approaches, because isolation studies and structure elucidation of unknown compounds add to the expense. On the other hand, the structural diversity provided by natural products is unsurpassed by traditional synthetic chemistry. Natural products already have a function in the environment so there is a greater likelihood that they have some desired biological activity. Natural products also frequently have drug-like properties (which we will discuss later in this chapter) so that they can be absorbed, distributed, and metabolized appropriately in the body. Consequently, natural products are excellent sources of novel compounds for activity against challenging biological targets.

Rational Design

Scientists often struggle with the problem of deciding which compounds to synthesize from thousands of possible molecules. Rational design was the first approach to overcome this problem by focusing on a few promising structures. A fundamental assumption of rational design is that drug activity depends on molecular binding of the drug to a biomolecule, usually a target protein. The steps in rational design are target identification, designing a molecule to bind to the target, and then synthesizing the compound in the laboratory.

Target Identification

The first step in rational design is to understand the molecular biology of the disease or illness and to search for target proteins that play a role. If there is a

Taxol

The first plant-derived anticancer drug was Taxol (generic name paclitaxel), isolated from the bark of the Pacific yew or *Taxus brevifolia,* a slow-growing tree found in old-growth rain forests in the northwestern United States. Interest in paclitaxel revealed major supply problems, because many groups wished to conduct clinical trials and required large quantities of the drug. Because of the low concentration of paclitaxel in the bark, more than 25,000 trees were needed for early clinical trials. Once the bark is removed from the tree, the tree dies. The Pacific yew is an environmentally protected species and is also one of the slowest growing trees in the world. Isolation of the compound from the bark involved killing the tree, and the quantities available by this method were very small. It was clear that harvesting of *Taxus brevifolia* bark was not a viable long-term option for Taxol production on a large scale.

An analog of paclitaxel called baccatin III was discovered in leaves of the English yew *Taxus baccata.* Baccatin could be converted to paclitaxel in the laboratory. Removal of the leaves had no detrimental effect on the health of the tree, and the leaves regenerated relatively quickly, so it was unnecessary to cut down the trees. Although the extraction and subsequent conversion of baccatin to paclitaxel were difficult, the source was renewable and sufficient quantities were obtained to carry out clinical trials. Paclitaxel is now made by a modified version of this semisynthetic procedure.

The success of Taxol stimulated interest in preserving biodiversity and deriving value from it. It brought together several groups united in an effort to advance new drug discovery and simultaneously preserve the yew and the rain forest.

---

relationship between the suppression (or reinforcement) of a protein function and the symptoms of a disease, the protein is identified as a target protein for drug discovery efforts.

Once a target has been established and characterized, rational design begins. The first consideration is that the designed molecule must complement the active site of the target. Steric, electrostatic, and hydrophobic complementarity must be established, and the pharmacophore must be presented to the active site for recognition and binding to occur. The aim is to find a molecule that binds to the target protein with suitable affinity and selectivity. If reinforcement of the protein's function is desired, the molecule must be an *agonist,* whereas if suppression is needed the molecule should be an *antagonist* (or *inhibitor* if the target is an enzyme).

The optimal combination of atoms and functional groups to complement the target is often the natural, endogenous ligand that binds to it. Unfortunately, this is usually an unacceptable candidate as a drug, because the natural ligand is almost always an agonist, or a compound that cannot be patented, or lacks appropriate ADME requirements for an administered drug, or has other side effects. Therefore, alternative chemical structures must be devised.

Computational tools can predict the binding of a hypothetical molecule to a target protein and are used routinely to study drug–receptor complexes and to calculate properties of small molecule drug leads. The computer analyzes the interactions between the proposed compound structure and the target active site to design molecules that give an optimal fit.

Direct and Indirect Rational Design

Depending on whether the sequence and three-dimensional structure of the target protein is known or not known, rational design may be approached directly or indirectly. If the structure is known, medicinal chemists can directly determine an optimum ligand structure that can be placed inside the target active site in a conformation that results in a good fit. This is referred to as *docking* the relative orientation and fit of the target protein to a potential drug molecule. Docking is a function of the conformation of each partner in the interaction. Looking for a compound that can dock appropriately with a target is like searching for a key that fits a given lock. Once the computer models predict a suitable structure for a drug, the compound can be synthesized in the laboratory as a lead.

Often, the structure of the active site is unknown. In fact, the three-dimensional structure of relatively few receptors has been determined, although this number is increasing. In such cases, scientists use indirect approaches to obtain information about the target. One way is to study the binding of the target to several small molecules. Using the geometric structure and the chemical characteristics of the molecules that show strong binding, scientists can deduce some information about the structure of the active site. This is analogous to using a given key to search for other fitting keys without knowing the lock. Once the pharmacophore is identified, a suitable lead compound can be identified and further refined.

Once a promising compound structure or series of structures have been identified by computational analysis, the compounds can be synthesized in the laboratory and screened for activity in animals, cells, or binding assays, as discussed earlier.

De Novo Design

The concept of generating virtual lead compounds entirely through computer simulation is termed de novo design. Compound structures are both identified and screened for activity using computers. High-performance computers are first used to search for structures that fit the proposed active site of the target protein. Then automated robotic systems and advanced algorithms are used to screen compounds entirely *in silico*, meaning that experiments are carried out not in the laboratory, but on the computer by a process called virtual screening. Virtual screening is the evaluation of virtual, or hypothetical, compounds for binding to a virtual receptor protein. Virtual libraries of three-dimensional compound structures and three-dimensional protein structures are available in several computer databases. High-speed computing highlights the properties of compounds that appear to bind to a receptor and models their characteristics. As a result, researchers can identify structures that are worth investigating.

Although computers have become faster, the number of calculations needed to accurately predict the binding of a de novo generated structure to its target in a useful time frame still requires significant approximations. An additional difficulty is predicting how the chemical structure will behave in real life. Chemical compounds are inherently flexible structures and can assume many different conformations and orientations. Predicting how any structure will actually interact and bind with a target in the physiological environment is very uncertain. Another major deficiency of de novo drug design is that the entire structure is created from scratch. There are a nearly infinite number of potential combinations of atoms, which leads to the generation of many useless chemical structures. Undesired structures are those that will have toxicity, chemical instability, or synthetic difficulty.

De novo design may not be feasible yet, but such computational techniques are valuable in optimizing hits and lead compounds into potent drugs. Although computers cannot substitute for a clear understanding of the system being studied, they are an important tool to gain better insight into the chemistry and biology of the problem at hand. Modern drug discovery combines the power of computational chemistry with other approaches to further speed up the identification of new drugs.

The Combinatorial Approach

Both random screening and rational drug design use traditional wet chemistry methods, in which a synthetic procedure is designed to make one compound at a time in the laboratory. The compound is then purified and analyzed, also one at a time. It is then tested in a biological assay to see whether it binds to a target protein, cell, or tissue. High-throughput screening and combinatorial chemistry have changed this traditional approach dramatically, and have revolutionized the capacity of pharmaceutical companies to identify potential new drug leads.

High-Throughput Screening

High-throughput screening (HTS) uses miniaturized, robotics-based technology to test large compound libraries for binding to a target to identify potential new drugs or leads. The advent of HTS allowed scientists to screen large numbers of compounds in a short time. High-throughput screening depends on the development of a quantitative, pharmacologically relevant assay for the identified target, which can then be reproduced across a large number of samples. Recently, technological advances have allowed screening of up to 100,000 compounds per day for binding to a protein target.

Classic methods of drug synthesis, however, could not make the large numbers of compounds for which screening capability was available. A new approach was needed to significantly increasing the throughput of chemical synthesis, both in terms of the number and the diversity of compounds; this new approach is combinatorial chemistry.

Combinatorial Chemistry

Combinatorial chemistry (often called combichem) is the use of a small set of chemical building blocks or reagents, combined together in multiple ways using standard synthetic chemical reactions, to make libraries of compounds. A library in this context is a mixture of several compounds made from the same building blocks. As with traditional drug design, combinatorial chemistry relies on organic synthesis. The difference is the scope—instead of synthesizing a single compound, combinatorial chemistry exploits automation and miniaturization to synthesize large compound libraries. Many different compounds are made simultaneously by assembling the same set of reagents in different ways; the resulting compound library contains all possible chemical structures that can be produced by combining the building blocks. Thus, combinatorial organic synthesis is not random but systematic and repetitive, using sets of chemical building blocks to form a diverse set of molecular entities.

The concept of combinatorial chemistry has many counterparts in nature. For example, our body is able to synthesize a variety of proteins from the same amino acid building blocks by assembling them in different sequences.

One can envision the process as shown in Figure 7.3, which depicts the library created by combining four different building blocks once. If all the reactions proceed successfully, 16 different reaction products will be present in the final mixture, with the shaded compound being active. If this mixture is screened and found active, it will indicate that at least one of the compounds has biological activity. The challenge is to identify the active compounds in the library. One way is to make each individual compound and test it for activity, but this would be very inefficient. Another is to synthesize and screen eight sets of compounds, each set representing either a row or a column from Figure 7.3. Two sets will show activity, and the only common compound in each will be the active compound β-γ.

The large number of compounds that can be generated by several such reactions is illustrated as follows. A mixture of 10 amino acids is coupled with another mixture of 10 amino acids to make a mixture of 100 possible dipeptides. These are then reacted with another 10 amino acid mixtures to create a combinatorial library of 1,000 different tripeptides. As the length of the peptide chain is increased in this manner, the number of compounds in the library increases exponentially.

Combinatorial libraries are screened as a group by HTS for binding to target proteins to identify one or more lead compounds. A new compound that binds to the target is called a *hit;* when biological activity is found for a particular library, one can trace back and find the structure of the active compound as discussed above. New combinatorial libraries can then be created to focus on the specific functional groups and structural features of the initial hit, and to develop the hit into a lead.

A crucial aspect of combinatorial chemistry is being able to identify the compounds produced in a combinatorial scheme. Not all the possible reactions work, and not all possible compounds are actually present in the mixture. It is important to know not just what reactions were run, but whether the compounds are actually present in the library. Detecting the presence of an active component in a mixture of thousands of compounds and then correctly identifying its structure is a challenge and has opened up new approaches in high throughput analytical characterization.

Rational Combinatorial Chemistry. Traditional combinatorial chemistry without any preconceived biological basis results in very large libraries, with compounds that may not have any chance of being developed into a drug. In the rational combinatorial approach, the advantages of rational drug design and combinatorial chemistry are combined to reduce the number of compounds in the library and give them a greater chance of being useful drugs. The starting reagents or building blocks are selected on the basis of structural properties that are believed to have the best probability of biological activity, the result being a *targeted library.* Often, the resulting library consists of systematic variants of one chemical structure or scaffold or template. The scaffold structure contains a portion that remains constant, whereas a number of functional groups are allowed to vary using a combinatorial approach. The process of making a targeted library based on a scaffold is illustrated in Figure 7.4. Natural products are

	α	β	γ	δ
α	α-α	α-β	α-γ	α-δ
β	β-α	β-β	β-γ	β-δ
γ	γ-α	γ-β	γ-γ	γ-δ
δ	δ-α	δ-β	δ-γ	δ-δ

Figure 7.3. An example of a combinatorial library resulting from four reacting components α, β, γ, and δ. If all the reactions proceed, 16 different products will be present in the final mixture. The shaded compound, β-γ, is active.

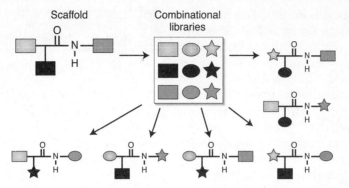

Figure 7.4. Rational combinatorial chemistry approach in making a targeted library of compounds based on a peptide scaffold.

becoming important scaffolds for building such targeted libraries, because scientists recognize that natural compound starting points have a higher degree of probability of being drug-like.

Optimization of the Lead Compound

Once a lead compound is identified, it almost always requires modification to improve its pharmacokinetic, pharmacodynamic, and safety properties. ADME properties need to be optimized for a lead compound to become a successful drug. Although the pharmacophore is responsible for biological activity, a multitude of modifications are possible in the vector groups of the molecule. Many potential drug leads that look excellent in the laboratory can become expensive failures later because of poor ADME properties or unacceptable toxicity.

Selectivity and Toxicity

The ability of a drug compound to be selective in binding to its target is important to avoid toxicity. A lead compound may show excellent affinity to the target,

Virtual Combinatorial Chemistry

For speed and convenience, some combinatorial compound libraries begin as virtual libraries. For example, if 200 amines are reacted with 200 amino acids, the library would contain 40,000 amides, and considerable time and money would be spent in synthesizing even some of these compounds. In a virtual approach, the library is made using computational techniques. The virtual compounds are docked to their targets on the computer to identify structural features that give the best fit. Only the compounds that meet all desired properties, such as solubility, stereochemistry, and fit into the target active site, are selected. Multiple virtual experiments can be done on the same virtual compounds using different conditions to give faster and cheaper information. A smaller, more focused combinatorial library is then synthesized in the laboratory based on the structural features identified.

but if it is not at least somewhat selective, its suitability as a drug is diminished. An important step in lead optimization is screening for selectivity against other similar proteins, to ensure that the lead compound binds to the target with much greater affinity than to nontarget proteins. A selective compound is less likely to show toxicity as development proceeds.

Other screens for general cellular toxicity are also carried out at this time to make sure that the compound is relatively safe when in contact with the body's cells.

Drug Likeness

The first step in lead optimization is to predict whether the compound has appropriate physicochemical properties to make it a good drug. Even though chemical structures of drugs differ greatly because each one is targeted to a different protein, successful drugs on the market share similarities in their physicochemical properties. This is particularly true for orally administered drugs. Druglike characteristics are those that increase the probability that the drug will have favorable ADME properties. A well-known approach is that of Lipinski, who performed statistical analyses of about 2,000 drugs. This study established a set of empirical criteria that are generally valid for the majority of the drugs. The set of criteria is known as the rule of five, shown in Table 7.1. The rule of five identifies characteristics that make a compound undesirable as a drug, particularly with regard to ADME properties.

Because all parameters can be easily calculated from the structure, the rule of five has become the most widely applied filter in selecting compounds for development. It is particularly useful in modifying structures of lead compounds to impart desirable physicochemical properties. Compounds that cannot be ruled out by the rule of five are considered

TABLE 7.1. The Rule of Five to Eliminate Leads With Undesirable ADME Properties[a]	
Property	Value Above Which Compound Is Undesirable as a Drug
Log P	>5
Molecular weight	>500
Number of H-bond donating groups	>5
Number of H-bond accepting groups (−N and −O)	>10

[a]Compounds not ruled out are considered drug-like and are predicted to have satisfactory ADME (absorption, distribution, metabolism, and excretion) behavior after oral administration.

drug-like, meaning that they are predicted to have satisfactory ADME behavior after oral administration. Obviously, this simple rule is not always correct in identifying drug-like compounds. More complex analyses using artificial neural networks and fragment screening have been proposed and used, but these are outside the scope of our discussion.

Once the drug likeness of the lead is established, several analogs of the lead are synthesized. An analog is a compound with the same or similar pharmacophore as the lead, but with differences in other parts of the molecule. If analogs differ in structure by a simple and constant increase in one part of the molecule (such as the length of an alkyl chain), they are part of a homologous series. The objective of making analogs is to retain pharmacological activity of the lead but to minimize or eliminate unwanted properties. Analogs are then tested in the laboratory to select the compound that will proceed to animal testing and ultimately into human clinical trials.

Some important questions addressed in making analogs are as follows. Can the structure of the compound be simplified without loss of activity? Does the partition coefficient or solubility need to be improved? Do vector groups need to be altered to prevent or change metabolism? Some logical approaches to modifying lead compounds have been more successful than others.

Bioisosterism

On the basis of the analysis of drug likeness, structural changes are often needed to improve physicochemical properties without significantly changing biological properties of a lead compound. In other words, the pharmacophore needs to be kept relatively unchanged while vector groups are modified to improve lipophilicity, water solubility, or susceptibility to metabolism.

Chemical isosterism is the similarity in physicochemical properties of ions, compounds, or elements because of similarities in their electronic structures. This concept was first introduced for atoms: elements in the same vertical row of the periodic table have similar outer shells of electrons, giving them the same electronic properties. In these rows, atoms with the same size and mass also have similar physicochemical properties. A similar trend is seen for neighboring atoms in horizontal rows of the periodic table. Thus, if one atom or group of atoms in a molecule is replaced with its *isostere*, the physicochemical properties of the compound do not change significantly. Chemical isosteric equivalents can

be used to synthesize different compounds with the *same* physicochemical properties.

Bioisosterism is an application of isosterism to biological systems and guides molecular modification of drugs without dramatic changes in their biological properties. The underlying principle is that if a modified compound is to interact with the same target as the original lead to give the same action, then the modification cannot be too drastic. Small structural changes may be achieved by replacing specific atoms or groups of atoms with their bioisosteres. The reason for making bioisosteric modifications is to synthesize similar compounds that retain biological activity, but have improved physicochemical properties and better pharmacokinetic behavior. This approach is widely used in the synthesis of improved drugs based on a lead compound.

Bioisosteric Equivalents

Classic bioisosteres are subdivided by equivalence into several categories such that atoms or functional groups within a category are interchangeable. Examples are shown in Table 7.2. Substitution with a bioisosteric equivalent usually changes one or more physicochemical properties of the drug. A few classic examples of bioisosterism are shown in Figure 7.5.

TABLE 7.2. Examples of Bioisosterically Equivalent Functional Groups[a]	
Category	*Examples*
Monovalent atoms or groups	$-Cl$, $-Br$, $-I$
	$-XH_n$, where X is C, N, O, or S
Divalent atoms or groups	$R-O-R_1$; $R-NH-R_1$; $R-CH_2-R_1$, $R-Si-R_1$
Trivalent atoms or groups	C and N in $R-CH=R_1$ and $R-N=R_1$
Tetravalent atoms or groups	$=C=$; $=N^+=$; $=P=$
Ring equivalents	$-CH=CH-$; $-S-$; $-O-$; $-NH-$; and $-CH_2-$

[a]The groups in each category can be substituted for one another on a drug molecule without significant changes in biological activity.

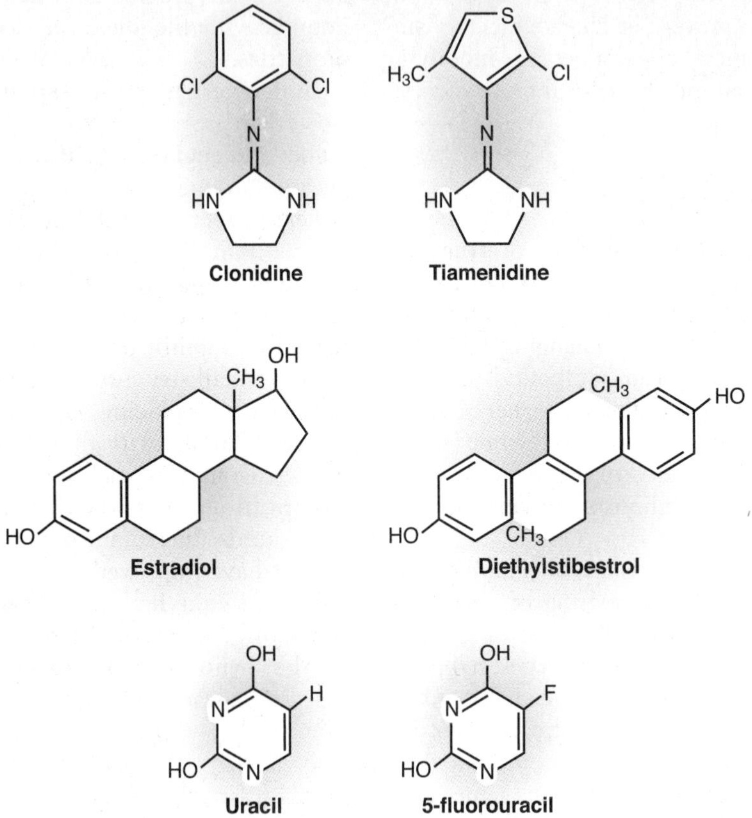

Figure 7.5. Examples of bioisosteres. On the left is the parent compound and on the right is the bioisostere.

Structure–Activity Relationships

A structure–activity relationship (SAR) is the relationship of the molecular structure of a compound with a biological property. The basic assumption behind these relationships is that different structures must give different activities or different degrees of the same activity. Relationships between structure and behavior can be found for a drug's pharmaceutical properties (solubility, stability, dissolution), its pharmacokinetic properties (absorption, distribution, metabolism, and excretion), or its pharmacodynamic properties (interaction between drug and target). These correlations may be qualitative (simple SAR) or quantitative (quantitative SAR, or

QSAR). In general, they are a set of rules that predict whether a compound will be active, and to what extent. Structure–activity relationships can then be used to predict which analogs will have the most desirable properties.

Qualitative predictions are based on a comparison of the properties of one or more analogs (i.e., structurally similar compounds) with the compound of interest. For example, terms such as "similarly active," "less active," or "more active" would be used in a qualitative SAR assessment for the biological activity of a series of analogs compared with the lead compound. An example is the SAR for analogs of the anticancer drug cisplatin, as shown in Figure 7.6.

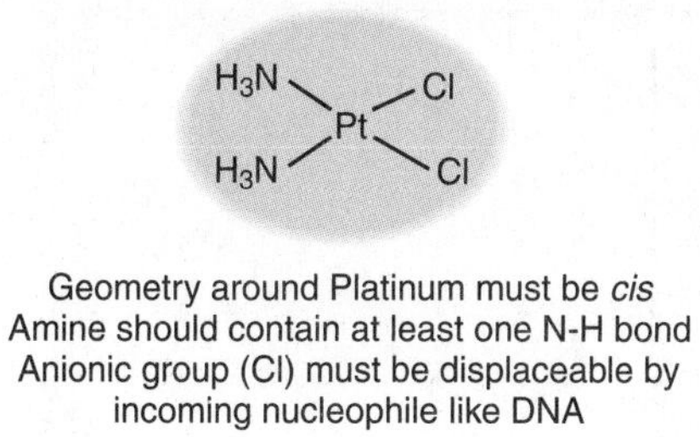

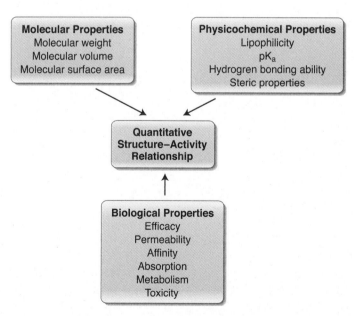

Geometry around Platinum must be *cis*
Amine should contain at least one N-H bond
Anionic group (Cl) must be displaceable by
incoming nucleophile like DNA

Figure 7.6. Structure–activity relationship rules for analogs of the anticancer drug cisplatin.

Quantitative predictions, on the other hand, are usually in the form of an equation that relates some property of the compound to specific structural features of the compound. They also give some estimation of the degree of biological activity expected. Researchers have attempted for many years to develop drugs based on QSAR, and there have been numerous attempts to mathematically correlate drug structure with pharmacological activity. Many parameters enter into the development of a QSAR as illustrated in Figure 7.7. Classic QSAR analyses consider only two-dimensional structures whereas the newer three-dimensional QSAR approach is much more complex and takes into account three-dimensional properties.

Equations have been developed to correlate activity with physicochemical properties such as partition coefficient, pK_a, hydrogen bonding ability, or other structural features such as steric effects and electronic properties of the drug. These properties may be determined experimentally, but are increasingly being calculated by computational methods. In fact, QSAR of biological activity has evolved into what we discussed as rational drug design or computer-assisted drug design.

The QSAR equation is a model that relates variations in a biological parameter to variations in values of computed (or measured) properties for a series of molecules. QSAR relationships are often presented as graphs of variation in a compound property versus biological effect, and a systematic relationship is often observed. The relationship is usually linear but is sometimes nonlinear, as shown in Figure 7.8.

Molecular Properties
Molecular weight
Molecular volume
Molecular surface area

Physicochemical Properties
Lipophilicity
pK_a
Hydrogren bonding ability
Steric properties

**Quantitative
Structure–Activity
Relationship**

Biological Properties
Efficacy
Permeability
Affinity
Absorption
Metabolism
Toxicity

Figure 7.7. An illustration of the concept of quantitative structure–activity relationships. The relationship is established by correlating molecular or physicochemical properties of a drug with its biological or pharmacological behavior.

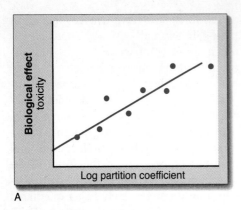
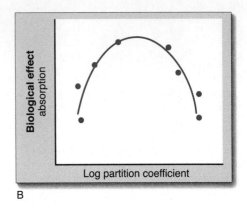

A   B

Figure 7.8. An example of linear (A) and nonlinear (B) structure–activity relationships between a biological property and a physicochemical property such as partition coefficient. The circles represent data from compounds. From such a graph, the optimal partition coefficient can be selected depending on the particular requirements.

Developing a quantitative structure–activity relationship is difficult. Molecules are typically flexible, and it is possible to compute many possibly useful properties that might relate to activity. For the method to work efficiently, compounds selected to define the equation should be diverse; the quality of any QSAR will only be as good as the quality of data used to derive the model. Once the relationship is defined, it can be used to aid in prediction of new or unknown molecules. QSAR has been surpassed by rational drug design as a technique for lead identification, but it continues to be an important tool for lead modification and optimization to predict structures that have better ADME properties than the lead compound.

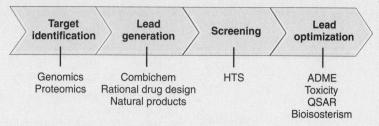

Figure 7.9. A summary of the steps involved in new drug discovery. The target is identified and selected based on information about genes or proteins involved in the disease process. Leads are generated and synthesized using several approaches. The leads are screened for biological activity, and then optimized to make the compounds more drug-like. ADME, absorption, distribution, metabolism, and excretion; HTS, high-throughput screening; QSAR, quantitative structure–activity relationship.

KEY CONCEPTS

A drug's structure can be divided into the pharmacophore, the portion that fits into the target active site, and vector groups that control ADME properties.

- The lead compound serves as an initial prototype for drug discovery, but must be optimized to make it drug-like.

- Biological screens identify compounds that can serve as leads.

- Leads are discovered through random screening of synthetic compounds, or by screening natural products or combinatorial libraries.

- High-throughput screens are capable of rapidly testing combinatorial libraries.

- Lead compound structures are optimized by retaining the pharmacophore and modifying vector groups to make the compound more drug-like.

- Poor drug candidates can be rejected using Lipinski's rule of five.

- Bioisosteric principles and SAR are used to modify the structure of the lead compound to provide suitable ADME properties while retaining biological activity.

- The overall process of drug discovery discussed in this chapter is summarized in Figure 7.9.

ADDITIONAL READING

1. Krogsgaard-Larsen P, Liljefors T, Madsen U (eds). Textbook of Drug Design and Discovery, 3rd ed. Taylor and Francis, 2002.

2. Abraham DJ (ed). Burger's Medicinal Chemistry and Drug Discovery, 6th ed. Wiley-Interscience, 2003.

3. Ng R. Drugs—From Discovery to Approval. Wiley-Liss, 2003.

4. Silverman R. The Organic Chemistry of Drug Design and Drug Action, 2nd ed. Academic Press, 2004.

REVIEW QUESTIONS

1. What is the difference between lead identification and lead optimization in drug discovery? Why is a promising lead not always a good drug?
2. Discuss the roles of the pharmacophore, the carrier groups, and the vulnerable groups in determining the fate and action of a drug.
3. Explain why random screening is still used for the identification of lead compounds.
4. Why are natural products attractive sources for new drugs?
5. Describe the steps involved in rational design of lead compounds. What role does the computer play in this method of drug discovery?
6. Explain de novo design in drug discovery. What are its advantages and limitations?
7. Discuss how high-throughput screening opened the door to the combinatorial approach to drug discovery.
8. What is a combinatorial library? How is such a library made?
9. How is a single lead identified from a combinatorial library?
10. Discuss the concept of drug likeness and the rule of five.
11. How is bioisosterism used to modify a lead compound into a useful drug?
12. What is the role of structure–activity relationships in optimizing the structures of lead compounds?

Transport Across Biological Barriers

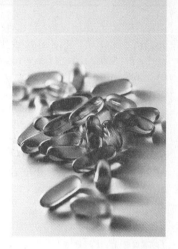

We know that cell membranes have many structural features designed to control the passage of molecules in and out of the cell. Furthermore, cells in epithelial and endothelial tissues are packed in a fashion to regulate transport of molecules from cell to cell, and between cells from the basolateral to the lumenal side and vice versa.

When a drug is administered, it often has to cross an epithelial tissue before it can enter the bloodstream. From the bloodstream, the drug must leave capillaries through the capillary endothelium and enter various organs and tissues, including the site of action. Drugs with membrane receptors may remain in the extracellular fluid at the site of action; drugs with intracellular targets must cross cell membranes of cells at the site of action before they can exert their action. Many endogenous ligands must also travel from their site of synthesis to reach their targets; this may involve crossing the capillary endothelium and other cell membranes.

Thus, the transport of drugs from site of administration to site of action and the transport of endogenous ligands from site of synthesis to site of action are important factors in physiological function and drug action.

Multiple Biological Barriers

After it is administered, a drug will encounter many tissue and cell membrane barriers. Most drugs have to reach targets that are some distance away from the site of administration. The effectiveness of a drug, at least in part, depends on how much reaches its site of action and how fast that occurs. Thousands of compounds can kill the AIDS virus in test tubes, but few are viable drugs because most cannot effectively cross our body's biological barriers.

Tissue Barriers

Consider a hypothetical orally administered drug designed to work in the brain. The types of tissue barriers this drug will encounter on the way to the brain and on its eventual way out of the body are illustrated in Figure 8.1. When a tablet containing the drug is administered orally, it must dissolve in the stomach and small intestines and release the drug. The drug then has to travel from the intestines, through the intestinal epithelium (*barrier*

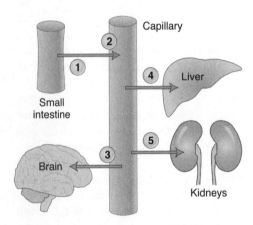

Figure 8.1. Barriers encountered by a drug whose site of action is the brain. Numbers denote the barriers. Barrier 1 is the intestinal epithelium; barrier 2 is the peripheral capillary endothelium; barriers 3–5 are the capillary membranes in the brain, the liver, and the kidneys, respectively. Each of the membranes that make up these barriers has different properties.

1), through the capillary endothelium (*barrier 2*), and into capillaries. This overall transport of the drug from the administration site (the gastrointestinal tract in this case) into the bloodstream is called absorption. The drug is now in the circulation and is carried by the bloodstream. It leaves capillaries through the capillary endothelium and enters various tissues and organs, a process called distribution.

The drug eventually arrives at the site of action (the brain in this case); only when it has crossed the brain capillary endothelium (*barrier 3*) and entered brain tissue can the drug exert its action. The drug must eventually leave the site of action by reentering capillaries. The blood carries the drug to the sites of *elimination,* which remove the drug from the body. For this to occur, the drug must leave the bloodstream through the capillary endothelium at the sites of biotransformation (liver; *barrier 4*) and excretion (kidney; *barrier 5*) for ultimate removal from the body.

Tight junctions between epithelial and endothelial cells play an important role in regulating and controlling transport through tissues, as we will see later in this chapter.

Cell Membrane Barriers

If the target of a drug is inside cells at the site of action, the drug must be able to cross the cell membrane to achieve adequate intracellular concentrations. The lipid bilayer and membrane proteins may provide passage to some drugs. In addition, drugs that cannot traverse epithelial tissue through tight junctions may be able to cross the tissue by passing through epithelial cells, as explained below.

Mechanisms of Transport

When a solute encounters a cell or tissue that it has to cross, it can either travel

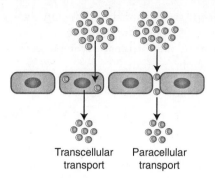

Transcellular   Paracellular
transport   transport

Figure 8.2. Diagram showing the two major transport routes of solutes across a multicellular (epithelial or endothelial) membrane. This membrane is composed of a single layer of cells. Paracellular transport occurs when the molecules travel between the cells, through cell junctions. Transcellular transport involves the drug molecules going through the cells, across the cell membrane.

it. Cell membranes are **semipermeable** and have *selective permeability,* which means that they allow certain solutes to cross more easily than others and may prevent the passage of some solutes. In this way, cells can transport desirable substances such as nutrients, signaling molecules, and other vital materials necessary for survival, but keep out toxic compounds.

Cell membranes have several transport mechanisms to enable materials to enter or leave cells. The four primary mechanisms for transport of a substance across a cell membrane are:

1. Passive diffusion
2. Facilitated diffusion
3. Active transport
4. Transcytosis

The first three processes are able to transport small molecular weight solutes (such as drugs), whereas transcytosis is primarily for transport of macromolecules (such as proteins) and small particles (such as viruses and bacteria). These processes exist to transport materials necessary for the cell's survival. Drugs that are similar to these substances can also use these transport mechanisms.

through the cells, or between the cells through tight junctions. These two pathways are illustrated in Figure 8.2 for transport through epithelial cells from the apical to basolateral side or vice versa.

When molecules travel *through* cells the process is called **transcellular** transport. This is a two-step process: entry into the cell and exit out of the cell. The molecules thus have to cross the cell membrane on the way in and on the way out of the cells in their path.

On the other hand, **paracellular** transport involves the passage of a solute *between* cells through cell junctions (such as tight junctions). Here, molecules do not cross cell membranes nor enter cells in their path. Paracellular transport is possible only for solute molecules smaller in size than the junctions between cells in a particular tissue.

Transcellular Transport

During transcellular transport, a solute crosses the cell membrane to move in and out of cells. **Permeability** is a property of a membrane that describes its ability to allow solutes to move through

Passive Diffusion

Diffusion is the natural tendency of molecules to move from a region of higher concentration to a region of lower concentration until the two regions reach the same concentration. It is a process by which a system tries to achieve equilibrium, and is a result of the random kinetic movement of molecules in a medium. **Passive diffusion** describes a diffusion process that is not energy-dependent; a source of energy is not required for diffusion to occur. Passive diffusion proceeds as long as there is a concentration difference, or *concentration gradient,* between the two regions. When the concentrations in the two regions become equal and equilibrium is reached, there is no further *net* change in concentration of the two regions. Exchange of molecules between the two regions continues at equilibrium, but at the same rates.

The diffusion coefficient (D) is a constant that measures how well a solute can diffuse in a particular medium. It is defined as the rate at which a diffusing solute is transported between two regions when there is unit concentration gradient between them. D depends on size (or molecular weight) of the molecule, the medium in which it is diffusing, and temperature. The larger the molecular weight, the lower the diffusion coefficient.

A barrier such as a membrane often separates the regions of high and low concentration. For diffusion to occur, the membrane must be permeable to the diffusing solute. Diffusion will not occur if the membrane is impermeable to the solute, even if a concentration gradient is present.

Consider passive diffusion of a solute with diffusion coefficient D diffusing in or out of a cell. The two regions (intracellular fluid and extracellular fluid) are separated by the cell membrane. The concentration on one side of the membrane is C_1 and on the other side of the membrane is C_2 (assume $C_1 > C_2$). If the membrane is permeable to the solute, transport will occur from the side with high concentration (the *donor* side) to the side with lower concentration (the *receiver* side); the concentration gradient ($C_1 - C_2$) is the driving force for passive diffusion.

Fick's law of diffusion is a mathematical expression that describes the passive diffusion process. It states that the rate of passive diffusion (called *flux*, or change in donor side concentration with time, with units of concentration/time) is:

- directly proportional to concentration gradient ($C_1 - C_2$) of solute (mg/mL)
- directly proportional to surface area (A) of membrane exposed to solute (cm^2)

- directly proportional to diffusion coefficient (D) of solute (cm^2/sec)
- inversely proportional to thickness (h) of membrane (cm)

$$\frac{dC}{dt} \propto \frac{A \cdot D (C_1 - C_2)}{h} \quad \text{(Eq. 8.1)}$$

Recall that cell membranes are composed of a lipid bilayer with embedded peripheral and transmembrane proteins. A solute, depending on its properties, may cross the cell membrane by diffusion through the lipid bilayer of the membrane, or through hydrophilic channels created by transmembrane channel proteins.

Passive Diffusion Through Hydrophilic Channels. Channels created by channel proteins allow small solutes (such as water) to diffuse through if they are smaller than the channel diameter (less than 0.7 to 1 nm), as illustrated in Figure 8.3. Small molecules may pass through these channels by passive diffusion driven by a concentration gradient between intracellular and extracellular regions; no energy is required. Small ions may also pass passively through such channels. Ion transport through channel proteins, however, is usually an active transport process, as we shall discuss later in this chapter.

Most drugs and endogenous ligands are too large to be transported through cell membrane channels. Thus, this is not an important pathway for ligand or drug transport in and out of cells.

Passive Diffusion Through the Lipid Bilayer. The lipid bilayer of cell membranes is permeable to lipophilic molecules, and solutes with a large enough partition coefficient are able to passively diffuse across the lipid bilayer. This pathway is the primary mode of transport of drugs into and out of cells and across epithelial tissue. The drug dissolves in the lipid bilayer on one side of the membrane, diffuses through, and leaves the

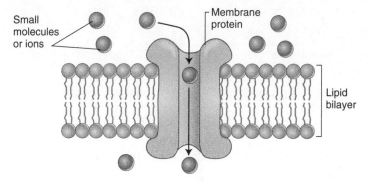

Figure 8.3. Illustration of the transport of very small solutes and ions through hydrophilic protein channels in the lipid bilayer of a cell membrane. Transport may be driven by a concentration or electrochemical gradient.

lipid bilayer on the other side. If extracellular solute concentration is higher, drug will be transported into the cell, whereas if intracellular concentration is higher, drug will be transported out of the cell.

Uncharged lipophilic molecules have a high enough partition coefficient and are able to dissolve in and diffuse through the lipid bilayer readily. Hydrophilic molecules, including ions, cannot dissolve in the lipid bilayer to any significant extent. Therefore, ionized forms of weak acid and weak base drugs cannot cross cell membranes by passive diffusion. Only nonelectrolyte drugs and the un-ionized forms of weak acid and weak base drugs can diffuse passively through cell membranes. This is analogous to partitioning of compounds between *n*-octanol and water—only un-ionized neutral forms can partition from the aqueous phase into *n*-octanol.

Rate of Passive Diffusion Across the Lipid Bilayer. The rate at which a solute diffuses across the lipid bilayer of cell membranes is also governed by Fick's law (Eq. 8.1), but the rate of diffusion will now also be directly proportional to the partition coefficient of the compound between the lipid bilayer and water. In practice, we use the partition coefficient between *n*-octanol and water to approximate this term.

Figure 8.4 illustrates passive diffusion of a solute with partition coefficient P and diffusion coefficient D across a cell membrane of thickness h and exposed surface area A. Extracellular concentration of the un-ionized or neutral form of the solute is C_1 and its intracellular concentration is C_2. The concentration of the un-ionized form rather than total concentration is used because the lipid bilayer is permeable to the un-ionized form only.

Assume that $C_1 > C_2$, so that transport occurs from the extracellular donor side to the intracellular region receiver side. The rate of passive diffusion is given by:

$$\frac{dC}{dt} = -\frac{P \cdot A \cdot D\,(C_1 - C_2)}{h} \quad \text{(Eq. 8.2)}$$

The negative sign denotes a decrease in donor side concentration with time. In reality, molecules are continuously diffusing both in and out of the cell. However, the transport rate for diffusion into the cell is greater than the rate for diffusion out because of the higher extracellular concentration. The overall direction of transport will be the net result of transport rates in and out of the cell.

Permeability. Consider how transport rate is influenced by terms in Equation 8.2. If the solute is in contact with a large membrane surface area, A, then transport will be faster. If the solute diffusion coefficient D is large, the solute can move rapidly in the medium (smaller molecules

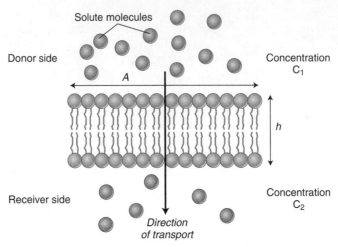

Figure 8.4. Schematic representation of passive transcellular diffusion of a solute across the lipid bilayer of a cell membrane. The direction of transport is from a region of high concentration (donor side) to a region of lower concentration (receiver side). The thickness of the membrane is h, and the area of membrane exposed to the drug is A.

have larger diffusion coefficients), resulting in a high transport rate. If the solute partition coefficient P is large it means that the solute is hydrophobic, dissolves readily in the lipid bilayer, and will have a high transport rate. A large cell membrane thickness, h, makes the diffusion path longer and results in slower transport.

The inherent permeability of a given membrane for a particular solute is given by:

$$\text{Permeability} = \frac{P \cdot D}{h} \quad \text{(Eq. 8.3)}$$

Thus, permeability depends both on properties of the solute (partition coefficient and diffusion coefficient in the lipid bilayer) and on properties of the membrane (thickness). The units of permeability are centimeters per second.

Diffusion coefficients of most small molecule solutes (molecular weights 100 to 500) are similar, and the thickness of cell membranes is also relatively constant. Thus, lipophilicity of the solute is the major determinant of cell membrane permeability.

Balance Between Lipophilicity and Hydrophilicity. Equation 8.2 also shows that transport rate is influenced by the concentration gradient ($C_1 - C_2$). Therefore, a solute that can achieve higher concentrations on the donor side will initially be transported faster than one that attains lower concentrations. Because the medium on the donor and aqueous sides is aqueous, solutes with higher aqueous solubility (greater hydrophilicity) will be able to achieve higher concentrations and thus will be transported faster. This appears to contradict the statement that solutes with greater lipophilicity are more permeable.

The reality is that both hydrophilicity and lipophilicity are important in drug transport, and good drugs need a balance between these properties. Solutes that are very hydrophilic (usually with a very low partition coefficient) will partition slowly from water into a lipid membrane. If the receptor is in or beyond the membrane, this molecule will have a low probability of reaching it in the desired time. Conversely, highly lipophilic molecules (with a very high partition coefficient) will readily partition into the first series of lipid membranes they encounter, but will tend to remain there; this will prevent them from reaching the target receptor in a timely manner. Hence, drugs of intermediate partition coefficient achieve optimum transport, where neither entry into nor departure from the lipid membrane is too slow.

Passive Diffusion of Nonelectrolytes.

Consider a situation in which a nonelectrolyte solute is initially present in extracellular fluid but not in intracellular fluid. Therefore, $C_2 = 0$ initially, and the concentration gradient = C_1.

Diffusion begins, and the solute is transported passively into the cell. As C_2 begins to increase, the concentration gradient $(C_1 - C_2)$ begins to decrease, progressively slowing diffusion rate. Eventually $C_1 = C_2$, the concentration gradient becomes zero, and passive diffusion stops because equilibrium has been reached. However, if the solute is consumed in the cell or can somehow leave the cell, C_2 may remain small and passive diffusion will continue.

Thus, transport rate is high if the concentration gradient is large; the concentration gradient is large if C_1 is large and C_2 is small. Transport continues as long as a concentration gradient is maintained, as when solute continues to be added to the donor side or is allowed to leave from the receiver side.

Although we have considered transport *into* the cell, remember that passive diffusion can occur from the intracellular to the extracellular region if the concentration inside the cell is higher than that outside. In this case, the intracellular region is the donor and the extracellular region is the receiver.

Passive Diffusion of Weak Acids and Bases.

In the previous example, we assumed that the solute behaved as a nonelectrolyte on both donor and receiver sides. Therefore, all solute molecules were capable of diffusing through the lipid bilayer, i.e., C_1 = total solute concentration on the donor side and C_2 = total solute concentration on the receiver side. The pH of the donor or receiver sides has no influence on the transport rate of nonelectrolytes, and the total concentration of the solute on the donor and receiver sides is equal at equilibrium.

The situation is different when the solute is either a weak acid or weak base. These solutes can ionize, with concentrations of ionized and un-ionized forms dependent on the pK_a of the compound and pH of donor and receiver fluids. Ionized molecules cannot enter the lipid bilayer and therefore cannot diffuse passively through cell membranes. The concentration gradient of the permeable species is the driving force for passive diffusion. Therefore, the driving force for diffusion of weak acids and bases ($C_1 - C_2$) is the *concentration gradient of the un-ionized form*, as depicted in Figure 8.5.

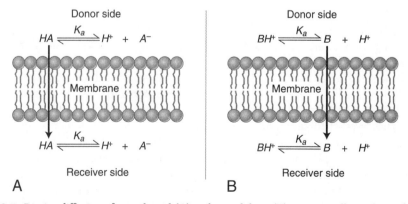

Figure 8.5. Passive diffusion of a weak acid (**A**) and a weak base (**B**) across a cell membrane from higher concentration (donor side) to lower concentration (receiver side). The concentration gradient of the un-ionized form (and not the total concentration of drug) is the driving force for diffusion.

Influence of pH and pK$_a$ on Passive Diffusion

Consider a weak acid drug *HA* of pK$_a$ 7. Initially, assume that total drug concentration on the donor side [HA]$_{total}$ is 0.1 M, and that there is no drug on the receiver side. Also assume that the pH of the donor and receiver sides is 7. The drug on the donor side is 50% un-ionized (determined using the Henderson–Hasselbalch equation), so the concentration of the un-ionized form [HA] is 0.05 M (Fig. 8.6A). Because there is no drug on the receiver side, the concentration gradient of [HA] is = 0.05 M − 0 M = 0.05 M.

Because a driving force for diffusion is present, HA will begin to diffuse passively through the lipid bilayer. Once some HA appears on the receiver side, it will ionize to satisfy the Henderson–Hasselbalch relationship. This means that drug appearing on the receiver side will be 50% ionized and 50% un-ionized. Now, the concentration of HA on the receiver side is no longer zero, and the concentration of HA on the donor side is still less than 0.05 M. Because there is still a favorable concentration gradient of HA across the membrane, diffusion will continue but at a progressively slower rate.

Eventually, equilibrium will be reached when *the concentration gradient of the permeable species* (un-ionized HA) is zero, which is the same as saying that the concentration of un-ionized HA is the same on both the donor and receiver sides. At the same time, the Henderson–Hasselbalch relationship must be satisfied on both the donor and receiver sides; in this case, the drug on both sides has to be 50% ionized. This condition is satisfied when the concentrations of all the species are as shown in Figure 8.6B. A similar outcome would be obtained if the drug were a weak base.

This was a simple example in which the pK$_a$ of the drug was the same as the pH of the extracellular and intracellular fluids. Figures 8.7 and 8.8 illustrate the situation in which the pK$_a$ is not the same as the pH of the environment. Figure 8.7 shows the equilibrium state for passive diffusion of 0.1 M of a weak acid of pK$_a$ 6, and Figure 8.8 shows it for 0.1 M of a weak base of pK$_a$ 8.

For passive diffusion of a weak acid or base across a cell membrane when the pH of both the receiver and donor sides is the same, we can say that

- Concentration gradient of the un-ionized form drives diffusion.
- Concentration of the un-ionized form depends on the pH of the environment, the pK$_a$ of the solute, and its total concentration.
- Concentration of the un-ionized form on the two sides will be the same at equilibrium.

- Concentration of the ionized form on the two sides will be the same at equilibrium.
- Total concentration of solute (ionized + un-ionized) on the two sides is the same at equilibrium.

Ion Trapping. The attainment of equilibrium is more complex when the pH of donor and receiver fluids is different, i.e., when the intracellular contents have a different pH than the extracellular fluid. In such situations, equilibrium is reached when the concentration of *un-ionized*

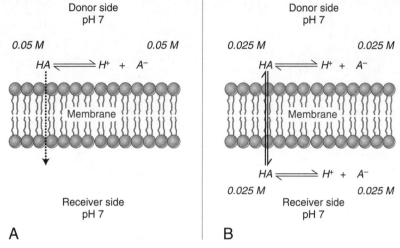

Figure 8.6. Initial (A) and equilibrium (B) conditions for the passive diffusion of a weak acid of $pK_a = 7$ across a cell membrane. The pH of the donor and receiver sides is 7.

solute (the permeable species) is the same on both sides. However, the difference in pH between the donor and receiver sides means that the concentration of *ionized* solute is different on the two sides: higher on the side where the pH favors greater ionization. The total solute concentration is consequently higher on the side where the solute is more ionized. The solute is *trapped* on the side of greater ionization.

If this happens to be the intracellular fluid, a drug can be concentrated in the cell, achieving higher intracellular concentrations than otherwise expected.

Ion trapping of drugs occurs in many instances, and could be desirable or undesirable. The pH of cytoplasm of cells is around 7, and the pH in the cells' endosomes, lysosomes, and other intracellular particles is acidic, around 5. This acidity

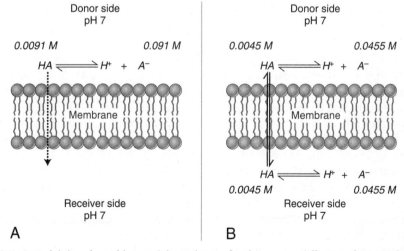

Figure 8.7. Initial (A) and equilibrium (B) conditions for the passive diffusion of 0.1 M of a weak acid HA of $pK_a = 6$, across a cell membrane. The pH of the donor and receiver sides is 7. Note that the initial concentration gradient is much smaller than that in Figure 8.6, so it will take longer for this system to reach equilibrium.

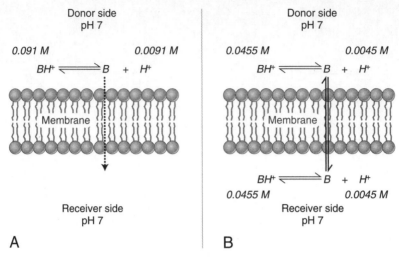

Figure 8.8. Initial (**A**) and equilibrium (**B**) conditions for the passive diffusion of 0.1 M of a weak base of $pK_a = 8$ across a cell membrane. The pH of the donor and receiver sides is 7.

is maintained by proton pumps (an active transport mechanism) in the endosomal membrane, which are similar to the proton pumps in the stomach. When a weak base drug enters the cell, it will be concentrated in a ratio of 100 to 1 inside endosomes compared with the cytoplasm. This type of ion trapping is well known for the basic drug chloroquine used to treat malaria.

Many anticancer drugs, such as doxorubicin, mitoxantrone, and other drugs in these families are weak bases. Ion trapping of these drugs in endosomes decreases their concentration in the cytoplasm, so that less drug is available at the site of action, usually DNA. Scientists are working to see whether they can decrease this sequestration of drug in the endosomes so that more drug is able to reach its target. One approach being tried is to use a proton pump inhibitor such as omeprazole to increase the pH in endosomes.

Another important illustration of ion trapping is placental transfer of weak base drugs such as local anesthetics from mother to fetus. The pH of the fetal circulation is lower than maternal plasma pH. Therefore, un-ionized local anesthetics cross the placenta into the fetal circulation and are converted to their ionized form, thus trapping them in the fetus and leading to fetal distress.

It should be apparent from the above discussion that the pH of the donor and receiver sides is an important issue for ionizable drugs only. For drugs that do not ionize under physiological conditions, the pH has no effect on passive diffusion.

Carrier-Mediated Transport

The above discussion has treated the cell membrane as a simple semipermeable barrier that allows lipophilic solutes to diffuse passively through the lipid bilayer. Many hydrophilic solutes, however, are also able to cross the cell membrane and to enter and leave cells. Because the protein aqueous channels in the cell membrane are too small to allow most ligands or drugs to cross, other transport mechanisms have to be present that make this possible.

The body has specialized processes to transport essential solutes that have difficulty crossing the lipid bilayer by passive diffusion. One process is carrier-mediated

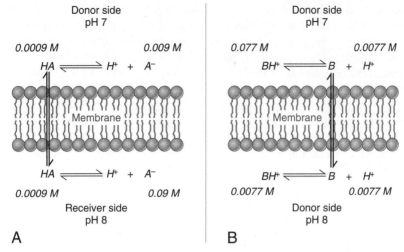

Figure 8.9. Equilibrium conditions for passive diffusion across a cell membrane when the pH of the donor and receiver sides is different. **A.** Ion trapping of a weak acid ($pK_a = 6$) on the receiver side. **B.** Ion trapping of a weak base ($pK_a = 8$) on the donor side.

Ion Trapping

A weak acid of pK_a 6 crosses a cell membrane by passive diffusion, from a donor side of pH 7 to a receiver side of pH 8 (Fig. 8.9A). Initially, before diffusion starts, the situation on the donor side is the same as in Figure 8.6A. Once transport begins and some un-ionized HA diffuses to the receiver side, it is ionized to a greater extent on the receiver side because the pH is higher. Using the Henderson–Hasselbalch equation, we can calculate the ratios of ionized and un-ionized forms on the two sides:

$$\frac{[A^-]_{donor}}{[HA]_{donor}} = 10 \text{ and } \frac{[A^-]_{receiver}}{[HA]_{receiver}} = 100$$

The objective is to calculate the concentrations on the donor and receiver sides at equilibrium.

If we designate $[HA]_{donor} = X$, then $[HA]_{receiver} = X$, by the definition of equilibrium. Simultaneously, to satisfy the Henderson–Hasselbalch equation, $[A^-]_{donor} = 10X$, and $[A^-]_{receiver} = 100X$. Now we need to solve for X to determine the individual concentrations of all the species. The total drug concentration in the system is 0.1 M; in other words

$$[HA]_{donor} + [HA]_{receiver} + [A^-]_{donor}$$
$$+ [A^-]_{receiver} = 112X = 0.1 M$$

Solving for X, we obtain $X =$ approximately 0.0009 M. Now, looking at *total* (un-ionized + ionized) drug concentrations on the donor and receiver side, we find that there is 0.0099 M drug on the donor side, but 0.0909 M drug on the receiver side (Fig. 8.9B). In other words, most of the drug is on the receiver side after the passive diffusion process.

transport in which the molecule to be transported binds to and hitches a ride on a membrane protein called a carrier or transporter. Drugs with appropriate structures may also make use of these carriers to cross cell membranes.

Transporters. Transporters are integral membrane proteins with one or more active sites for a particular molecule or ion. The transporter binds to this substrate on one side of the cell membrane and transports it through the lipid bilayer to the other side. Recall that the cell membrane is fluid in nature and allows the movement of membrane proteins. Transporters have the ability to recognize (often through attached carbohydrates) and bind to particular substrates that they are designed to transport. Many transporters show specificity and stereoselectivity; for example, D-glucose is transported but not L-glucose. Carrier-mediated transport does not require the substrate to be lipophilic; both hydrophilic and lipophilic solutes can be transported in this manner. Transporters, depending on their function, can carry molecules into or out of cells. A representation of carrier-mediated transport is shown in Figure 8.10.

Cell membranes contain specific transporters to transport solutes needed for homeostasis. Drugs similar in structure to these natural substrates may also bind to and be transported by these transporters. Scientists have known for a while that transporters present in the kidney, liver, intestines, and other tissues play a role in elimination, distribution, and absorption of many drugs. However, only recently have some of these mechanisms been carefully examined and understood. Studies show that many drug transporters are somewhat nonselective, being able to transport drugs with diverse structures. In particular, transporters capable of binding to organic cations are important in transporting several amine drugs in their protonated forms. The total number of drug transporters is still unknown, and the functions of many known transporters have not yet been fully defined. Genetic variation of these transporters is also being shown to account for the variability among individuals in handling certain drugs.

Transporters may also be good drug targets for certain diseases. Many pathogens depend on their hosts to provide essential nutrients such as amino acids and vitamins. Bacterial transport proteins are attractive targets in designing drugs that can prevent the transport of essential nutrients, resulting in death of the pathogen.

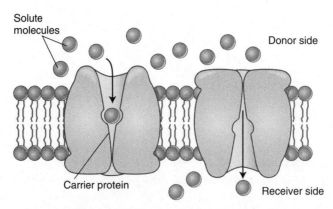

Figure 8.10. Representation of carrier-mediated transport. A solute molecule binds to the carrier on the donor side of the membrane. The drug then dissociates from the complex and is released on the receiver side. Carrier-mediated processes can transport drugs in or out of cells.

Nucleoside Transporters

Nucleosides are precursors of nucleic acid synthesis, which is fundamental to the control of growth and metabolism in all living systems. The purine nucleoside adenosine is also a powerful neuromodulator that regulates a variety of physiological processes including neurotransmission and cardiovascular activity. Nucleosides are hydrophilic, and passive diffusion across cell membranes is very slow; therefore, cells have evolved complex transport systems consisting of multiple carrier proteins known as the nucleoside transporters.

Numerous nucleoside analogs are used routinely as drugs in the treatment of cancer, viral infections, and many other pathophysiological conditions. Examples are the antiviral agents acyclovir, zidovudine (AZT), and didanosine (ddI), and the antineoplastic drugs mercaptopurine, fluorouracil, and thioguanine. Many of these drugs rely on nucleoside transporters to enter cells and reach their cellular targets at clinically relevant concentrations. Conversely, nucleoside transporters themselves could serve as drug targets. Nucleoside transporter inhibitors such as dipyridamole and dilazep have long been used in the treatment of heart and vascular diseases.

Rate of Carrier-Mediated Transport. After binding of the substrate to its transporter on the donor side of the membrane, the resulting substrate–transporter complex undergoes a change in conformation. This complex, which is now soluble in the lipid bilayer, diffuses to the receiver side and releases the substrate. The transporter then regains its original conformation and transports another substrate molecule to continue the carrier-mediated process.

The rate of carrier-mediated transport is governed by the principles of protein–substrate binding and Michaelis–Menten kinetics, discussed in Chapter 4, Rates of Pharmaceutical Processes. Recall that the Michaelis–Menten equation is written as:

$$V = \frac{V_{max}\,[S]}{K_m + [S]} \qquad \text{(Eq. 8.4)}$$

In the present context V is the rate of transport, K_m is the Michaelis–Menten constant, V_{max} is the maximum rate of transport, and [S] is the concentration of the substrate being transported.

A low K_m implies a high affinity between transporter and substrate and a fast transport rate, and vice versa. K_m can be different on the two sides of the cell membrane, so that the substrate is easily released on the receiver side of the membrane. Such a difference in K_m also favors transport in one direction over the other. V_{max} is related to the total number of transporter molecules present and to the mobility of the transporter in the cell membrane.

At low substrate concentration ([S] << K_m), the rate of transport is first-order and directly proportional to substrate concentration. The first-order rate constant is V_{max}/K_m.

$$V = \frac{V_{max}}{K_m}\,[S] \qquad \text{(Eq. 8.5)}$$

At high substrate concentration ([S] >> K_m), the transporter becomes *saturated* and the rate of transport is zero-order, independent of substrate concentration.

$$V = V_{max} \qquad \text{(Eq. 8.6)}$$

Types of Carrier-Mediated Transport.
The two major types of carrier-mediated transport processes are facilitated diffusion and active transport. The difference between the two lies in the absence or presence of an external energy source.

Facilitated Diffusion. Facilitated diffusion is a carrier-mediated process that occurs only when there is a concentration gradient between the donor and receiver sides. In other words, the transporter can only transport substrate from a region of high concentration to a region of low concentration, in the direction of the concentration gradient. Like other diffusion processes, facilitated diffusion does not require an energy source and ceases when equilibrium is reached. The transporters involved are called uniporters (Fig. 8.11A), which transport one molecule at a time. An example of this type of transporter is GLUT1, a widely distributed glucose transporter that transports glucose in and out of cells depending on the direction of the concentration gradient.

The rate at which a solute is transported by facilitated diffusion depends on

- concentration gradient of the solute
- concentration of transporter molecules in the membrane
- affinity $(1/K_m)$ between transporter and substrate

In general, the rate of facilitated diffusion is greater than that of passive diffusion. At low substrate concentrations, increasing concentration on the donor side increases the concentration gradient and hence the transport rate. However, if substrate concentration on the donor side is sufficiently large, there may not be enough transporter molecules in the cell membrane to bind to the substrate. Increasing the concentration beyond this value exhibits no further increase in transport rate because the transporter is saturated.

A transporter is usually specific for its intended substrate. However, the transporter may also bind to other compounds (such as inhibitors) that are structurally similar to the substrate. Recall that an inhibitor is a molecule that represses or prevents the substrate from binding to its target. Inhibition causes the transporter to

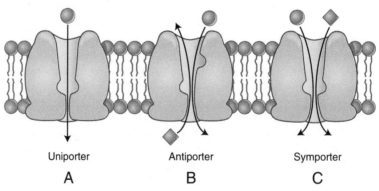

Uniporter   Antiporter   Symporter

A   B   C

Figure 8.11. Different types of transporters involved in carrier-mediated transport. **A.** Uniporters move one molecule at a time, and can be involved in either facilitated diffusion or active transport. **B** and **C.** Antiporters transport one solute across the membrane in one direction while simultaneously transporting a second solute across the membrane in the opposite direction. Symporters simultaneously transport two solutes across the membrane in the same direction. Both of these are active processes.

be partially occupied by the inhibitor, resulting in a decrease in the transport rate of the substrate. A large concentration of the inhibitor may saturate the transporter and completely inhibit transport of the substrate. Examples of drugs that are transported by facilitated diffusion across one or more membranes in the body are penicillin, furosemide, morphine, and dopamine.

Active Transport. Active transport is very similar to facilitated diffusion in that it requires a transporter molecule, is saturable, and can be inhibited. However, active transport processes are able to transport a substrate *against* a concentration gradient, i.e., from a region of low concentration to a region of high concentration. This is not a simple diffusion process and requires a source of energy from the cell. This active involvement of the cell in the transport gives this process the name *active* transport.

In addition to uniporters, two other types of transporters are involved in active transport, as illustrated in Figure 8.11B and 8.11C. Antiporters transport one solute across the membrane in one direction while simultaneously transporting a second solute across the membrane in the opposite direction. Symporters simultaneously transport two solutes across the membrane in the same direction. Energy is required for both of these transporters to function. Substances called metabolic poisons can deplete the energy source, resulting in reduced active transport.

Examples of drugs that use active transport to cross membranes are intestinal absorption of 5-fluorouracil and some cardiac glycosides, absorption of α-methyldopa into the brain, and secretion of certain drugs into the bile and urine.

Drug Efflux. Just as some transporters assist a substrate in entering cells, other transporters pump substrates out of cells; these are called efflux proteins or *efflux pumps*. Efflux is usually an energy-driven

active transport process that works to keep intracellular concentrations of drug low.

Multidrug efflux is a phenomenon in which a single type of transporter (multidrug resistance, or MDR, transporter) recognizes and pumps many drugs, with no apparent common structural similarity, out of cells. The major mechanism of efflux is dependent on proteins that derive their transport energy from the hydrolysis of ATP. Many of these transporters belong to the ABC (ATP-binding cassette) superfamily of membrane transporters. MDR transporters are transmembrane proteins that detect and bind to substrates as they cross the lipid bilayer passively on their way into the cell. The substrate is then transported back out into the extracellular environment, thus preventing it from entering the cell (Fig. 8.12). This restricts entry of certain substrates into cells, or at least slows down their transport. The consequence is a lower than expected intracellular concentration of the substrate. Also, during absorption of drugs across an epithelial membrane, both passive diffusion and an opposing efflux pump may together determine how much of the drug is allowed to go from the apical to the basolateral side or vice versa.

Members of the ABC family of transporters include the clinically significant

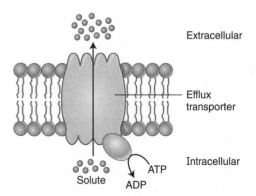

Figure 8.12. Illustration of multidrug efflux out of a cell via a membrane transporter protein. Note that energy from the cell (conversion of ATP to ADP) is required for this process.

multidrug resistance pump P-glycoprotein (P-gp) and the multidrug resistance protein (MRP). Related transporters are also found in a number of pathogenic bacteria and fungi, and parasitic protozoa, in which they confer resistance to antimicrobial drugs. In humans, these efflux transporters are expressed in cells of the small and large intestines, liver, kidney, and pancreas, and in the blood–brain barrier.

An important characteristic distinguishing MDR transporters from other mammalian transporters is their wide substrate specificity; unlike other selective (classic) transporters, multidrug transporters recognize and handle a wide range of substrates. In normal tissues MDR transporters may function as protective mechanisms against toxins and as transporters of endogenous materials out of cells.

Multiple drug resistance as a result of MDR transporter efflux is known to develop in bacterial and cancer cells; drugs that were once effective become ineffective, presumably because cells that express more of the transporter survive and become more efficient at pumping out the drug. Research is under way to improve activity of existing antibiotics by binding to and inhibiting bacterial multidrug transporters.

Transcytosis

Transcytosis, also called *vesicular transport,* is a process by which specific substances (usually macromolecules such as proteins, polysaccharides, polynucleotides, and antibodies) are transported across cells by the formation of vesicles. This mode of transport is usually seen in epithelial and endothelial cells.

The transported substance is taken into the cell by endocytosis, a process in which vesicles form at the cell membrane and internalize extracellular materials into the cell. This intracellular vesicle fuses with the cell membrane on the other side of the cell and expels its contents

into the extracellular fluid, a process known as exocytosis. Endocytosis and exocytosis can occur against a concentration gradient and require cellular energy as in active transport. The transcytosis process for transport of materials through the capillary endothelium is illustrated in Figure 8.13.

Endocytosis. Endocytosis can be further classified as pinocytosis (cell drinking), in which fluids and dissolved materials are internalized by a cell, and phagocytosis, in which cells engulf large particles such as bacteria and viruses.

Endocytosis is frequently receptor-mediated, meaning that cells internalize materials only after their recognition by a specific receptor protein on the cell membrane. The cellular uptake of large molecule drugs such as insulin, growth hormone, erythropoietin, and the interleukins is believed to be related to receptor-mediated endocytosis.

Exocytosis. Cells use exocytosis to expel proteins, secreted substances, and wastes from the cell. Many signaling molecules secreted by cells, such as insulin secreted by the pancreas and neurotransmitters secreted by neurons, are released extracellularly by exocytosis.

Rate of Transcytosis. Transcytosis is a relatively slow process compared with

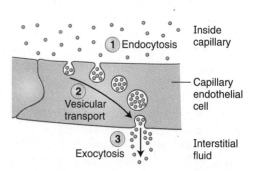

Figure 8.13. Illustration of transcytosis for transporting material through a cell. In this case, the substances are moving through a capillary endothelial cell.

other transport mechanisms we have discussed. Thus, transport by transcytosis is negligible for solutes that can be effectively transported by passive diffusion or carrier-mediated processes. However, transcytosis becomes important for materials that cannot cross the cell membrane by another mechanism. For example, many proteins (such as antigens, botulinus toxin, and oral vaccines) are able to enter the bloodstream after being orally ingested. Transcytosis through intestinal epithelial cells is presumed to be the mechanism of transport in these cases. The amounts of macromolecules transported in this way are extremely small, but sufficient to elicit their biological response.

It is not completely clear whether transcytosis contributes significantly to drug transport. However, based on the relative slowness of this process and the very small amount of material that is transported, we assume that transcytosis probably does not play a role in the transport of most small molecule drugs across biological membranes.

Paracellular Transport

A substance must cross an epithelial membrane to move from the external environment into the bloodstream; it must cross the capillary endothelium to move from blood into tissues.

One way that molecules can move through epithelial and endothelial membranes is using the transcellular mechanisms just discussed, in which the drug crosses the cell membranes of the various cells in its path. However, it is also possible for molecules to diffuse passively through cell junctions of an epithelial or endothelial membrane by a process called paracellular transport. This is a *passive diffusion* process that occurs as a result of a concentration, electrochemical, or hydrostatic (pressure) gradient.

Molecules that are smaller in diameter than the junction can cross the membrane paracellularly, thus avoiding the lipid bilayer of the cell membranes. Solute lipophilicity is not a requirement for passive paracellular transport, whereas lipophilicity was an important

Transcytosis by Intestinal M Cells

The intestinal epithelium is composed of epithelial cells called *enterocytes*, scattered among which are a few specialized cells called *M cells*. The function of an M cell is to "sample" ingested pathogens in the intestines so that the body can mount a defense. An M cell engulfs the microbe or particle on the lumenal side and passes it to the basolateral sides by transcytosis. Here it is released into the bloodstream, where it enters cells of the immune system. This activity normally stimulates secretion of antibodies into the bloodstream, which destroy the invading pathogen.

Certain bacteria and viruses exploit this pathway to infect the body. One example is poliovirus, which traverses M cells by transcytosis and enters lymphocytes in the bloodstream; these ferry the virus to the nervous system. Oral polio vaccine is a disabled virus that also uses this route. M cells are also known to transport HIV in rectal tissue and transfer the virus to lymphocytes. Another example of M cell transcytosis is the transport of an invasive form of *Salmonella,* which causes fever and gastroenteritis.

criterion for passive transcellular diffusion. Ions and small molecules such as water can move relatively easily across tissues by a paracellular mechanism.

Paracellular Transport Through Epithelial Membranes

Epithelial membranes are barrier membranes designed to protect the body from foreign substances, and are usually found at sites of administration and absorption of drugs (skin, intestinal wall, and so forth). Most epithelial membranes have tight junctions (less than 1 nm in diameter) between their cells, so that paracellular transport of drugs or ligands (particularly those with molecular weights greater than about 200) through epithelial cell junctions is next to impossible. Paracellular transport cannot occur through such tissues, and drugs must cross epithelial tissue transcellularly to enter the bloodstream.

Paracellular Transport Through the Capillary Endothelium

Cells of the capillary endothelium are more loosely packed and allow most drugs and other small molecules to diffuse through cellular junctions if there is a concentration gradient. Thus, once the drug has entered the bloodstream, movement of individual drug molecules in and out of capillaries proceeds freely regardless of polarity or lipophilicity of the drug. Paracellular diffusion of uncharged molecules is proportional to their diffusion coefficient, as predicted by Fick's law. The diffusion of positively charged molecules is observed to be somewhat slower than that predicted by the diffusion coefficient, presumably owing to repulsion by positive charges on membrane proteins in the endothelial junctions. Lipophilic drugs may be additionally transported by passive transcellular diffusion through the endothelial cells.

The size of endothelial junctions is in the range of 5 to 30 nm. Generally, molecules with molecular weights up to about 20,000 to 30,000 can diffuse paracellularly through the capillary endothelium. Proteins and blood cells, which are larger than the capillary endothelial junctions, are not capable of paracellular diffusion.

Blood–Brain Barrier. The **blood–brain barrier** (BBB) is the specialized system of capillary endothelial cells that protects the brain from harmful substances in the bloodstream while supplying it with essential nutrients for proper function. Unlike peripheral capillaries that allow relatively free exchange of molecules between blood and tissues, the BBB strictly limits transport into the brain through both physical (tight junction) and metabolic (enzyme) barriers. Capillaries bringing blood to the brain contain endothelial cells that are very tightly packed, similar to tight junctions in epithelial tissue. Cell-to-cell contacts between adjacent endothelial cells are essentially sealed, forming a continuous blood vessel. These tight paracellular junctions do not allow drugs and other small molecules to move between the blood and the brain; molecules can enter and leave the brain capillaries by transcellular pathways only.

The BBB has a number of highly selective carrier-mediated mechanisms to transport nutrients and other essential molecules into the brain. For example, receptor-mediated endocytosis occurs for endogenous macromolecules such as transferrin, insulin, and leptin.

The BBB is often the rate-limiting factor in determining permeation of drugs into the brain. The general rule is that the higher the lipophilicity of a substance, the greater its transcellular passive diffusion into the brain. Even if a drug molecule is lipophilic enough to diffuse transcellularly through the capillary endothelium, there are other processes that oppose uptake into the brain. One significant opposing process is carrier-mediated efflux, a major obstacle for many drugs with sites of action in the brain. Another is the presence of metabolizing enzymes in the capillary endothelium that break down the drug before it can enter the brain. Poor delivery into the brain remains a major challenge for many CNS drugs.

Filtration. In addition to a concentration gradient as a driving force for paracellular diffusion, solutes can cross capillary endothelial junctions paracellularly as the result of a pressure gradient. The pressure-driven movement of dissolved solutes through cell junctions is known as **filtration** or **convection**. When the hydrostatic pressure across an endothelial membrane is unequal, fluid moves from the area of high pressure to the area of low pressure through cell junctions. Dissolved solids will move along with the fluid if their size is smaller than the size of the junctions. For example, if pressure in blood vessels is larger than in surrounding tissues, bulk water flows out between the cells of the blood vessel. Solutes dissolved in the water will also be transported out at a rate much faster than simple diffusion. Even macromolecules such as plasma proteins may leak out of capillaries if the hydrostatic pressure in the circulation is high enough, compared with that of the surrounding tissue.

Filtration is the main driving force for fluid exchange in and out of capillaries. It is also important in the kidneys in which high arterial pressure and leaky capillaries allow drug and waste molecules to be filtered readily along with water to be excreted as urine.

Leaky Capillaries. Endothelial cells of some capillaries have larger junctions (diameter of 50 to 100 nm) than the peripheral capillaries; these openings are called *fenestrations* (meaning windows), and the capillaries are called **fenestrated capillaries**. The extent of the fenestration may depend on the physiological state of the surrounding tissue, i.e., fenestration may increase or decrease as a function of the need to absorb or secrete. Fenestra-

tions are found in the capillaries of organs that transport lots of water, such as the bowels, glomerular capillaries of the kidneys, and salivary glands. Fenestrations allow bulk flow of water and dissolved materials between blood and the tissue.

Fenestrations are even larger in some specialized capillaries and become discontinuous because they do not have a complete layer of endothelial cells lining them. Discontinuous capillaries form large irregularly shaped vessels called sinusoids or *sinusoid capillaries*. Many materials, including macromolecules and even cells, can diffuse paracellularly through sinusoids. Such capillaries are found where a very free exchange of substances between the blood and an organ is advantageous, such as in the liver, spleen, and bone marrow.

Rate of Paracellular Diffusion

The predominant way that solutes move through the paracellular junctions is by diffusion in the direction of a concentration gradient. Fick's law, discussed earlier for transcellular passive diffusion, also governs the rate of paracellular transport; the difference is that lipophilicity is not required for paracellular transport. In addition, molecular size is an important factor; transport will occur only if the size of the solute is smaller than the size of the junction. Thus, the rate of paracellular transport through junctions in the endothelial membrane is given by:

$$\frac{dC}{dt} = -\frac{A \cdot D \cdot (C_1 - C_2)}{h} \quad \text{(Eq. 8.7)}$$

Rate of paracellular diffusion depends on the concentration gradient $(C_1 - C_2)$, the surface area of the membrane A, the membrane thickness or length of the diffusion path h, and the diffusion coefficient D of the solute.

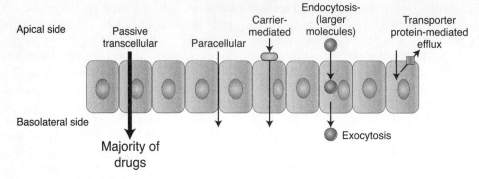

Figure 8.14. Summary of possible processes involved in transport of materials in and out of cells, and across an epithelial or endothelial barrier.

Multiple Transport Pathways

It is important to understand that a solute may be able to cross membranes using several transport pathways simultaneously. Consider a solute that has good lipophilicity, fits through the endothelial paracellular junction, and can bind to a specific transporter in the capillary membrane. This solute can be transported across the capillary wall by passive transcellular diffusion, carrier-mediated transport, and paracellular diffusion.

The dominant mechanism of transport for this solute may vary from membrane to membrane. For example, passive transcellular diffusion may be dominant for intestinal absorption of this solute, paracellular transport may be controlling for its distribution in and out of peripheral capillaries, and active transport may be important for its entry into the brain.

The different pathways involved in transport of materials across a cell or tissue membrane are depicted in Figure 8.14.

KEY CONCEPTS

We can summarize passive transcellular diffusion through a cell membrane as follows:

- Most drugs cross cell membranes and epithelial membranes by passive diffusion across the lipid bilayer.

- Only un-ionized, lipophilic drug molecules cross the lipid bilayer by passive diffusion.

- Ion trapping on either the donor or receiver sides can occur if their pHs are different.

- Most drugs cross endothelial membranes (e.g., the capillary endothelium) by paracellular diffusion through cell junctions.

- Specialized endothelia (blood–brain barrier or fenestrated capillaries) can restrict or enhance paracellular transport.

- Diffusion of drugs through hydrophilic cell membrane protein channels is insignificant.

- The rate of diffusion is governed by Fick's law.

- Most proteins cannot diffuse passively across the cell membrane because they are too large and too polar.

- Carrier-mediated processes and efflux pumps play an important role in determining intracellular drug concentrations.

ADDITIONAL READING

1. Washington N, Washington C, Wilson C. Physiological Pharmaceuticals: Barriers to Drug Absorption, 2nd ed. Taylor & Francis, 2001.

2. Amidon GL, Lee PI, Topp EM (eds). Transport Processes in Pharmaceutical Systems, 1st ed. Marcel Dekker, 2000.

3. Ritschel WA, Kearns GL. Handbook of Basic Pharmacokinetics, 5th ed. American Pharmaceutical Association, 1999.

4. Shargel L, Yu ABC. Applied Biopharmaceutics and Pharmacokinetics, 4th ed. McGraw-Hill/Appleton & Lange, 1999.

REVIEW QUESTIONS

1. What does the term *semipermeable* mean? Describe the features of a cell membrane that regulate the transport of small molecules across it.

2. How do most ions and very small solutes enter and leave cells?

3. How do most small molecule drugs enter and leave cells? What parameters control the rate of this transport?

4. What role do transport membrane proteins play in the transport of solutes in and out of cells? Why are only some solutes transported in this manner?

5. Discuss the Michaelis–Menten equation and its relevance to carrier-mediated transport.

6. What are efflux proteins and how do they reduce intracellular concentrations of drugs?

7. Explain the process of transport by transcytosis. What types of materials

are transported predominantly by this mechanism?

8. Which of the transport processes are saturable? Why?

9. How do most drugs cross epithelial barriers? How do most solutes cross the peripheral capillary epithelium?

10. What is the blood–brain barrier? What types of compounds can cross the blood–brain barrier?

11. Elaborate on the specialized capillary endothelium in the kidneys and liver and how it influences drug transport.

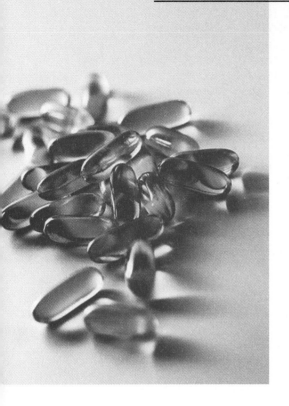

Section III • **Drug Delivery**

Chapter 9

Drug Absorption

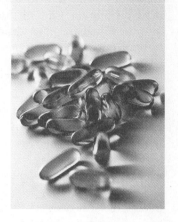

Systemic Versus Local Administration

Drugs are given to patients at locations of the body called sites of administration. The overall goal is for the drug to travel from the site of administration and reach its site of action in a timely and predictable manner, where it can perform its function. There are numerous ways to administer a drug to a patient, and drugs are available in a variety of *dosage forms*. The choice of administration method depends on, among other factors, the physicochemical properties of the drug, physiological limitations of the administration or absorption site, and the clinical situation.

The site of action is generally not a single location, or is difficult to reach. In such situations the drug is administered at some convenient location far removed from the site of action. The drug must be absorbed into the bloodstream so that the body's circulatory system can carry it to its site of action; this is called systemic administration. In some situations, the site of action is localized and is readily accessible; in these cases the drug can be administered very close to or right at this site. Such an approach to drug administration is termed *topical, nonsystemic,* or local administration.

The first step in the journey of a systemically administered drug to its site of action is absorption, in which the drug moves from the site of administration into the bloodstream. A drug given topically or nonsystemically needs merely to enter the desired tissue at the site of administration; absorption into the bloodstream is not necessary.

Table 9.1 summarizes the various routes of systemic and nonsystemic administration available for drug delivery. Some routes can be used for either systemic or nonsystemic dosing. For example, a drug can be applied to the skin for treating a local rash (nonsystemic application), whereas another drug can be applied to the skin (such as nicotine patches for smoking cessation) to elicit a systemic effect. In the latter case, the drug is absorbed into the bloodstream and carried to the site of action.

Systemic Administration

Systemically administered drugs may be absorbed from the site of administration; an example is found in transdermal patches, from which the drug is absorbed through the skin where it is administered. In other cases, the drug moves from the site of administration to a different region called the site of absorption. An example is orally administered drugs, which are administered in the mouth and swallowed; absorption usually occurs from the small intestines. Regardless of where the site of absorption is located, the drug must be in solution for absorption to occur. We will discuss the dissolution process in depth in Chapter 10, Drug Delivery Systems.

Dissolved drug molecules have to cross the epithelial tissue at the absorption site and the capillary endothelium to enter the bloodstream. Most drugs are small molecules and cross the capillary endothelium readily by paracellular passive diffusion regardless of their physicochemical properties. Thus, the slowest or *rate-limiting step* in absorption is usually the drug's ability to cross epithelial membranes at the absorption site.

Rate of Absorption

Rate of absorption into the bloodstream depends on physicochemical properties of the drug, permeability of the epithelial membrane at the site of absorption, surface area of the membrane exposed to drug at the absorption site, and concentration gradient of drug between the absorption site and the bloodstream. The equation for the rate of absorption is similar to Fick's law of diffusion:

$$\text{absorption rate} = \frac{P \cdot A \cdot D \cdot (C_a - C_p)}{h}$$

(Eq. 9.1)

The partition coefficient P and diffusion coefficient D depend on the structure of the drug. The term A refers to the surface area of the membrane, and the term h is the thickness of the epithelial membrane at the absorption site; this

TABLE 9.1. Classification of the Available Routes of Administration for Drugs	
Systemic	*Nonsystemic*
Oral	Oral
Parenteral	Parenteral
Intravenous	Intracardiac
Intramuscular	Intrathecal
Subcutaneous	Intralumbar
Intraarterial	
Rectal	Rectal
Sublingual/buccal	Buccal
Transdermal	Dermal
Pulmonary	Pulmonary
Nasal	Nasal
	Ophthalmic
	Vaginal/urethral

membrane may be composed of one or several layers of epithelial cells.

Let us look more closely at the concentration gradient term $(C_a - C_p)$. Here, C_a is the concentration of drug at the absorption (donor side) site and C_p is the concentration of drug in plasma or blood (receiver side). Obviously, the higher the concentration of dissolved drug at the absorption site, the faster the rate of absorption will be. This concentration is controlled by the *dose* of drug administered and its rate of dissolution. On the receiver side, if the absorptive tissue is well perfused (i.e., has good blood supply), blood flows through the absorption site so rapidly that drug is carried away in the circulation almost as soon as it enters. Consequently, the concentration of drug in the capillaries is very small relative to the concentration at the absorption site. This maintains a positive concentration gradient for continued absorption until all administered drug is absorbed.

If we assume that C_p is approximately 0, Equation 9.1 simplifies to

$$\text{absorption rate} = \frac{P \cdot A \cdot D}{h} C_a \quad \text{(Eq. 9.2)}$$

Combining D, A, P, and h to give a new constant k, we can write

$$\text{absorption rate} = k \cdot C_a \quad \text{(Eq. 9.3)}$$

This is a first-order expression, and k is the *first-order permeation rate constant*. Equation 9.3 shows that if the absorption site has good blood flow, absorption is a first-order process directly dependent on the concentration of dissolved drug at the absorption site. Therefore, fast dissolution of drug from the dosage form and good perfusion of the absorption site facilitate rapid and complete absorption of drug after administration.

The actual rate of absorption is often less than that predicted by Equation 9.3. One reason is the presence of efflux pumps in many epithelial cells. Consequently, many drugs are pumped out of epithelial cells at the absorption site as they are being absorbed and returned to the donor side. This protective mechanism contributes to the poor absorption of many drugs from the site of absorption.

The Oral Route

Oral administration, in which a drug product is administered by mouth and swallowed, is the most common and preferred route of systemic administration. The drug moves down the gastrointestinal (GI) tract, and can be absorbed in any of several regions. Oral administration is effective if the drug is able to cross the epithelial membranes of the GI tract efficiently.

Structure of the Gastrointestinal Tract

The primary organs of the GI tract are the stomach, the small intestine (made up of the **duodenum**, **jejunum**, and **ileum**), and the **colon** (large intestine); these are shown diagrammatically in Figure 9.1. The GI tract ends in the **rectum**. The various parts differ from each other in structure, size, secretions, and pH, all of which influence drug absorption. Although an orally administered product starts in the mouth and travels down the *esophagus*, the drug spends so little time here that the esophagus has no significant role in absorption of oral medications.

The GI tract is lined with four concentric layers of tissue. Starting from the *intestinal lumen*, successive layers are the *mucosa, submucosa, muscular tissue,* and *serosa.* The mucosa consists of three layers: a single layer of epithelial cells in contact with intestinal contents, an underlying *lamina propria* containing blood vessels and lymphatic vessels, and a layer of muscle fibers. Absorption of drugs takes place across the epithelial layer into the blood capillaries of the lamina propria, from which the drug is carried in the

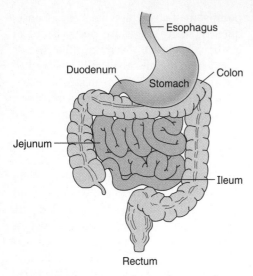

Figure 9.1. Diagram of the esophagus and gastrointestinal tract, showing the different parts.

bloodstream to the rest of the body. Epithelial cells of the mucosa are closely packed with very tight junctions. The diameter of these gaps has been estimated to be about 1.5 nm, too small for most drugs to cross paracellularly. The primary mode of transport of drugs across GI epithelial tissue is passive transcellular diffusion.

Several transporters are present in GI epithelial cell membranes, particularly in the small intestines. The primary function of these transporters is the absorption of nutrients from the GI lumen into the bloodstream. There is growing evidence, however, that these pathways may play a role in the absorption of some drugs. This is another reason why oral drug absorption cannot be predicted based solely on Equation 9.3.

The Stomach. An orally administered drug product arrives in the stomach after administration. The stomach is a pouch-like organ whose primary purpose is to grind food and mix it with acidic gastric fluid. The empty stomach contains approximately 100 mL of gastric fluid; its maximum capacity is about 1 L. The mucosa lining the stomach is composed of cells that secrete mucus, hydrochloric

acid, and digestive enzymes, all of which make up gastric fluid.

Gastric fluid pH lies in the range of 1 to 3 under normal conditions. Most weak bases are completely ionized in this pH range, whereas many weak acids are at least partially un-ionized in the stomach. Recall that ionization increases total solubility of a drug but reduces its apparent partition coefficient and, therefore, the observed permeability.

The main role of the stomach is as a site for drug dissolution. The permeation of drug from the stomach to the bloodstream is either modest or negligible. One reason is the short time that dissolved drug spends in the stomach; after dissolution from its dosage form, a drug is very quickly transported to the small intestines, allowing little time for significant absorption to occur in the stomach. A second reason is that the surface area of the stomach is relatively small, making permeation slow.

Therefore, although passive transcellular absorption could occur from the stomach given sufficient time, the stomach plays a negligible role in the absorption of most drugs under normal circumstances. The primary function of the stomach is to grind up a solid dosage form and facilitate release and dissolution of drug for subsequent absorption from the small intestines.

The Small Intestine. The intestinal epithelium, or *gut wall*, acts as a barrier between two compositionally distinct compartments—the gut lumen and blood. Maintenance of this barrier is required for protection of the body from pathogens and toxins.

The intestinal epithelium is designed for efficient absorption of nutrients, and is also the most important region for absorption of orally administered drugs. The primary reason for this absorptive capability is the extremely large surface area of epithelial tissue in the small intestines. Although the small intestine looks like a cylinder, its absorptive surface area is tremendously enhanced by its unique internal structure, as shown in Figure 9.2.

The intestinal mucosa is bent into folds called the *folds of Kerckring;* this alone increases surface area threefold over that of a simple cylinder. These folds are composed of further fingerlike protrusions called villi that increase surface area by another factor of 10. Villi are lined with epithelial cells (through which absorption takes place) and *goblet cells* (which secrete mucus). The surface of epithelial cells in contact with intestinal contents has brushlike projections called microvilli that increase absorptive surface area by another factor of 20. Because microvilli resemble a brush, the epithelial cell surface is often called the *brush border.* Consequently, the actual absorptive surface area of the small intestines is about 600 times what it would be if the small intestines were a simple cylinder. This extraordinarily large sur-face area and the relatively long time (about 4 hours) that a drug spends in the small intestines explain the excellent permeability and absorptive ability of this region.

Villi are well perfused by blood and lymph, further enhancing absorption from the small intestines. Within each villus is a network of capillaries, and a lymph duct called the *lacteal.* Most drugs are absorbed into blood in the capillaries and carried away by the portal vein. The main function of the lacteals is the absorption of digested fat; lipophilic drugs may also be absorbed with digested fats into the *lymphatic circulation.*

Intestinal fluid is a complex mixture. Cells of the intestinal membrane secrete mucus and digestive enzymes into the intestinal lumen. In addition, digestive juices from the liver (bile) and pancreas (pancreatic juice) empty into the duodenum as needed after a meal. The pH of small intestinal contents varies slightly in different

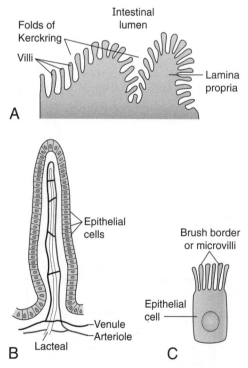

Figure 9.2. **A.** Layers of the small intestines and the folds of Kerckring. **B.** Schematic cross-section of a villus. **C.** Interpretation of the structure of the brush border of a single intestinal epithelial cell.

regions. The duodenum, the part closest to the stomach, is somewhat acidic (pH 5.5 to 6.5) owing to the influence of gastric juices emptying into it. In the jejunum and ileum, the pH is modified by the presence of alkaline pancreatic juice and bile, raising it to approximately 6.5 to 7.5.

The Large Intestine. The large intestine or colon is structurally similar to the small intestines but does not have villi on its inside surface, limiting the surface area available for absorption. The main absorptive function of the colon is absorption of water and electrolytes into the circulation. Nutrients are not generally absorbed from the large intestines, and this is not an important absorption site for most orally administered drugs. However, small amounts of some drugs that have not been absorbed earlier in the GI tract may be absorbed in this region; for example, theophylline is partially absorbed from the colon. In general, if a large amount of unabsorbed drug reaches the colon, it is excreted in the feces.

Oral Drug Absorption

As a result of surface area and residence time constraints, the small intestines are the main site for drug absorption. Most orally administered drugs are absorbed across the small intestinal epithelium by passive transcellular diffusion.

Passive Transcellular Diffusion. Only uncharged drugs and un-ionized forms of weak acids and weak bases can cross the intestinal epithelium by passive diffusion. The ionization of a drug will depend on its pK_a and the pH of the GI fluid. The composition, volume, and pH of GI fluids varies down the length of the tract; Table 9.2 lists the pH ranges of the various GI fluids.

Dissolution and absorption of weak acid and base drugs depend on their ionization state, which in turn depends on drug pK_a and the pH in the stomach and

TABLE 9.2. Typical pH Values of the Various Regions of the Human GI Tract	
GI Region	Normal pH
Mouth	6.5–7.0
Esophagus	5.0–6.0
Stomach	1.0–3.5
Duodenum	5.5–6.5
Jejunum	6.5–7.0
Ileum	7.0–7.5
Colon	6.0–7.0
Rectum	7.0–7.5

small intestine. In the stomach, a drug that exists predominantly in its ionized form will dissolve better (because of a higher solubility) than one that exists predominantly in its un-ionized form. Consequently, weak bases dissolve well whereas weak acids have difficulty dissolving in gastric fluid.

In the small intestines, a drug that exists predominantly in its un-ionized form will be absorbed faster than one that exists predominantly in its ionized form. Consequently, bases of pK_a 10 or higher and acids of pK_a less than 3 are poorly absorbed, because these are completely ionized at intestinal pH. In general, weak bases are absorbed better than weak acids. The ionization equilibrium of drugs is rapid. This means that as the un-ionized form of the drug is absorbed and leaves the intestinal lumen, equilibrium reestablishes to produce more un-ionized drug. Thus, if a drug has a high enough partition coefficient and is sufficiently unionized in the small intestines, it can be absorbed.

The dissolution and absorption of nonionizable drugs will not be influenced by pH in the GI tract. If such drugs have adequate intrinsic water solubility they will dissolve sufficiently in the stomach. If they also have adequate lipophilicity, they will be absorbed well from the small intestines by passive transcellular diffusion.

Biopharmaceutics Classification System (BCS)

The biopharmaceutics classification system is a scientific framework for classifying orally administered drugs on the basis of their aqueous solubility and intestinal permeability. The BCS takes into account three major factors that govern the rate and extent of drug absorption from solid oral drug products: dissolution, solubility, and intestinal permeability. According to the BCS, drug substances can be classified into the following categories:

Class 1: High solubility–high permeability (e.g., propranolol)
Class 2: Low solubility–high permeability (e.g., naproxen)

Class 3: High solubility–low permeability (e.g., cimetidine)
Class 4: Low solubility–low permeability (e.g., taxol)

Using this framework, the role of dissolution and permeability in drug absorption can be separated. Appropriate laboratory and clinical studies can then be designed to evaluate the influence of dissolution or permeability on drug absorption. The U.S. Food and Drug Administration uses the BCS in evaluation of dosage forms for new drug substances.

In general, the overall oral absorption of a drug depends on both dissolution and permeability. If absorption is poor as a result of inadequate water solubility and dissolution rate, the drug is said to have *dissolution-limited absorption*. On the other hand, if low lipophilicity compromises absorption, the drug is considered to exhibit *permeability-limited absorption*.

Carrier-Mediated Absorption. Many ions and nutrients (such as amino acids, small peptides, vitamins, minerals, and sugars) are absorbed from the GI tract via selective transporters present on the epithelial cell membrane and in the brush border region of the small intestines. These transporters may also help to absorb drugs that are structurally similar to the natural substrates. For example, the amino acid transporter in the small intestines absorbs many oral cephalosporins. Peptidelike drugs (such as β-lactam antibiotics and angiotensin-converting enzyme, or ACE, inhibitors) use relatively nonspecific transporters that mediate the absorption of a large variety of dipeptides and tripeptides. Nucleosides are believed to be absorbed into mammalian intestinal cells by sodium-dependent nucleoside transporters. Many antiviral and anticancer drugs are nucleoside analogs, e.g., zidovudine, cladribine, acyclovir, cytosine arabinoside, and dideoxycytidine; their absorption may at least in part be carrier-mediated.

Intestinal Drug Efflux. The role of nonspecific multidrug resistance (*MDR*) transporters as efflux pumps is becoming increasingly important in understanding the poor oral absorption of a variety of drugs. Epithelial cells of the small intestines express the multidrug transporter, which transports drug unidirectionally from the epithelial cell back into the intestinal lumen.

Hydrophobic drugs appear to be more susceptible to these efflux systems than hydrophilic drugs. For example, the HIV-1 protease inhibitors ritonavir, saquinavir and indinavir are poorly absorbed after oral administration because of P-glycoprotein (P-gp)–mediated efflux. Efflux transporters, being governed by Michaelis–Menten kinetics, can become saturated. Celiprolol, a cardiovascular drug, is absorbed in much greater proportion after an oral dose of 400 mg than after a dose of 100 mg; this difference can be explained by saturation of the efflux pump at higher doses. A greater proportion of the higher dose can escape efflux and reach the systemic circulation.

Transcytosis. Transcytosis is relatively uncommon for the absorption of drugs from the GI tract because most drugs are small molecules. However, it is believed that many orally administered vaccines are absorbed by this mechanism.

Nonoral Routes for Systemic Administration

Most patients prefer to take drugs orally than by other routes. It is not possible to administer a drug orally, however, if its properties or the patient characteristics are unfavorable or inappropriate. These are listed in Table 9.3. Some drugs may never be developed as oral products. Other drugs may be available in both oral and nonoral forms; the oral form may not be suitable for certain patients.

The Parenteral Route

In situations in which oral administration is not feasible, one option is to administer the drug parenterally. Although parenteral means "other than enteral," the term is usually reserved for drugs given *hypodermically,* by injection. Parenteral administration avoids epithelial barriers that are so difficult for some drugs to cross. The drug may be injected directly into the bloodstream by *intravenous (IV;* in a vein) or *intra-arterial* (in an artery) administration. Alternatively, the drug may be injected into a tissue from which it can reach the bloodstream, such as in *subcutaneous (SC;* under the

Drugs and Grapefruit Juice

The oral absorption of several drugs, including cyclosporine, is limited by P-gp efflux pumps in intestinal epithelial cells. Grapefruit juice contains various flavonoids that appear to have inhibitory effects on P-gp–mediated transport. A single glass of grapefruit juice can inhibit P-gp up to 24 hours. Therefore, when cyclosporine is coadministered with grapefruit juice, a large increase in cyclosporine absorption is observed. Because grapefruit juice is a natural product, there is wide variability, which makes these interactions very unpredictable in individual patients. The intensity of the effect depends on how much and how often the grapefruit juice is consumed, the timing of the grapefruit juice and the drug dose, the specific brand of juice, and how concentrated the juice is.

This type of interaction also provides a potential application to increase absorption of drugs like cyclosporine that are P-gp efflux substrates. The use of P-gp inhibitors to increase intracellular concentrations of chemotherapeutic agents in tumor cells is also being evaluated in patients with multidrug-resistant tumors.

TABLE 9.3. Drug or Patient Characteristics That Make Oral Administration Unsuitable

Drug Properties

- Instability in GI fluids and consequent rapid degradation
- Irritation of the gastric or intestinal epithelium
- Poor lipophilicity for passive transcellular diffusion
- Large molecular size resulting in a slow absorption rate

Patient Characteristics

- Unable or unwilling to swallow medications
- Needs immediate response; not provided by relatively slow oral absorption
- Suffering from GI distress (nausea, vomiting, diarrhea)
- Suffering from GI disease that may be exacerbated by oral administration, or that compromises drug absorption
- Taking another medication that is incompatible with drug

---

skin), *intramuscular* (*IM;* in a muscle), or *intraperitoneal* (*IP;* in the abdomen) administration.

Absorption is not an issue for IV and intra-arterial administration because the drug is placed directly in the bloodstream. These methods ensure that the entire dose of drug enters the bloodstream, and represent the fastest systemic ways of getting drug to the site of action. IV administration is more common because veins are easily accessible for administration.

In contrast, SC, IM, or IP administration requires drug to travel through the tissue at the administration site before it can enter the bloodstream. Fortunately, this entails crossing the more permeable endothelial barriers in the body rather than epithelial barriers with tight junctions. Therefore, drugs administered by SC, IM, or IP injections usually enter the bloodstream more readily than those administered orally, although there still is a *lag time* before the drug reaches the bloodstream. In some cases however, the absorption rate of a drug given IM or SC is no faster than when it is given orally.

SC, IM, or IP routes can be used to administer both lipophilic and hydrophilic drugs. Hydrophilic drugs will enter capillaries by paracellular transport through the large gaps in the capillary endothelium; lipophilic drugs can use both paracellular and transcellular diffusion mechanisms. Even small proteins can cross the capillary endothelium and enter the bloodstream after SC, IM, or IP administration. SC and IM injections are easier and more convenient to administer than IP injections.

The Rectal Route

Most drugs given orally can also be administered rectally. Rectal dosing of a drug product involves its administration through the anus into the rectum (lower portion of the large intestines). The medication is administered either by a *suppository* or by a *retention enema.* Drugs are absorbed from the rectum in the same way as from other parts of the GI tract—by crossing the epithelial membrane lining the rectum by passive transcellular diffusion.

Although the rectal region has a fairly good blood supply, it has a much lower surface area than the small intestines because of the absence of villi. Thus, absorption is much slower compared with the oral route and is often more variable. This method of systemic drug delivery is reserved for situations in which oral administration is difficult, such as in children or the elderly. It may also be used in patients who are vomiting or unable to take medications orally. An example is the rectal administration of diazepam to children having an epileptic seizure and in whom intravenous access is difficult.

The Buccal or Sublingual Route

These routes involve placing the medication in the mouth, without swallowing, enabling absorption through **buccal** (cheek) or **sublingual** (below the tongue) mucosal membranes. The oral mucosa is very well perfused and allows rapid absorption of lipophilic drugs by passive transcellular diffusion. These routes are generally used for drugs that are destroyed by the low pH in the stomach, decomposed by enzymes of the GI tract, or extensively metabolized by first-pass metabolism (discussed in Chapter 13, Drug Metabolism). Sublingual administration is used for nitroglycerin, a drug used to treat angina.

The Transdermal Route

Although many drugs are applied to the skin for treating local disorders, systemic absorption of drugs through the skin is possible. In transdermal delivery, the intention is to deliver drugs systemically through the skin into the bloodstream.

The skin is a formidable barrier that protects the body against entry of undesirable substances. It is composed of three main layers: *epidermis, dermis,* and *subcutaneous fat.* The outermost layer of the epidermis is the stratum corneum, made up of several layers of dead cells, which is the main barrier to drug absorption. If a drug is able to cross the stratum corneum, it can travel easily through the rest of the epidermis into the dermis. The dermis is well perfused; once a drug arrives in the dermis, it can readily enter the bloodstream. Therefore, if physicochemical properties of a drug are suitable for transport through the stratum corneum, systemic absorption of the drug can occur.

The dead cells of the stratum corneum are very tightly packed with junctions that do not allow paracellular drug transport. Thus, passive transcellular diffusion is the only means of transdermal drug absorption. Lipophilic drugs with small molecular size can penetrate the stratum corneum and be absorbed. The surface area for absorption is the area of the skin the drug is applied to, and is small compared with extensive absorptive surface areas for other routes of administration. Therefore, absorption through the skin is

usually a slow process, and transdermal administration is reserved for long-term therapy.

Scientists have been able to design effective sustained-release transdermal delivery systems so that once-daily or once-weekly therapies are possible. Once-weekly administration of estrogen in transdermal patches is used for hormone replacement therapy.

The Pulmonary Route

This route is also called the inhalation or *respiratory* route, in which drug is inhaled through the mouth into the lungs, where absorption takes place. The *trachea* divides into the *bronchial tree* that forms the lungs. The bronchial tree consists of the *primary bronchi,* which divide successively into smaller branches: the *bronchioles,* the *terminal bronchioles,* the *respiratory bronchioles,* and finally, clusters of tiny air sacs called *alveoli.* The alveolar epithelial membrane is very thin with a large surface area and an extensive blood supply. Once drug reaches the alveoli, it is rapidly absorbed into the bloodstream by passive transcellular diffusion through the alveolar epithelium. There is also some evidence that macromolecular drugs, such as insulin, are absorbed in the alveolar epithelium by vesicular transport and receptor-mediated endocytosis.

As the majority of the absorption occurs in the alveoli, substances must reach this region to be absorbed. If a drug can travel down the bronchial tree and get to the alveoli, its absorption will be rapid and complete. Inhaled gases and vapors (general anesthetics, for example) have no difficulty reaching this region, and are rapidly and completely absorbed after inhalation. However, drugs inhaled as solid particles or liquid droplets have a more difficult time reaching the lower bronchial tree. Drug particles have to be small enough to be able to fit through the increasingly smaller passages of the bronchial tree. Only particles less than 5 μm in diameter are small enough to reach the lower bronchial tree. Thus, although the lung is a great site for systemic absorption, getting a sufficient dose of the drug to the absorptive regions is a challenge.

The Nasal Route

Nasal delivery involves depositing drug in the nose, usually by a liquid spray or drops. The nasal mucosa is very permeable and has a good blood supply, so drugs are absorbed rapidly. Although nasal delivery seems like a convenient route for systemic administration, it has several limitations. The anatomical and physiological features of the nose are not ideal for drug administration for several reasons, and put considerable constraints on formulations and drug candidates. It is often difficult to get a large enough dose into a small volume of liquid to spray into the nose. The nasal mucosa has a relatively small surface area (150 cm^2) for absorption. The drug product does not remain in contact with the nasal mucosa long enough for complete absorption. Many drugs irritate the nasal lining and can damage it with long-term use. Therefore, the nasal route is not commonly used for systemic administration when alternative routes, especially oral, are available.

The nasal route is a good option when oral absorption is problematic. An example is nasal delivery of vitamin B_{12} to patients with Crohn's disease and irritable bowel syndrome. The nasal route is also very attractive for macromolecular drugs that are not orally absorbed. Peptide hormone analogs such as antidiuretic hormone and calcitonin are given as nasal sprays. These drugs are destroyed in the GI tract if given orally.

Recent findings also suggest that nasal delivery allows drugs to preferentially cross the blood–brain barrier and enter cerebrospinal fluid (CSF) directly. In the future, this approach may provide a new, noninvasive way of treating Alzheimer's disease, Parkinson's disease, stroke, and other important brain diseases and conditions.

Absorption of Macromolecular Drugs

Proteins and other macromolecules present a difficult delivery problem, not only because of their large size but also because of their extreme sensitivity to the surrounding environment. Parenteral administration is still the most common route of delivery. Noninvasive systemic delivery systems do not work well. Oral administration of proteins and large peptides is being studied, but no completely effective system has yet been developed. The hydrochloric acid and digestive enzymes in the stomach rapidly degrade proteins and peptides. Even if the molecules could somehow be protected, it is difficult for large molecules to cross the intestinal epithelium in sufficient quantities for therapeutic benefit. No acceptable transdermal delivery systems have been found because protein size and inherent physicochemical properties prohibit these large polar molecules from crossing the stratum corneum without the addition of potentially irritating penetration enhancers.

The pulmonary route has shown success with macromolecular drugs delivered either as solutions or fine powders. The properties and composition of lung fluid are similar to those of blood, so pulmonary delivery is very similar to injection into the bloodstream. The lungs can absorb many macromolecules and some small particles, presumably by transcytosis in the alveoli. Once absorbed in the deep lung, the drug passes readily into the bloodstream. The body's protective mechanisms, however, pose a problem in getting drug to the deep lung. Large molecules and particles are removed by metabolism and via *phagocytosis* by white blood cells. Nevertheless, if the drug is delivered efficiently to the lower pulmonary regions, a sufficient quantity can be absorbed into the bloodstream to exert a therapeutic effect. For example, the pulmonary delivery of insulin has been very successful, and that of other protein drugs is showing success in clinical trials.

Local Administration

Systemic administration is appropriate when the intention is to get drug to the site of action via the bloodstream. In nonsystemic or local administration, it is possible to administer the drug at or close to the site of action so that absorption into the bloodstream is unnecessary. The drug has to merely stay at the site of application or be transported a short distance through the tissue to exert its action. This does not mean, however, that absorption does not occur; some of the drug may enter the bloodstream (by the processes discussed above under Systemic Administration) and travel to the rest of the body. Thus, systemic side effects may occur with locally applied medications, particularly with inappropriate use.

Local administration is usually rather inefficient in that only 5 to 15% of applied drug reaches the site of action. Nevertheless, high local tissue concentrations are achieved, usually much higher than those possible by a systemic route. Therefore, a much lower dose is needed for local delivery compared with administration of the same drug systemically.

Many of the systemic routes discussed earlier can also be used to treat localized conditions. Although the *oral route* is most commonly used for systemic administration, orally administered drugs often treat ailments of the GI tract locally.

Delivery of Insulin

Insulin injections are considered undesirable by patients because of local discomfort and disruption of normal lifestyle. As a result, there has been a search for alternative routes of insulin delivery.

Two issues limit oral delivery of insulin. One is the instability of insulin at the low pH of the stomach and in the presence of the GI tract's digestive enzymes. The second is the poor permeability of the very large insulin molecule through the intestinal epithelium. Nasal delivery also suffers from several problems. Poor transport across mucous membranes of the nose requires either very large doses of insulin, or an excipient called a *penetration enhancer* to speed up insulin transport. Only a small fraction of the nasal dose is absorbed, making costs prohibitive. Additionally, penetration enhancers trigger nasal irritation and rhinorrhea, which can easily alter insulin absorption.

Inhaled insulin has finally become a possibility for the first time since injections were introduced 75 years ago. Insulin absorption into the bloodstream occurs through the thin alveolar wall. This novel pulmonary insulin delivery system has been demonstrated to have dose-to-dose consistency similar to injectable insulin with respect to the amount of insulin absorbed. The portable aerosol delivery system is about the size of a flashlight, and it converts a fine insulin powder into an aerosol. One or two inhalations provide a therapeutic dose. The packaged powder is stable at room temperature.

Examples are antacids to neutralize stomach acid and antibiotics for the treatment of GI infections. In these situations, the drug needs to remain in the GI tract for action and does not need to be absorbed into the circulation.

Local *parenteral* delivery involves injecting the drug near the site of action, as in *intracardiac* (in the heart), *intrathecal* (in the cerebrospinal fluid), or *intralumbar* (in the lumbar space) application. These routes are only used in specialized situations, when other routes of administration cannot achieve adequate concentrations of drug in these tissues.

Examples of *buccal* delivery for local treatment are sprays applied to gums, mouth, and throat for local infections or pain, and lozenges for dissolution in the mouth to soothe the mouth and throat regions.

Suppositories and enemas given *rectally* are used for relief of constipation and for clearing out the lower intestines before surgical procedures. Ointments and creams are applied rectally for the relief of hemorrhoids and itching.

Dermal delivery involves application of medications to the skin for local treatment. Medications can be applied to skin for protection (e.g., sunscreens), to fight infection (e.g., antibacterials and antibiotics), or to modify properties of the skin (e.g., anti-acne products, anti-aging products, or chemical peels). Many of the latter are considered cosmetics rather than drug products, but the distinction is often blurred.

Pulmonary delivery of drugs is more common for local treatment than for systemic application. It is widely used to treat local conditions such as asthma, chronic pulmonary diseases such as emphysema, and pulmonary infections. *Nasal* delivery is also more common for treatment of local conditions. Nasal allergies and nasal congestion are frequently treated with drops or sprays applied in the nostrils.

The *ophthalmic* route is reserved for local application to the eye only and is generally not used for systemic administration. This is because the eye is a very delicate organ and is easily irritated and damaged by introduction of foreign substances. Therefore, medications are applied to the eye only when necessary to treat ophthalmic diseases. Eye infections and inflammatory conditions can be treated by the placement of eye drops or ointments in the eye. Ophthalmic products can also be used to treat glaucoma, with the drug traveling through the cornea into the aqueous humor.

Vaginal and *urethral* application is also reserved for treating local conditions, vaginal application being more common. Solution, creams, or tablets can be applied to the vagina for contraception or to treat infections. Small tablets can also be used for treating urethral infections.

KEY CONCEPTS

- Drugs can be administered either systemically or locally.
- Absorption rate is influenced by drug physicochemical properties and the physiological conditions at the site of absorption.
- Absorption rate depends on the dissolution rate of drug as it arrives at the absorption site, and the permeability of drug through the membranes at the absorption site.
- Most drugs are absorbed by passive transcellular diffusion. Only the un-

ionized form of the drug diffuses through epithelial barriers at absorption sites.
- Carrier-mediated absorption enhances the absorption of some drugs, whereas opposing efflux pumps limit the absorption of others.
- Local administration does not require drug absorption into the bloodstream; however, absorption may occur.

ADDITIONAL READING

1. Shargel L, Yu ABC. Applied Biopharmaceutics and Pharmacokinetics, 4th ed. McGraw-Hill/Appleton & Lange, 1999.

2. Dipiro JT, Talbert RL, Yee GC, Matzke GR, Wells BG, Posey LM (eds). Pharmacotherapy: A Pathophysiologic Approach, 5th ed. McGraw-Hill/Appleton & Lange, 2002.

3. Banker GS, Rhodes CT (eds). Modern Pharmaceutics, 4th ed. Marcel Dekker, 2002.

4. Gennaro AR (ed). Remington—The Science and Practice of Pharmacy, 20th ed. Lippincott Williams & Wilkins, 2000.

REVIEW QUESTIONS

1. Differentiate between systemic and local (nonsystemic) drug administration, and list the routes used for each.
2. What is the primary mechanism for drug absorption across epithelial membranes? What parameters control the rate of absorption of a drug?
3. Discuss the role of transporters in increasing or decreasing drug absorption.
4. Describe the role of the esophagus, stomach, small intestines, and colon in oral drug absorption. Why are most drugs absorbed from the small intestines?
5. What influence does the pH of GI fluids have on the release and absorption of ionizable drugs?
6. When is it appropriate to use non-oral routes for systemic delivery? List the key features of each route.

Drug Delivery Systems

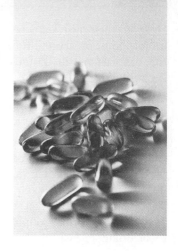

The development and therapeutic use of a new drug involve more than just the compound with intrinsic pharmacological activity. Of equal importance is the path the drug molecules take in getting from site of administration to site of action; the drug must somehow get to the right place at the right time. That is where drug delivery comes in. Once an appropriate route of administration, whether systemic or local, has been identified, scientists must design a drug product that facilitates transport of drug to its site of action and makes it available at the right concentration, at the appropriate time, for the appropriate duration. This is not a trivial issue; the development of an appropriate delivery system is often as complex as development of the drug compound itself.

The three important considerations in the design of a delivery system are release of drug, stability, and elegance. Drug release is necessary for drug absorption and action. Stability is important to ensure that a product retains its characteristics for a long duration and provides reproducible performance over its shelf life. Elegance is critical to make sure the product's appearance, smell, taste, and method of administration are acceptable to patients.

Dosage Forms

Drugs in their pure state exist as powders (amorphous or crystalline solids) or in rare cases as viscous liquids. In the past, such pure drug substances were often given directly to patients in preweighed quantities; this type of dosing is almost never used today. Drugs are now combined with a variety of inert substances called **excipients**, and these mixtures are processed into distinct products called **dosage forms**. Each excipient plays an important role in the overall performance of the dosage form. Excipients are added to facilitate release of the drug, to improve the stability of the drug in the product, to provide elegance, and to make the product easy to manufacture on a large scale.

Examples of dosage forms are tablets, capsules, suspensions, solutions, and ointments. Dosage forms can be administered to patients via several different *routes of administration* (e.g., oral, injectable, rectal), as discussed in Chapter 9, Drug Absorption.

Many dosage forms are provided in a specific or unique administration device, such as an inhaler, a nasal spray, or a transdermal patch. The complete system of dosage form and administration device is called the **drug delivery system**, or drug product.

Need for Dosage Forms

Dosage forms provide control and accuracy of dosing, improve convenience of dosing, and enhance stability and shelf life of a drug. They also make it possible for the drug to be delivered at a rate appropriate to the needs of the illness or condition.

We have already seen that structure and physicochemical properties play a critical role in a drug's ability to cross membrane barriers in the body and to reach the site of action. The therapeutic efficacy of a drug is also highly dependent on how the drug is delivered to the body and the design and properties of the dosage form into which it is formulated. An optimized drug product should deliver the drug in a manner that produces maximum effectiveness, safety, and reliability of the drug in the patient. The characteristics of an ideal drug delivery system are as follows:

- Releases drug at the appropriate location in the body
- Releases drug at a controlled, predictable rate that is unique to each drug
- Is not affected by physiological variability such as gastrointestinal pH, food, digestive enzymes, patient activity, patient health, and so forth
- Is convenient and easy for the patient to take
- Has a long shelf life when stored under various environmental conditions
- Is easy to manufacture on a large scale
- Is cost effective
- Is aesthetically pleasing to the patient (taste, smell, appearance)

Although it is not always possible to achieve all objectives for every drug, these considerations are important in designing drug products. The physicochemical properties of each drug, such as its solubility, pK_a, lipophilicity, particle size, and chemical stability, have to be taken into account when determining which dosage form and excipients will be best suited for a particular application. The science of the design, evaluation, and manufacture of drug delivery systems is called *pharmaceutics*.

Types of Dosage Forms

Dosage forms are broadly classified according to their gross physical nature as:

- Solutions
- Dispersions
- Semisolids
- Solids

The drug in the dosage form is often referred to as the active ingredient and is present along with several excipients.

Solutions are dosage forms in which drug is completely dissolved in a medium, usually aqueous. Excipients present in drug solutions may be buffers, preservatives, stabilizing agents, flavors, and colors. Solutions are commonly administered orally or by injection, or can be applied to the nose, ear, or eye. Nonaqueous solutions, although not common, are also available. Examples include drugs dissolved in oils for administration by injection, or dissolved in other lipids for dermal application.

Dispersions are products that contain two phases, one phase dispersed in a medium of another phase. The active ingredient is usually the *dispersed phase,* and the medium is called the *dispersion medium.* Examples are suspensions (solid drug dispersed in a liquid) and emulsions (liquid dispersed in a liquid). To keep the active ingredient uniformly suspended throughout the liquid, a suspending or thickening agent is usually added. Other excipients are similar to those found in solutions. Dispersions are often given orally or by injection, or can be applied to the nose, ear, eye, or skin. Specialized dispersions of drug in a nonaqueous medium also exist, e.g., metered-dose inhalers, which contain drug dispersed in a liquid propellant mixture.

Semisolids such as ointments, creams, and gels are dosage forms generally meant for application to the skin. They may also be applied to the eye as ophthalmic ointments, and rectally or vaginally as suppositories. In addition to their active ingredient, semisolid dosage forms may contain oils or lipids, water, buffers, polymers for thickening, and preservatives for stability.

Solids are the most common types of dosage forms; examples are tablets, capsules, and powders. Solid dosage forms vary greatly in shape, size, weight, and many other properties. They are usually given orally, but powders may be designed for application to the skin or for inhalation.

Drug Release and Dissolution

In considering the factors involved in transport of drug across biological membranes, one of the main assumptions is that the drug is in solution. The drug has to first dissolve at the absorption or administration site before it can cross membranes or enter cells. The medium in which drugs must dissolve in the body is usually aqueous; this is why it is important for drugs to have adequate water solubility.

In solution dosage forms the drug is already dissolved when the product is administered to a patient. Thus, the drug is available for absorption immediately after administration. In other types of dosage forms, however, drug is present in its solid form, as in tablets, capsules, suspensions, and so forth. Before absorption can occur, drug must be released from the dosage form and dissolve in the fluids at the site of absorption, as shown in Eq. 10.1.

$$\text{solid drug} \xrightarrow{\text{dissolution}} \text{solution}$$
$$\xrightarrow{\text{absorption}} \text{blood} \qquad \text{(Eq. 10.1)}$$

Even if the drug product is intended for local action and does not require systemic absorption, dissolution is necessary for the drug to exert its response. If the drug dissolves slowly or incompletely, the amount of drug available for absorption or action may be much less than the dose administered.

Dissolution Rate

Dissolution is a process by which a compound goes from the solid state into solution in a solvent. The dissolution of a solid particle can be broken down into two consecutive steps, as shown in Figure 10.1.

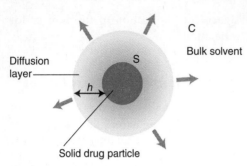

Figure 10.1. Schematic diagram of the dissolution process. S is the saturated solubility of the drug, and is the concentration of drug in the diffusion layer. C is the concentration of drug in the bulk solvent. h is the thickness of the diffusion layer.

1. Drug begins to dissolve at the surface of the solid particle, forming a thin film (called the diffusion layer, stagnant layer, or unstirred layer) around the particle containing a saturated solution of drug.
2. A concentration gradient develops, with a high drug concentration in the diffusion layer around the particle and a low concentration in the bulk solvent. Drug molecules diffuse through the diffusion layer into the bulk solvent, and more drug dissolves from the particle to maintain a saturated diffusion layer.

Using this model of the dissolution process, the dissolution rate of a drug is given by the modified Noyes–Whitney equation, derived from Fick's first law of diffusion:

$$\text{dissolution rate} = \frac{D \cdot A(S-C)}{h} \quad \text{(Eq. 10.2)}$$

A is the surface area of solid drug exposed to the dissolution medium, S is the drug solubility in the dissolution medium, C is the concentration of the drug in the bulk dissolution medium, D is the diffusion coefficient of the drug, and h is the thickness of the diffusion layer. Thus, $(S - C)$ is the concentration gradient that drives the dissolution

process. A plot of this concentration gradient is shown in Figure 10.2.

Equation 10.2 is often written as:

$$\text{dissolution rate} = k \cdot A(S-C) \quad \text{(Eq. 10.3)}$$

The constant k is called the *intrinsic dissolution rate constant* of the drug in the medium. It is directly proportional to diffusion coefficient D of the drug, which in turn depends on drug molecular weight. k is also inversely proportional to thickness h of the diffusion layer. Diffusion layer thickness can be reduced by stirring the medium or by decreasing its viscosity.

Solubility and Dissolution Rate

The solubility, S, of a drug is an important parameter in determining dissolution rate. In Chapter 3, Solubility and Lipophilicity, we saw that intrinsic water solubility depends on the solid state crystal structure of the drug, and that total solubility of weak acids and weak bases further depend on pH of the medium. Consequently, dissolution rate is influenced by these factors as well.

As mentioned earlier, most physiological environments in which drug must dissolve are aqueous. Thus, solubility and dissolution rate in water are critical in determining the rate and extent of drug absorption. However, in some cases, water solubility does not help but hinders the absorption process. This is true for transdermal drug delivery in which the medium encountered by drug is non-aqueous, made up of lipids secreted by the skin. Consequently, lipid solubility rather than water solubility is important in controlling absorption after transdermal application.

Effect of Polymorphism on Dissolution. If a drug exhibits polymorphism, one polymorph will be the most physically stable, i.e., will have the strongest crystal lattice. All other forms will have weaker lattices and will be less stable. In general, the unstable or *high-energy* polymorphs

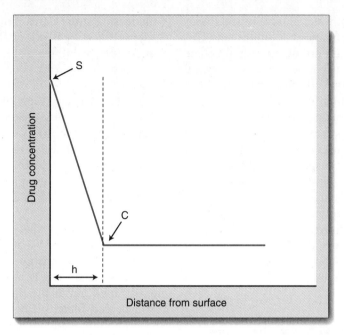

Figure 10.2. Plot of concentration gradient in the diffusion layer of a dissolving particle. The solubility of the solid is S, the concentration in the bulk solvent is C, and the thickness of the diffusion layer is h.

of a drug have higher intrinsic solubilities and faster dissolution rates compared with the stable polymorph, because their crystal lattices are more easily broken to get the drug into solution.

Unfortunately, unstable polymorphs revert to the stable, less soluble polymorph with time. This process is usually difficult to control and is nonreproducible. Thus, although high-energy polymorphs are attractive for dissolution purposes, they are not used frequently in drug delivery systems. Pharmaceutical companies like to identify and select the most stable polymorph for development. In general, the stable polymorph has the highest melting point, the lowest solubility, and the maximum stability.

Effect of pH on Dissolution. When dissolving in aqueous media, drugs dissolve faster if they can ionize because the ionized form has higher water solubility. Therefore, a higher total drug concentration is reached in the diffusion layer, increasing the concentration gradient for dissolution. This is important when we consider dissolution of drug at sites of administration and absorption. The local physiological pH has a tremendous influence on dissolution rate, and consequently could have a big influence on drug absorption.

For example, stomach fluids are acidic with pH in the range 1 to 3.5, whereas the small intestines have pH in the range 5.5 to 7.5. A weak acid drug has a lower solubility and dissolution rate in the stomach and a higher solubility and dissolution rate in the small intestines. The opposite is true for weak base drugs.

Salts of weak acids and bases often have faster dissolution rates than the parent acid or base. The faster dissolution rate is a reflection of higher water solubility of the salt because of a local pH effect; the salt effectively acts as its own buffer and facilitates ionization and dissolution. The type of salt, i.e., the counterion, influences dissolution rate; each type of salt of a given acid or base has a different water solubility and dissolution rate. Enhanced solubility and dissolution rate do not necessarily translate to better absorption. There are several reports of salts with differing solubilities behaving similarly with respect to absorption after administration.

Solid drugs may also be administered by nonoral routes of administration, such as powders or suspensions by inhalation. The pH of pulmonary fluids is close to 7.4, and drugs must dissolve in these fluids for absorption. However, we have seen that transcytosis of fine particles is also possible in deep lung tissue, and drugs may be absorbed without first dissolving in lung fluids.

Immediate-Release Products

The goal for most drug delivery systems is rapid dissolution of drug after administration; such formulations are called immediate-release systems. The objective with these is to get drug into the bloodstream and to the site of action as rapidly as possible. Rapid release and dissolution can be achieved by modifying key parameters as follows:

- increasing surface area A of drug particles (reducing particle size)
- increasing solubility S of weak acids and bases (altering the pH of the medium)
- reducing concentration of drug C in the bulk medium (constantly "removing" dissolved drug)
- decreasing thickness h of the diffusion layer (agitating the dissolution medium)
- using appropriate excipients (enhancing solubility of drug in diffusion layer)

From an *in vivo* perspective, the terms D and h in Equation 10.2 are fixed by the drug and the administration route and site. If dissolved drug is absorbed or removed rapidly from the dissolution site, C can be considered to be zero. Thus S (drug solubility) and A (surface area of solid exposed to the dissolution medium) are the prime drivers for dissolution. Increasing either or both increases dissolution rate and may consequently increase rate of absorption.

Figure 10.3 illustrates the drug release and dissolution process from a typical dosage form, an oral tablet. For rapid dissolution, most tablets are designed to undergo rapid disintegration to granules and

Dissolution Testing of Drug Products

Dissolution testing is a very important tool during drug development and quality control in the pharmaceutical industry. Although traditionally developed for solid oral dosage forms, the use of dissolution testing has been widened to a variety of other dosage forms. Much research is being done to develop dissolution tests that better predict performance of drug formulations in the body. A number of studies have been published that successfully establish a correlation between the dissolution behavior of a drug product in a laboratory test and its *in vivo* behavior. Such *in vitro–in vivo* correlation (IVIVC) continues to be of importance from both developmental and regulatory aspects. An appropriate dissolution test can serve as a surrogate to the extensive, expensive, and time-consuming *in vivo* testing of the absorption of drugs from dosage forms in humans.

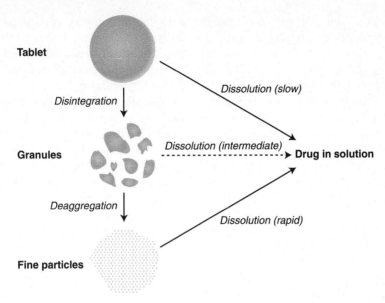

Figure 10.3. The processes involved in dissolution of a drug from a tablet in the presence of fluids. Although dissolution can occur from the whole tablet, granules, and fine particles, the large surface area of the granules and even larger surface area of the fine particles give faster dissolution rates.

subsequent deaggregation to fine particles. This provides a larger surface area exposed to the dissolution medium, resulting in a faster dissolution rate. Excipients that facilitate disintegration (*disintegrants*) and deaggregation (*surfactants*) are usually included in immediate-release solid dosage forms.

With each dose of an immediate-release product, the concentration of drug in the bloodstream rises rapidly, peaks very soon after administration, and then declines. If the peak concentration is too high, the drug may exhibit undesirable side effects. If the decline in blood concentration is very rapid, the product may have to be dosed very frequently to maintain therapeutic blood levels. Such a large fluctuation in blood concentration may not be suitable for some drugs.

Controlled Drug Delivery

As the term implies, a controlled-release drug delivery system is one that supplies drug to the body in a manner precisely controlled to suit the drug and the condition being treated. The primary aim is to achieve a therapeutic drug concentration at the site of action for the desired duration of time. Controlled release implies a degree of predictability and reproducibility in drug dissolution from the dosage form.

The term *controlled release* is often used to refer to a variety of methods that modify release of drug from a dosage form. This term includes preparations labeled as "extended release," "delayed release," "modified release," or "sustained release." Unlike immediate-release products from which the entire dose of drug is rapidly released after administration, controlled-release products are designed to gradually release specific amounts of drug for a longer time period. Major benefits include less frequent dosing, improved pharmacokinetics (less fluctuation of drug concentration in the blood) and pharmacodynamics (better efficacy and fewer side effects), and better patient compliance.

Sustained Release

The most common application of controlled release is sustained release, in which dissolution rate is deliberately reduced to achieve extended absorption of drug for a long time. In such cases, the delivery system is manipulated to obtain a dissolution rate that matches the removal of drug from the bloodstream (by elimination processes), so that a constant effective concentration of drug is maintained in the blood.

Ideally, the dissolution rate of the drug from a sustained release dosage form should be constant, or *zero-order*. Releasing drug at a slow, constant rate can maintain drug concentration within the therapeutic range for a long time, decrease fluctuation in blood levels, and reduce the need for frequent dosing. When patient convenience is increased by reducing the number of doses to be ad-

ministered, compliance is automatically enhanced. Sustained drug release can also minimize unwanted side effects, and reduce the amount of drug required to maintain the desired therapeutic effect.

A number of sustained-release systems have been developed for almost every route of administration. Many marketed sustained-release products are designed for oral administration. Oral sustained-release dosage forms use a few common techniques for achieving slow and extended dissolution.

Coated systems are made up of beads, granules, or microspheres surrounded by a slowly dissolving polymer. The thickness of the coat determines when a particular set of granules will dissolve. By using different coating thicknesses, the granules

Controlled Release of Methylphenidate

Methylphenidate hydrochloride is a mild CNS stimulant with actions similar to the amphetamines. It is used to treat attention-deficit disorder (ADD)/attention-deficit hyperactivity disorder (ADHD) and narcolepsy. Several sustained-release oral products are available for methylphenidate.

Ritalin SR is one product in which methylphenidate is incorporated into a water-insoluble cetyl alcohol wax matrix, allowing for the gradual diffusion of methylphenidate as the tablet passes through the gastrointestinal (GI) tract. The water-soluble ingredients (methylphenidate, lactose) are released gradually as the GI fluids penetrate the tablet and create pores. Ritalin SR has a duration of action of approximately 8 hours.

Concerta is an osmotic controlled-release product (OROS) of methyl-

phenidate. The tablet has an immediate-release overcoat that provides an initial dose of methylphenidate within 1 hour after administration. The overcoat covers a trilayer core. The trilayer core is composed of two layers containing the drug and excipients, and one layer of osmotic components. As water from the GI tract enters the core, the osmotic components expand and methylphenidate is released. The initial dose of methylphenidate is released from the outer coating over 1 to 2 hours, and the remainder is released at a controlled rate for 10 hours. Therefore, the total methylphenidate dose is released during 12 hours. For example, the 18-mg tablet releases 4 mg initially from the outer layer of the tablet, then releases 14 mg over the course of 10 hours from the core. The tablet shell, along with insoluble core components, is eliminated from the body in the stool.

dissolve progressively over time. Matrix systems are made up of a polymer (water soluble or water insoluble) or wax in which drug is dissolved or embedded. The soluble matrix dosage forms erode slowly in water, releasing drug from the surface. The insoluble matrix forms rely on diffusion of water into the matrix to form pores; the drug gradually dissolves in the water and leaves through these pores. Reservoir systems contain a core of drug surrounded by a water-insoluble polymer coat. The coat allows water to diffuse in and dissolved drug to diffuse out slowly. Osmotic devices are made up of a tablet coated with a semipermeable polymer coat; water can diffuse in but drug cannot diffuse out. As water diffuses in and dissolves the drug, an osmotic pressure is created in the tablet. A hole in the polymer coat allows the osmotic pressure to be relieved by allowing the drug solution to come out.

Sustained-release products contain a much larger total amount of drug than a single therapeutic dose of an immediate-release product, because they are expected to maintain a therapeutic concentration for a prolonged period. This poses one of the biggest problems in using such products—the danger that inappropriate manufacture or use may result in a large amount of drug being released and absorbed rapidly, causing toxicity.

Not all drugs can or should be formulated in sustained-release systems. The physicochemical or absorption, distribution, metabolism, and excretion (ADME) properties of the drug may make sustained-release delivery unfeasible. Additionally, constant blood levels may not be pharmacodynamically or therapeutically desirable for some drugs or disease states.

Targeted Drug Delivery

The next level of sophistication after controlled release is site-specific delivery or targeted delivery. The objective is to localize and concentrate drugs to a desired therapeutic site, avoiding all other tissues in the body and, consequently, achieving the desired pharmacological response at the selected site without undesired actions at other sites. The therapeutic potential of many of today's highly potent drugs is limited by the severity of their side effects; examples are cancer chemotherapeutic drugs that are toxic to normal cells.

Ideally, true targeting can be achieved by designing selective drugs that bind to only the desired receptor subtype. This is difficult in practice, however, and most drugs not only distribute into many body tissues but also bind to many receptors. Therefore, another way to reach the same goal is by designing drug delivery systems that localize the drug at the site of action.

Three main approaches exist for targeted delivery:

- restrict drug distribution to the site of action only (organ or tissue)
- selectively deliver drug to specific cells only (e.g., tumor cells)
- design drug release at predetermined intracellular sites only

Targeted delivery often involves the association of a drug with a carrier system, allowing modulation of the drug's ADME properties. The drug–carrier delivery system is injected into the bloodstream and carried to the site of action, where the drug is then preferentially released.

One approach has been to attach the drug molecule to a macromolecule designed to "hone in" on the desired site, such as a tumor. The most commonly used macromolecule has been a *monoclonal antibody* to which the drug is covalently bound. On injection, the drug–antibody conjugate is preferentially concentrated at the tumor site, and the drug is then released in or near the tumor.

Another approach is to trap the drug in very small particles of polymers, called *nanoparticles*, which are then injected

Targeting to the Brain

Getting drugs into the brain is a formidable challenge because the blood–brain barrier (BBB) prevents many therapeutic molecules from crossing from brain capillaries into the brain in sufficient quantities. A particularly important problem in the treatment of human brain tumors is the need to deliver therapeutic agents to specific regions of the brain, and target them to brain tumors. Molecules that might otherwise be effective in diagnosis and therapy either do not cross the BBB in the region of the tumor, or do not cross the blood–tumor barrier (BTB) in adequate amounts. The expression of efflux transporters at the BBB and BTB further exacerbates the problem; these actively efflux chemotherapeutics from the brain back to the blood. This is partly why most classic chemotherapeutic molecules used to treat cancer outside the CNS are ineffective in the treatment of brain tumors.

Overcoming this problem will have a profound effect on the treatment of many neurological disorders, allowing larger water-soluble molecules to pass into the brain. Transport vectors, such as endogenous peptides, modified proteins, or peptidomimetic monoclonal antibodies, are one way of tricking the brain into allowing these molecules to enter. These use existing active transporters in the brain to gain entry across the BBB, and thus do not need to have the high lipophilicity usually required for crossing the BBB.

into the bloodstream. These particles are preferentially taken up by the liver, lungs, and spleen and can be used to target drugs to these organs. Drugs may also be trapped in phospholipid bilayer vesicles called *liposomes*. These vesicles protect the drug from degradation in the body, and also show enhanced uptake into cells, resulting in higher intracellular concentrations. Drug-loaded erythrocytes and viruses are also being studied as carriers for drugs.

Drug Stability

A good drug product should maintain its performance (effectiveness, safety, and reliability) for a long time. Unfortunately, the performance of most drug products changes with time. The shelf life is the time period during which a drug product will give consistent performance, within specified limits, when stored under the recommended conditions. Ideally, we would like drug products to have a long shelf life; in other words, we would like them to be stable or to have good stability. The major types of stability that are of concern in a drug product are:

- Chemical stability
- Microbiological stability
- Physical stability

Chemical Stability

Chemical stability refers to the change in concentration or amount of the active ingredient in the product with time. The drug in a drug product can degrade with time as a result of chemical reactions such as hydrolysis, oxidation, or photolysis; this results in a decrease in the amount of drug in the dosage form, and therefore, a decrease in the dose provided to the patient. Additionally, the degradation products can be harmful or toxic. Thus, chemical instability results in a gradual decline in the effectiveness and safety of a drug product.

Hydrolysis is probably the most significant reaction for chemical instability of drugs. This is because many drugs have functional groups (ester, amide, lactone, lactam) that are prone to hydrolytic attack, and because the other reactant, water, is present to some extent in most drug products and in the environment. Hydrolysis rates depend on the pH in the drug product, the temperature at which the product is stored, and excipients in the product.

Oxidation, particularly oxidation catalyzed by light (*photooxidation*), is the next most common degradation reaction of drugs. Oxidation is often catalyzed by heavy metal ions.

Degradation reactions are generally fastest in solutions and slowest in solid dosage forms. Therefore, solid dosage forms of a drug are usually more stable than its liquid dosage forms.

Excipients are frequently added to drug products to improve chemical stability. Appropriate buffers and cosolvents can reduce hydrolysis rates, whereas chelating agents and antioxidants reduce oxidation rates. Additionally, solid dosage forms may be coated with a protective film to slow the entry of moisture and oxygen into the product.

The package in which the product is provided also plays a role in drug product stability. Hydrolysis and oxidation rates can be reduced by using airtight containers and seals. The use of desiccants (such as silica) in the product container helps to reduce moisture content and, therefore, hydrolysis rates. Opaque containers protect products from light and reduce photooxidation.

Chemical Shelf Life

Almost all drugs chemically degrade to some extent with time, resulting in a decrease in the concentration of the active ingredient. The accepted limit of chemical decomposition for most drug products is $\pm 10\%$, i.e., drug products should contain 90 to 110% of the active ingredient claimed on the label. The chemical shelf life is the time period after initial manufacture for which the drug concentration remains within these limits. When the active ingredient concentration goes outside these limits, the product is considered to have *expired.*

Microbiological Stability

The **microbiological stability** of a drug product is a measure of its resistance to microbial (bacterial and fungal) contamination from the environment during storage and use. Such contamination and subsequent growth of microbes can seriously compromise the safety of a drug product. Microbial growth is especially likely in products with high moisture content such as solutions, dispersions, and water-based semisolids. The inclusion of an antimicrobial preservative in the formulation is essential for such products. Most solid dosage forms contain relatively small amounts of water and may not require an antimicrobial agent.

Certain pharmaceutical products, such as injectables, are also required to be *sterile* (free from contaminating microorganisms) throughout their shelf life. If these products are intended for a single use (such as a prefilled syringe for injection), an antimicrobial preservative may not be necessary. However, sterile multidose products need to be preserved to maintain sterility during use.

Physical Stability

Many physical characteristics of dosage forms change with time. Examples of physical characteristics are dissolution rate, uniformity, appearance, taste, and odor. These changes also influence effectiveness, safety, and reliability of the product. The effect of a changing dissolution rate on drug absorption and effectiveness is obvious. However, a patient's perception of the effectiveness and safety of a drug product is also influenced if a product's color, taste, odor, or other appearance changes with time. Thus, even if a drug product has good chemical and microbiological stability, these physical changes may result in a shorter overall shelf life.

Macromolecular Drugs

Advances in biotechnology have made possible the development of biopharmaceutical drug products based on very large molecules such as proteins, peptides, and strings of nucleic acids. These new drugs present unique delivery and stability issues. Although they offer a new approach to therapy, macromolecules pose many challenges in designing safe, stable, and effective drug products that are convenient to administer.

Delivery Systems for Macromolecular Drugs

The large molecular size of biopharmaceuticals makes it difficult for them to cross epithelial membranes and be absorbed into the bloodstream. Consequently, most macromolecular drugs have to be administered as injectable solutions. Unfortunately, injectable delivery has poor patient acceptance because of inconvenience, discomfort, and the potential for infection at the injection site. An example is the administration of insulin injections to patients with diabetes, in which patient compliance and long-term complications are serious problems. With the introduction of many new chronically administered macromolecular drugs such as interferons and growth factors, there is a need for the development of alternative, noninvasive, and more convenient methods of administration.

Stability of Macromolecular Drugs

Most of the previous discussion applies to the stability of macromolecular drugs as well. However, biopharmaceutical products have additional considerations with regard to stability, which will be discussed in Chapter 21, Biopharmaceuticals. Special excipients and packaging approaches need to be used for optimum stability of protein drugs. A detailed discussion is outside the scope of this book.

KEY CONCEPTS

- Design of a good drug delivery system is important in optimal drug therapy.
- Excipients are added to drug products to enhance release, stability, elegance, or manufacturability.
- Drug dissolution is a necessary first step before absorption.
- Dissolution rate is described by the Noyes–Whitney equation.
- The rate of dissolution must be programmed to match the needs of the clinical application.

- Immediate-release products are designed to dissolve fast for rapid absorption.
- Sustained-release products dissolve slowly to maintain steady blood levels.
- The chemical, microbiological, and physical stability of a drug product together determine its shelf life.

ADDITIONAL READING

1. Gennaro AR (ed). Remington—The Science and Practice of Pharmacy, 20th ed. Lippincott Williams & Wilkins, 2000.

2. Ansel HC, Popovich NG, Allen LV. Pharmaceutical Dosage Forms and Drug Delivery Systems, 8th ed. Williams & Wilkins, 2004.

3. Aulton ME (ed). Pharmaceutics: The Science of Dosage Form Design, 2nd ed. Churchill Livingstone, 2001.

4. Banker GS, Rhodes CT (eds). Modern Pharmaceutics, 4th ed. Marcel Dekker, 2002.

REVIEW QUESTIONS

1. What are the advantages of using a delivery system to administer drugs? What are the characteristics of an ideal delivery system?
2. Discuss the mathematical expression describing the dissolution of a solid drug particle. What parameters can be changed to increase or decrease dissolution rate?
3. What are polymorphs of a solid drug? Why do pharmaceutical companies prefer to use the most stable polymorph in marketed products?
4. What are the differences between immediate-release and sustained-release products? When are sustained-release products a better therapeutic option?
5. Describe the meaning of targeted or site-specific delivery. What are the approaches to achieving site-specific delivery?
6. What is meant by the shelf life of a drug product? Discuss the various aspects of stability of a drug product.
7. What are the unique delivery challenges of macromolecular drugs?

Section IV • **Drug Disposition**

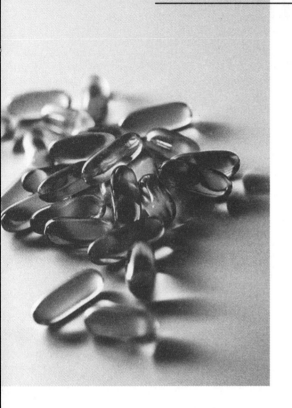

Drug Distribution

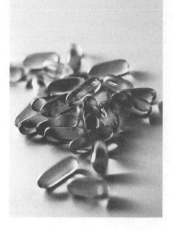

Systemic administration of drugs relies on blood and the circulatory system to physically transport the drug to its site of action and to other tissues in the body. After absorption into blood, most drugs must leave the bloodstream to exert their action. When a drug is administered topically or nonsystemically, entry into or exit from the blood is not necessary. In such applications, the drug merely has to move from its site of administration (i.e., the skin surface for dermal administration) to its site of action (i.e., dermis). Drugs applied topically, however, may enter the systemic circulation. Drug distribution is the reversible transfer of drug from one location in the body to another.

The body can be viewed as being composed of two distinctive fluids: vascular and extravascular. Vascular volume (i.e., blood) includes the fluid in the heart and vascular system of the body. Extravascular volume is everything outside the vascular space and includes many fluids such as cellular, interstitial, and lymphatic fluids. For our discussion in this chapter, distribution is the reversible transfer of drug between the vascular space (after absorption or entry of drug into blood) and the extravascular space.

A drug's pattern of distribution depends on the efficiency of blood circulation, physicochemical properties of the drug, and properties and composition of each tissue. Distribution is generally uneven throughout the body because of differences in blood perfusion, tissue binding, regional pH, and permeability of cell membranes. The dynamic nature of the drug distribution process also means that drug concentrations in blood and tissues are constantly changing as drug is absorbed, distributed, metabolized, and excreted.

Systemic Circulation

The cardiovascular system is the major conduit for distributing drug through the body. It has three distinct parts: pulmonary circulation for oxygenation of blood, coronary circulation for nourishment of the heart, and **systemic circulation** for nourishment of all other tissues. The latter is most relevant to our discussion of drug distribution.

The primary function of the heart is to generate and sustain an arterial blood pressure necessary to provide adequate blood flow to organs. The heart achieves this by contracting its muscular walls around a closed chamber to create sufficient pressure to propel blood from the cardiac chamber (e.g., left ventricle) through the aortic valve and into the aorta.

Cardiac Output

The heart pumps blood through a system of vessels that carries blood to the rest of the body. The volume of blood pumped by the heart per minute is called **cardiac output**, the product of heart rate and stroke volume.

$$\text{cardiac output} = \text{heart rate} \times \text{stroke volume} \quad (\text{Eq. } 11.1)$$

In healthy adults, stroke volume at rest in the standing position averages between 60 and 80 mL of blood per ventricular contraction. Therefore, cardiac output at a resting heart rate of 80 beats per minute varies between 4.8 and 6.4 L/min. The average adult body contains about 5 L of blood, which means all the blood is pumped through the heart about once every minute.

Blood Vessels

The systemic circulation is composed of a branching system of arteries and veins (Fig. 11.1) leading to and from all parts of the body. Arteries carry blood away from the heart and progressively become more finely divided into arterioles. Blood then flows into a system of capillaries, the smallest division of our vascular system, where its exchange functions take place. The vessels get larger again, forming venules that join and enlarge to form veins that carry blood back to the heart. The distinction between arteries and veins is made by direction of blood flow, not oxygen content.

Arteries and arterioles have many elastic fibers and smooth muscle cells that enable these vessels to withstand high pressures and to change their diameter, altering their resistance and thus blood flow. Veins, on the other hand, are not elastic and often contain unidirectional valves to prevent back-flow of blood.

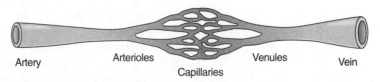

Figure 11.1. The branching arrangement of arteries, capillaries, and veins that make up the blood vessels of the circulatory system.

Capillaries are very small tubes, 7 to 9 μm in diameter, whose walls are composed primarily of endothelium, and the basement membrane on which the endothelium rests. There is no smooth muscle in the walls of capillaries; this distinguishes them from arterioles.

Capillary Exchange

With rare exceptions, blood does not come into direct contact with the cells it nourishes, but fluid readily exchanges between vascular and extravascular spaces. When blood enters the arteriole end of a capillary, it is still under pressure produced by contraction of the heart. This pressure allows a substantial amount of water to filter paracellularly through the walls of capillaries into the tissue space.

Blood cells and most plasma proteins are too large to leave the capillary space through cell junctions, but some plasma proteins are forced out with water. The resulting fluid, called interstitial fluid, bathes cells in the tissue space. This fluid brings essential substances to tissue cells.

Near the venous end of capillaries, blood pressure is reduced. Although interstitial fluid composition is similar to plasma, it contains a smaller concentration of proteins. This difference sets up an osmotic pressure that allows much of the interstitial water to reenter the capillary. This exchange of fluids between blood and tissues is illustrated in Figure 11.2. Waste products and other substances secreted by cells also diffuse into capillaries and are carried away in veins.

Capillaries may be of three major types: continuous, fenestrated, and discontinuous. Capillaries with a continuous endothelium are the most common in the body and are present in many tissues such as the skin, nervous system, and muscle. Their endothelial cells form a continuous internal lining. Recall that these endothelial cells are generally loosely packed with cell junctions in the range of 5 to 30 nm. Thus, small molecules can readily move paracellularly across continuous capillary endothelium. A continuous capillary endothelium with very tight junctions is found in the central nervous system (the blood–brain barrier, BBB); these capillaries have the lowest paracellular permeability.

Fenestrated capillaries are made up of endothelial cells pierced by pores or fenestrations that extend through their full thickness and provide channels across the capillary wall. A fenestrated capillary endothelium is present in exocrine glands, renal glomeruli, and intestinal mucosa, resulting in relatively high permeability. Continuous and fenestrated capillaries are shown in Figure 11.3.

Discontinuous capillaries (sinusoidal capillaries or sinusoids) are larger and more irregularly shaped than other capillaries. Unusually large gaps are present between their endothelial cells that allow leakage of material into and out of these vessels. A discontinuous capillary endothelium is found in liver, spleen, and bone marrow.

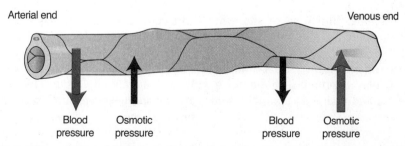

Figure 11.2. The exchange of fluids between circulating blood in capillaries and interstitial fluid. At the arterial end, there is a net movement of fluid out of capillaries. At the venous end, the balance of pressure sends fluid back into capillaries.

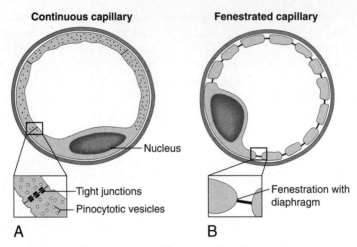

Figure 11.3. A comparison of continuous and fenestrated capillaries. Continuous capillaries (**A**) are lined by endothelial cells that form a continuous lining. The endothelial cells rest on a basement membrane. Fenestrated capillaries (**B**) are made up of endothelial cells with cell membranes pierced by pores or channels.

Lymphatic Circulation

There is net movement of fluid from vascular to extravascular compartments in most capillary systems of the body. In other words, the volume of fluid leaving the capillaries is greater than the volume reentering capillaries. This would cause fluid accumulation in the interstitium if it were not for the lymphatic system of vessels that removes excess fluid from the interstitium and returns it to the vascular space.

The lymphatic system is a subsystem of the circulatory system and works primarily as a drainage system. Its microscopic dead-end capillaries extend into most tissues, paralleling blood capillaries.

The principal functions of the lymphatic system are to:

- collect and return interstitial fluid, including plasma proteins, to the vascular space and thus help maintain fluid balance
- defend the body against disease by producing lymphocytes
- absorb lipids from the intestine and transport them to the blood

Lymph capillaries differ from blood capillaries in important ways. A blood capillary has an arterial and a venous end, whereas a lymph capillary has no arterial end. Instead, each lymph capillary originates as a closed tube; thus, lymphatic vessels only carry fluid away from tissues. Flow of this fluid is much slower than blood because of the absence of a pumping mechanism like the heart. The endothelium of lymph capillaries is more permeable than that of blood capillaries; larger paracellular junctions allow movement of larger molecules in and out of lymph capillaries.

Interstitial fluid that enters a lymphatic capillary is referred to as lymph. It is similar in composition to plasma and also contains particles such as viruses, pathogens, and cell debris. Certain lipophilic compounds, including long-chain fatty acids, triglycerides, cholesterol esters, lipid-soluble vitamins, and xenobiotics such as DDT (dichlorodiphenyltrichloroethane), are transported preferentially via the lymphatic system.

Lymph capillaries join to form larger vessels called lymphatics or lymph veins with one-way valves to direct lymph away from the tissue and eventually back into the systemic circulation. About 2 to 4 L of lymph is returned to the vascular circulation per day.

Drug Distribution Equilibria

The overall distribution of a drug between blood and extravascular space can be viewed as a series of processes as illustrated in Figure 11.4:

- movement of drug out of the bloodstream into interstitial fluid
- movement of drug from interstitial fluid into tissue cells
- movement of drug from cells into interstitial fluid
- movement of drug from interstitial fluid back into blood

Consider each of the distribution steps above in turn after a drug has been administered and absorbed, and is in the circulation.

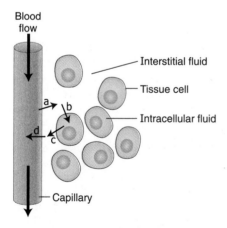

Figure 11.4. Dynamics of drug distribution processes. Drug molecules can move out of a capillary into the interstitial fluid (a), from the interstitial fluid into the intracellular fluid of tissue cells (b), and from the intracellular fluid back into the interstitial fluid (c) and return to the capillary (d). The extent to which each of these steps can occur depends on the physicochemical properties of the drug.

Drug Distribution Out of Capillaries

The rate of movement of a drug or other solute in and out of capillaries depends on hydrostatic pressure in the capillaries, physicochemical properties of drug, binding of drug to plasma and tissue proteins, properties of the capillary endothelium in each tissue, and rate of blood flow through the tissues.

At the arterial end of capillaries, hydrostatic pressure contributes significantly to distribution of solutes along with bulk water flow. As the pressure decreases at the venous end, diffusion processes become predominant for drug distribution.

Physicochemical Properties of Drug

Most small molecules diffuse easily out of capillary cellular junctions as a result of the pressure gradient coupled with a favorable concentration gradient. Generally, substances with molecular weights up to about 20,000 can move through paracellular gaps in the capillary endothelium. Lipophilic, un-ionized molecules can concurrently diffuse through capillary endothelial cells transcellularly. Macromolecular drugs are generally too large to enter interstitial fluid in significant amounts, and tend to be retained in blood. For this reason, drugs bound to plasma proteins are also retained in the blood. Only "free" drug molecules are able to leave capillaries.

Lipophilic Compounds. Solutes with good lipophilicity move rapidly through capillary endothelium by passive transcellular diffusion. The primary reason for this fast transport is the very large surface area of the capillary network in most tissues and the small thickness of the endothelial membrane. Although lipophilic solutes may also diffuse paracellularly through the capillary endothelium, passive transcellular diffusion is believed to be faster and is considered to be the predominant mechanism of distribution of

Lymphatic Transport of Drugs

The lymphatic system plays an important role in absorption and transport of lipids and associated drugs. Major products of intestinal lipid digestion—fatty acids and 2-monoglycerides—enter the enterocyte by passive diffusion across the cell membrane and also via a specific fatty acid transporter protein in the membrane. Once inside the enterocyte, fatty acids and monoglycerides are transported into the endoplasmic reticulum where they are used to resynthesize triglycerides. These in turn are packaged with cholesterol, lipoproteins, and other lipids into particles called chylomicrons.

Chylomicrons are excreted from the basal side of the enterocyte. Being too large to enter intestinal blood capillaries, chylomicrons are taken up exclusively by lymphatic capillaries that enter intestinal villi. Chylomicron-rich lymph then drains into the lymphatic system, which eventually flows into blood. Chylomicrons are rapidly disassembled in blood and the constituent lipids used throughout the body.

Lipophilic compounds in the intestinal lumen can be trapped and absorbed along with lipids into the lymphatic circulation as chylomicrons. Thus, the lymphatic system plays an important role in the absorption and transport of orally administered lipophilic drugs.

---

these solutes out of capillaries. Differences in distribution rates between various lipophilic solutes can be directly related to differences in their partition coefficients. If there is a pH difference between blood and tissue fluid, ion trapping may either favor or hinder distribution of acidic or basic drugs, as discussed in Chapter 8, Transport Across Biological Barriers.

Hydrophilic Compounds. Solutes with poor lipophilicity cannot diffuse efficiently through capillary endothelial cells and therefore use the paracellular pathway. The molecular size must be smaller than the size of the endothelial junction, which is the case for most drugs. Distribution rates for hydrophilic solutes can be directly linked to their molecular size (small molecules diffuse faster than large molecules) and the concentration gradient as defined by Fick's law. Hydrophilic solutes generally have slower overall distribution rates than lipophilic compounds.

Macromolecular Compounds. Large molecules like proteins are too polar for transcellular diffusion and too large for paracellular diffusion through endothelial junctions. However, even these substances may distribute out of capillaries to some extent by filtration as a result of arterial hydrostatic pressure, and by transcytosis (vesicular transport).

Blood Flow and Distribution

The amount of drug reaching a tissue during distribution may depend on the rate of blood flow, or perfusion, of the tissue. The rate at which blood flows to different organs varies widely. The highest perfusion rates are seen in the brain, kidney, liver, and heart. Drug distribution is, therefore, fastest to these organs.

For drugs that can cross the capillary wall rapidly, rate of distribution will depend on how quickly new drug molecules are available for distribution, i.e., distribution will depend on perfusion. This behavior is called *perfusion-controlled distribution* because blood flow determines the rate of distribution to the tissue. Distribution of perfusion-controlled drugs may be dramatically affected when the rate of blood flow to the organ is altered, as in certain diseases or under physiological states such as after eating or during exercise.

Conversely, if the capillaries in a particular tissue are poorly permeable to a drug and transport across the capillary endothelium is slow, changes in blood flow will not significantly affect distribution to that tissue. This behavior is termed *permeability-controlled distribution*. Conditions that change blood flow do not significantly alter distribution of such drugs to these tissues.

For situations in which filtration is the mechanism of distribution, such as in the kidney, blood flow will control the hydrostatic pressure difference that is the driving force for filtration. A reduction in blood flow will decrease the pressure gradient and decrease distribution to the organ.

Distribution in Special Tissues

The above discussion applies to distribution in and out of capillaries into most tissues in the body. As we have seen, however, in certain tissues the structure of the capillary endothelium is specialized for a specific function. In these cases, distribution of solutes can follow a different pattern from that in the rest of the body.

Distribution to the Kidney. The kidney has arterial glomerular capillaries that are fenestrated. Additionally, blood in these capillaries also has a higher hydrostatic pressure than in the rest of the body, making filtration a dominant mechanism for distribution of drugs from blood into the kidney. Consequently, glomerular capillaries filter water and dissolved solutes at rates 100 to 400 times faster than those in other tissues. This aids in excretion of drugs and metabolites in the urine.

Blood cells and platelets are larger in size than fenestrae, and are not filtered out of the bloodstream in glomerular capillaries. Many proteins present in blood are smaller than the size of fenestrae, yet very little protein is filtered out of renal capillaries. This is believed to be a consequence of the negative charge on most proteins slowing their movement through negatively charged protein pores in the basement membrane of capillaries.

Drug molecules bound to plasma proteins will also remain in blood and will not be filtered out in the glomerulus. This becomes important in slowing the excretion rate of protein-bound drugs.

Distribution to the Liver. Capillaries in the liver form *sinusoids* with a discontinuous endothelium with large cavities. Small solutes such as drugs can diffuse readily in and out of these sinusoids regardless of lipophilicity. Sinusoids are also large enough to allow diffusion of proteins (and protein–drug complexes) as well as blood cells out of capillaries. Consequently, even large molecules and particles can distribute into the liver through the discontinuous endothelium.

Distribution to the Brain. Endothelial cells of the brain capillary membrane are very closely packed with tight junctions. The *glial membrane*, closely attached to the capillary wall, is made up of cells called *astrocytes;* long projections from astrocytes completely cover the capillary endothelium.

A solute in blood must cross both the capillary endothelium and surrounding *astrocyte sheath* before entering the brain. Paracellular transport through tight junctions between endothelial cells is impossible even for small solutes. This means transcellular transport (either by passive diffusion or by a carrier-mediated process) or transcytosis are the only mechanisms for distribution of solutes into the brain. Even transcellular diffusion is slowed down considerably by the astrocyte sheath.

The unique structure of brain capillaries forms an effective blood–brain barrier that restricts and controls entry of solutes into the brain. Lipophilic compounds are able to enter the brain by passive transcellular diffusion, but polar drugs have a very difficult time entering brain tissue unless transported by a specific carrier-mediated process.

In addition, distribution of lipophilic drugs to the brain is restricted by the presence of efflux pumps in the lumenal membrane of the brain endothelium. These efflux pumps actively drive drugs such as chemotherapeutics from the brain back to the blood and may thereby prevent significant distribution of antitumor agents in the brain. Metabolizing enzymes in the capillary endothelium may also break down a drug before it can distribute into the brain.

Thus, distribution is a formidable challenge when the site of action of a drug is in the brain. It is partly for these reasons that most classic chemotherapeutic drugs used to treat cancer outside the central nervous system are ineffective in treatment of brain tumors.

Distribution from Mother to Fetus. Exchange of solutes between the maternal and fetal blood circulations takes place in the placenta. Maternal blood enters large cavities, or *sinuses,* in the placenta. Fingerlike projections from the fetus, called villi, also enter the sinuses. Villi are lined with epithelial cells and contain fetal capillaries. Thus, transport of drugs from the mother occurs through the epithelial membrane of placental villi, and subsequently through the endothelial membrane of fetal capillaries, and onward into the fetal circulation. Drugs cross the placental membrane by passive transcellular diffusion. The placental membrane has very tight junctions, so lipophilic solutes are transported and distributed faster than hydrophilic solutes. The

large surface area of fetal villi, however, allows even hydrophilic drugs to cross into the fetal circulation to some extent.

The fetal blood has fewer plasma proteins, so more of the drug is present as free fraction in the fetal circulation. Additionally, the other membrane barriers in the fetus are not as well developed as those in the mother, and drug may distribute into fetal tissues (such as the brain) more readily.

Distribution Into Breast Milk. The drug concentration in milk is related to the maternal plasma concentration, and is often described by the milk-to-plasma drug concentration (M/P) ratio. Most drugs pass into milk from maternal plasma by passive transcellular diffusion across an epithelial barrier. The M/P ratio is therefore influenced by the composition of the milk (aqueous, lipid, protein, and pH) and the physicochemical characteristics of the drug (protein binding, lipophilicity, and pK_a). Milk contains substantially more lipid and less protein than plasma, and is slightly more acidic. Therefore, drugs that tend to concentrate in milk are weak bases with low plasma protein binding and high lipid solubility. Secretion of drugs into breast milk is often considered a mode of drug excretion because it removes drug from the body of the mother.

Distribution Into Intracellular Water

Proteins and protein–drug complexes remain in plasma and cannot distribute into tissues (except into tissues with sinusoids) because of their large size. Smaller solutes can leave capillaries and enter interstitial fluid by diffusion processes.

When distribution between plasma and interstitial fluid reaches equilibrium, there is no net transport in or out of capillaries, and drug concentration in the interstitial fluid will be equal to the *free* drug concentration in plasma. Interstitial fluid and plasma are together called extracellular water, because together they make up the body's extracellular fluids.

Lipophilic solutes can diffuse from interstitial fluid, through cell membranes of tissue cells, into the intracellular fluid inside cells. For such solutes, intracellular drug concentration will be equal to extracellular drug concentration at equilibrium. Additionally, solutes that have transport proteins in cell membranes will be able to enter cells by carrier-mediated processes. This may lead to higher drug concentrations in the intracellular fluid, allowing drug to concentrate in the cell. Extracellular water and intracellular water together represent the entire fluid volume in the body; this is collectively called total body water.

Just as drugs bind to plasma proteins, they may bind to tissue proteins as well. This binding will influence the concentration of free drug in tissue cells. The overall distribution of drugs between vascular and extravascular spaces is illustrated in Figure 11.5.

Distribution from Tissues to Plasma

Distribution is a dynamic process influenced not only by transport of solute into tissues but also by transport of solute from tissues back into blood. This reverse process is important for removal of drugs and metabolites from the body. The transport mechanisms are passive paracellular and transcellular diffusion as before, which now occur in the opposite direction. The driving force is the concentration gradient of free solute between tissue and bloodstream. Drug (or metabolite) concentration in the tissue must be higher than in blood for drug (or metabolite) to be returned to blood. Drugs extensively bound to tissue proteins will tend to remain in tissues because free drug concentration in tissues is low and not enough to create a favorable concentration gradient. Lipophilic drugs, because

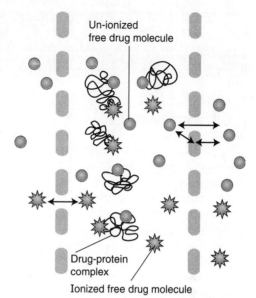

Figure 11.5. Distribution of a protein-bound drug across the capillary endothelium. Only free drug is able to cross the capillary endothelium. Ionized molecules (※) can only cross paracellularly, whereas un-ionized, lipophilic molecules (●) can cross paracellularly or transcellularly.

of their high partition coefficients, can also accumulate in organs or sites with adipose (fat) deposits.

Volume of Distribution

A quantitative analysis of distribution is necessary to understand pharmacokinetics of a drug. An average adult has about 0.04 L of plasma per kilogram of body weight. A 70-kg individual has approximately 5 L of blood, comprising 3 L of plasma and 2 L of blood cells. After entering the vascular fluid, a drug may distribute into the interstitial fluid and, further, into the intracellular fluid. Relative volumes of these fluids are shown in Figure 11.6.

On intravenous (IV) injection, a drug mixes with blood, equilibrates swiftly in plasma, and is transported throughout the body. At an average cardiac output of 4.8 to 6.4 L/min, it is reasonable to

Distribution of Opioids

The term *opioid* or *opiate* refers to all natural and synthetic drugs with morphinelike properties. They are classified as naturally occurring opium alkaloids (morphine, codeine, and papaverine), semisynthetic derivatives (oxycodone, hydromorphone, and heroin), and synthetic opioids (fentanyl, meperidine, and methadone). Opiates are used to provide both pain relief (analgesia) and sedation. They are agonists at opioid receptors in the brain and spinal cord. Multiple subtypes of these receptors have now been identified, with some receptors more involved in analgesia and others associated with side effects.

Opioids are lipid soluble and rapidly and extensively distribute to tissues, including the brain, after administration. Synthetic and semisynthetic opioids have higher lipid solubility than morphine, enabling them to cross the blood–brain barrier more quickly, resulting in a more rapid onset of action. Administration of repeated or large doses of many opioids leads to accumulation in adipose and muscle tissues, which further results in prolonged therapeutic and adverse effects.

---

assume (for most drugs) that distribution is complete very shortly after IV administration. If a blood sample is removed and analyzed immediately after IV administration, drug concentration in plasma will depend on amount of drug administered (dose) and extent of drug distribution out of the vascular space. If the blood sample were to be taken later, plasma concentration will be diminished as a result of elimination processes.

Apparent Volume of Distribution

Each solute will distribute differently into tissues depending on its physicochemical properties. A drug can, therefore, be characterized by the volume of fluids into which it distributes. Because the exact volume of tissue fluids cannot be easily measured, we simplify the analysis by assuming that the body is a tank of fluid into which the drug is placed. If the total amount of drug (dose) put into the tank (body) is known, and the concentration of drug in the tank is measured, the volume of fluid in the tank can be calculated. This volume is called the **apparent volume of distribution, V_d,** of the drug. The term *apparent* signifies this is not a real volume (because the body is not a uniform tank), but a calculated number that helps us to model the distribution process and to compare different drugs.

The apparent volume of distribution of a drug may be determined by administering a known dose by IV bolus and measuring plasma drug concentration immediately after injection. V_d can be calculated using the equation:

$$V_d = \frac{dose}{plasma\ concentration} = \frac{X}{C_p}$$

(Eq. 11.2)

where X is the dose of drug and C_p is drug concentration in plasma.

The volume of distribution depends on the drug's physicochemical properties, which control its ability to enter extravascular fluids and tissues. This is best

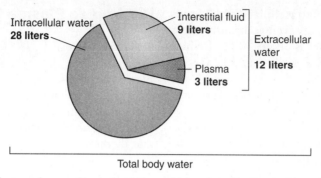

Figure 11.6. Relative volumes of body fluids into which a drug distributes. The volume of blood in the body is 5 L, of which plasma constitutes 3 L. The volume of blood cells (2 L) is included in the volume of intracellular water. Plasma and interstitial fluid together constitute extracellular water. The extracellular water and intracellular fluid together make up the *total body water.*

illustrated by examining distribution behavior of three types of compounds.

Macromolecular Drugs

X milligrams of a protein drug (e.g., *heparin*) is injected intravenously, an initial blood sample is taken, and V_d is calculated using Equation 11.2. Macromolecules like heparin are not able to distribute out of capillaries and remain confined to the vascular volume. The calculated V_d will be the volume of plasma in the individual, usually around 0.04 L/kg, or approximately 3 L in a 70-kg individual. Insulin is another example of a drug confined to plasma because of its large molecular size.

Polar Small Molecule Drugs

X milligrams of a polar, small molecule compound (e.g., mannitol) is injected intravenously and the initial plasma concentration (C_p) measured as before. Mannitol does not bind to plasma proteins and can, therefore, leave plasma and distribute into interstitial fluid. Mannitol is not lipophilic enough to enter intracellular fluid and is thus confined to the vascular and interstitial fluids. For an average healthy adult, the volume of *extracellular water* (plasma + interstitial fluid) is 0.18 L/kg of body weight. For a 70-kg individual, extracellular water volume is about

12 L, of which about 3 L is plasma and 9 L is interstitial fluid.

For such solutes at equilibrium, drug concentration in interstitial fluid can be assumed to be equal to plasma drug concentration C_p. Thus, it is not necessary (nor convenient) to measure concentration of solute in all tissue fluids. We can now calculate the total volume of fluid into which mannitol distributes:

$$V_d = \frac{\text{dose}}{\text{concentration in extracellular water}}$$

$$= \frac{X}{C_p} \qquad \text{(Eq. 11.3)}$$

This expression is the same as Equation 11.2. As mannitol can distribute into extracellular fluid but not into intracellular fluids, the V_d calculated will be approximately 0.17 L/kg, or 12 L in a 70-kg individual.

Lipophilic Small Molecule Drugs

Consider a lipophilic drug that can diffuse into cells in various tissues; most drugs fall into this category. Assume the drug does not bind to plasma proteins. Thus, the drug can distribute into interstitial fluid and intracellular fluid. Extracellular fluid (plasma + interstitial fluid) together with intracellular fluid is total body water. In an average healthy adult, total body water is about 40 L, of which 28 L is intracellular water and 12 L is extracellular water.

If X milligrams of this drug is given IV, drug concentrations in extracellular and intracellular fluids will be equal at equilibrium (assuming no ion trapping), and will be equal to plasma concentration C_p. Although this is not strictly true, it is a reasonable assumption for our purposes. Thus, the volume of distribution of such a drug will also be given by:

$$V_d = \frac{\text{dose}}{\text{concentration in total body water}}$$

$$= \frac{X}{C_p} \qquad \text{(Eq. 11.4)}$$

The V_d calculated in this case will be close to the volume of total body water (approximately 0.57 L/kg, or about 40 L in an average 70-kg individual). Examples of drugs that distribute in total body water are phenytoin, methotrexate, diazepam, and lidocaine.

Plasma Concentration and Volume of Distribution

In examining these three types of drugs, it is clear that as the drug is able to distribute into a larger volume of body fluids, its initial plasma concentration will be lower and the V_d calculated will be larger. Conversely, the V_d of a drug provides a measure of its permeability into various fluids and tissues. A word of caution is necessary here. Although some general patterns of distribution may be deduced based on the numerical value of V_d, it is incorrect to equate a given range of V_d too closely with a certain anatomical region of the body. Many factors such as drug binding to proteins and to other physiological components can complicate interpretation of V_d.

Binding to Plasma Proteins

The discussion of V_d so far assumes that the solute (or drug) is not bound to plasma proteins. However, most drugs bind to plasma proteins, and this affects their distribution. Proteins are macromolecules; they cannot leave capillaries and therefore remain in plasma.

Protein Binding Equilibrium

Many drugs bind reversibly to plasma proteins in blood to form drug–protein complexes. Consequently, the drug is present partly as free (unbound) drug and partly as protein-bound drug. Plasma proteins that complex with drugs to a significant extent are serum albumin, α_1-acid glycoprotein, lipoproteins, and globulins.

Plasma proteins are relatively nonspecific in their binding behavior. Albumin, which makes up more than half of all plasma proteins, is the most significant contributor. It interacts with and binds with most weak acid drugs in plasma. α_1-acid glycoprotein interacts with many weak bases, and various lipoproteins bind both basic and neutral drugs. Several endogenous ligands such as steroids and vitamins are bound to globulins, as are metal ions.

The binding equilibrium between drug and plasma proteins can be written as:

$$\text{drug} + \text{plasma protein} \rightleftarrows$$
$$\rightleftarrows \text{protein} - \text{drug complex} \qquad \text{(Eq. 11.5)}$$

Some drug is bound as the complex whereas the rest of the drug remains *free* or unbound. Another way of expressing this equilibrium is:

$$\text{free drug} + \text{plasma protein} \rightleftarrows$$
$$\rightleftarrows \text{bound drug} \qquad \text{(Eq. 11.6)}$$

The equilibria shown in Equations 11.5 and 11.6 are analogous to the formation of an enzyme–substrate complex in our discussion of Michaelis–Menten kinetics in Chapter 4, Rates of Pharmaceutical Processes. The main difference is that plasma proteins bind nonspecifically so that binding does not occur at a unique active site on the protein.

The total plasma concentration of drug is given by the sum of free and bound drug concentrations:

$$\text{total plasma concentration} = [\text{free drug}] + [\text{bound drug}] \quad \text{(Eq. 11.7)}$$

The ratio of free drug concentration to total drug concentration in plasma is called the free fraction, or fraction unbound (f_u), and is given by:

$$f_u = \frac{[\text{free drug}]}{[\text{total drug}]} = \frac{[\text{free drug}]}{[\text{free drug}] + [\text{bound drug}]} \quad \text{(Eq. 11.8)}$$

The free fraction is a unitless quantity.

Protein–drug complexes are too large to leave capillaries through the capillary endothelium. Thus, plasma protein bind-ing serves to retain drug in the bloodstream and decrease its distribution into interstitial fluid. As free drug leaves capillaries, some of the complex will dissociate to release free drug and maintain equilibrium in blood.

Drugs may bind to tissue proteins as well, reducing concentration of free drug in tissues. The distribution of a protein-bound drug is shown in Figure 11.7.

Physicochemical properties of the drug and protein are important in determining which drugs will be bound to which proteins and the extent of that binding. Generally, the higher the lipophilicity of a drug, the greater is its affinity for plasma proteins and tissue components. Binding of drugs to plasma proteins is the norm rather than the exception. Many drugs are greater than 90% bound to plasma proteins in healthy adults. Table 11.1 lists the extent of protein binding of selected drugs.

Protein Binding and Volume of Distribution

The protein–drug complex is too large to leave the vascular volume, but free drug

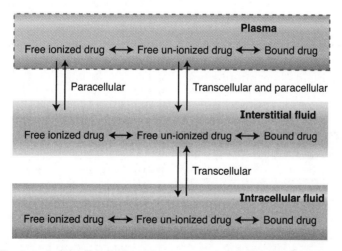

Figure 11.7. Illustration of the distribution of a protein-bound drug. Only free drug is able to cross the capillary endothelial membrane or cell membranes. Ionized molecules can only cross paracellularly across the capillary endothelium, whereas un-ionized, lipophilic molecules can cross both paracellularly and transcellularly. Furthermore, only un-ionized, lipophilic molecules can cross the cell membrane by passive transcellular diffusion to enter intracellular fluid. Exceptions to this are molecules with carrier-mediated transport pathways.

can distribute out of plasma. Drugs extensively bound to plasma proteins have a low free fraction of drug, f_u, and are less extensively distributed to tissues. Drugs with less extensive plasma protein binding have a higher free fraction of drug, f_u, diffuse more readily out of the vascular space, and generally have higher apparent volumes of distribution. Because both protein binding and lipophilicity influence V_d, the situation is more complex than the last statement implies.

Nevertheless, it is free drug in extravascular fluids (where the site of action is usually located) that influences pharmacological effect. Extensively protein-bound drugs may not be able to achieve a high enough concentration at the site of action to give adequate biological activity. Consequently, a high dose of drug may have to be administered to attain the desired concentration at the receptor. Because only free drug can be excreted by the kidney, plasma acts as a reservoir for protein-bound drugs, prolonging the time during which such drugs remain in the body. Thus, protein binding has to be taken into account when determining dose and frequency of administration of a drug.

Plasma protein concentrations are usually similar in most healthy adults, so determination of dose and dosing frequency can be standardized. However, plasma protein concentrations can change significantly in some disease states. In such situations, the dose needs to be adjusted to avoid either overdosing or underdosing. When several drugs that bind to the same protein are given together, one drug may displace another from protein-binding sites. This may result in higher free drug concentrations of the displaced drug, again requiring dosing adjustment. In some cases, such drugs should not be given together.

Many drugs can bind to tissue proteins as well, making tissue concentrations of these drugs higher than expected and increasing apparent volume of distribution. Such binding may be slow, and the distribution pattern of drug may be significantly different after several doses than it is after a single dose. In such situations, multiple dosing of the drug is carried out until the drug has equilibrated in all fluids; this condition is termed *steady state*. Measuring V_d at steady state rather than after a single dose gives a more physiologically relevant value.

Influence of Binding at Other Sites

Drugs can also bind to nonprotein components of tissues into which they distribute. The main result of this is storage of drug in the body for prolonged periods because only free drug in plasma can be metabolized or eliminated. One example of such a site is adipose or fat tissue, which stores many lipid-soluble drugs. Because adipose tissue is not well perfused, both uptake and release of drug into and from the tissue are slow. Drugs that partition into adipose tissue often have very large apparent volumes of distribution, often larger than the volume of total body water. Other sites where binding is seen are bone tissue and teeth. These tissues contain high concentrations of calcium, and drugs that chelate calcium (e.g., tetracyclines) often accumulate in bone and teeth.

TABLE 11.1. Extent of Plasma Protein Binding of Select Drugs	
Drug	*% Bound*
Gentamicin	3
Digoxin	25
Lidocaine	51
Phenytoin	89
Propranolol	93
Furosemide	96
Diazepam	99
Warfarin	99

TABLE 11.2. Examples of Apparent Volumes of Distribution of Select Drugs in a 70-kg Individual	
Drug	*V_d (L)*
Furosemide	8
Gentamicin	18
Phenytoin	45
Lidocaine	77
Propranolol	270
Digoxin	440
Nortriptyline	1,300

Many un-ionized acidic drugs, such as warfarin and salicylic acid, are highly protein-bound and thus have a small apparent volume of distribution. Many un-ionized basic drugs such as amphetamine and meperidine are extensively bound in tissues and thus have an apparent volume of distribution larger than the volume of the entire body. Table 11.2 lists apparent volumes of distribution of selected drugs.

KEY CONCEPTS

- Drug distribution follows drug absorption.
- Distribution occurs via the circulatory system, which transports drug throughout the body.
- Distribution is a dynamic process, and concentrations of drug in plasma and tissues are constantly changing as drug is absorbed and eliminated from the body.
- Distribution patterns depend on physicochemical properties of

drug, nature of the capillary endothelium in the tissue, perfusion of the tissue, and drug–protein binding.
- Only free, unbound drug is able to distribute across membranes.
- The apparent volume of distribution characterizes the extent to which a drug leaves vascular space and distributes into tissues.

ADDITIONAL READING

1. Shargel L, Yu A. Applied Biopharmaceutics and Pharmacokinetics, 4th ed. McGraw-Hill/Appleton & Lange, 1999.

2. Ritschel WA, Kearns GL. Handbook of Basic Pharmacokinetics, 5th ed. American Pharmaceutical Association, 1999.

3. Dipiro JT, Spruill WJ, Blouin RA, Pruemer JM, Hermann J. Concepts in Clinical Pharmacokinetics, 3rd ed. American Hospital Association, 2002.

4. Rowland M, Tozer TN. Clinical Pharmacokinetics: Concepts and Applications, 3rd ed. Lippincott Williams & Wilkins, 1995.

REVIEW QUESTIONS

1. What physicochemical properties allow a drug to easily leave the vascular space? What types of drugs cannot leave the vascular space?
2. What are the primary transport mechanisms for drug distribution in and out of capillaries?
3. How does the blood–brain barrier prevent entry of drugs into the brain? What types of drugs can enter the brain readily?
4. How is the apparent volume of distribution of a drug measured? What assumptions are made in this calculation?
5. How can the numerical value of the apparent volume of distribution be interpreted? What does it tell us about the drug?
6. Why does plasma and tissue protein binding of drugs influence drug distribution?
7. When is the apparent volume of distribution after multiple dosing a better measure of distribution than after a single dose?

Drug Excretion

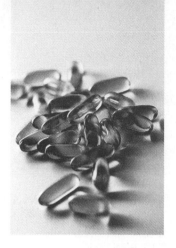

After a drug has been administered and is distributed, the body begins to remove the drug by several processes. The sum of these processes of drug loss from the body is known as drug elimination. A substance can be removed from the body either in its unchanged form (excretion), or as metabolites after being chemically altered (biotransformation or metabolism). Elimination starts soon after a drug is absorbed into the bloodstream and begins to distribute out of the plasma. As elimination continues, drug is progressively removed from the bloodstream and tissues and, thereby, from the site of action. The consequence of elimination is generally a progressive decrease in the pharmacological action of the drug.

Excretion is a process by which a substance is eliminated from the body without further chemical change. The kidney, the most important organ for drug excretion, makes a fluid called urine in which many substances are excreted. Polar, water-soluble solutes can be eliminated largely unchanged by excretion in urine. On the other hand, lipophilic solutes must first be metabolized to water-soluble compounds or metabolites before they can be excreted in urine. We will discuss the process of drug metabolism in the

TABLE 12.1. Examples of Drugs Excreted Primarily in the Unchanged Form and Primarily as Metabolites

Excreted Mostly Unchanged	Excreted Mostly as Metabolites
Digoxin	Phenacetin
Streptomycin	Morphine
Amphetamine	Chloramphenicol
Ampicillin	Isoniazid
Guanethidine	
Penicillin	
Tetracycline	

next chapter. The kidney is the primary site of excretion of both water-soluble drugs and metabolites of drugs. Table 12.1 lists examples of drugs excreted primarily in unchanged form and those excreted primarily as metabolites.

The liver may also serve as an organ for excretion of certain drugs. These drugs are excreted unchanged in bile, a fluid made by the liver. Bile empties into the digestive tract, from which drugs can be removed in feces or reabsorbed into the bloodstream and recycled. Other drugs may be excreted in saliva, sweat, breast milk, and exhaled air. Generally, the contribution of these alternative excretion routes is small, except for excretion of volatile anesthetics in exhaled air. Although excretion via breast milk may not be a significant route of excretion for the mother, the presence of drug in breast milk is important to the suckling infant, as discussed in Chapter 11, Drug Distribution.

Excretion by the Kidney

Although the kidney is the predominant organ of drug excretion, its main function is to maintain homeostasis by regulating fluid and electrolyte balance in the body. It is a selective organ that makes a fluid called urine, adjusting urine composition to reflect the needs of the body by removing waste products from blood and returning water and other essential substances back to blood. Although the kidney removes wastes from blood, it also re-

moves normal components of blood present at greater-than-normal concentrations. When excess water, sodium ions, calcium ions, and so forth are present, the excess quickly passes out in urine. On the other hand, the kidney steps up reclamation of these same substances when they are present in blood at less-than-normal amounts. Thus the kidney continuously regulates the chemical composition of blood within narrow limits.

To understand urinary excretion, we need to review the basics of renal physiology and the process of urine formation.

Renal Physiology and Urine Formation

The anatomical and functional unit of the kidney is the nephron, shown diagrammatically in Figure 12.1; each kidney contains about a million nephrons. A nephron is made up of Bowman's capsule with a long tubule leading from it. Bowman's capsule is a cup-shaped structure that is the filtering unit of the kidney. The tubule is divided into four functional parts: the *proximal tubule, loop of Henle, distal tubule,* and *collecting duct.* The kidneys' extraordinary excretory and regulatory functions are achieved through processes of glomerular filtration, tubular reabsorption, and tubular secretion.

Glomerular Filtration

Blood containing waste products (including drugs and their metabolites) enters the

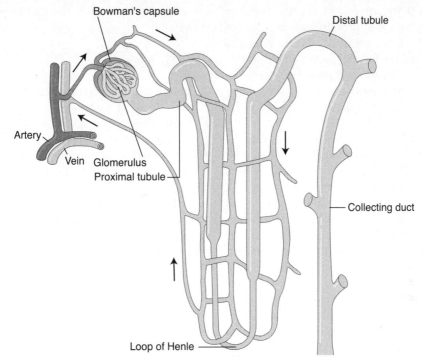

Figure 12.1. Schematic view of a nephron, composed of Bowman's capsule, tubules (proximal tubule, loop of Henle, and distal tubule), and collecting duct. Blood supply to the nephron is also shown, with arrows indicating the direction of blood flow.

kidney through the renal artery. An average adult man with a cardiac output of 6 L/min has a normal renal blood flow of about 1.2 L/min. Thus, the kidney is constantly fed about 20% of the cardiac output, a very substantial portion of the total blood flow.

The renal artery branches several times, ultimately forming a network of capillaries called the glomerulus nestled inside Bowman's capsule. After passing through glomerular capillaries, blood leaves Bowman's capsule to enter a second capillary network surrounding the tubules, and then leaves the kidney via renal venules.

The endothelium of glomerular capillaries is in intimate contact with Bowman's capsule. The glomerular endothelium is fenestrated (as discussed in earlier chapters), permitting paracellular transport of most solutes (except proteins and other macromolecules) from the glomerulus into Bowman's capsule. This process is greatly assisted by the high hydrostatic pressure within the glomerulus created by the pumping action of the heart. This pressure forces fluid out of the glomerular capillary and results in a large volume of fluid (along with dissolved substances) being filtered out of the vascular space.

The "effective pore size" of the glomerular filter is a complex concept and depends on a range of factors such as size, shape, and charge of filtered substances as well as the characteristics of the glomerulus itself. There is no barrier to filtration for molecules up to a molecular weight of about 5,000, but above that charge and shape become progressively more important determinants of filtration.

As blood passes through the glomerulus, continued loss of water by filtration lowers the hydrostatic pressure but at the same time leaves plasma proteins in the capillary. As filtrate leaves without concomitant protein loss, the relative concentration of protein increases and so does osmotic pressure. Thus, filtration pressure is a balance between these two effects. Hydrostatic pressure predominates at the arteriolar end of the capillary but becomes dissipated toward the venous end.

Liquid collected in Bowman's capsule as a result of glomerular filtration is called the glomerular filtrate, which can be viewed as an ultrafiltrate of plasma, i.e., protein-free plasma. All solutes up to a molecular weight of approximately 5,000 are present in the glomerular filtrate at the same concentration found in plasma, with the exception of those bound to plasma proteins. Essentially, the glomerular filtrate is no different in composition from interstitial fluid.

Approximately 10% of plasma flowing through the glomerulus is converted into filtrate by the two kidneys. This is a very large volume, and the body would become dehydrated if all this fluid were excreted as urine.

Tubular Reabsorption

The renal tubules are lined with a single layer of epithelial cells in close contact with the renal capillary network. As glomerular filtrate travels down the tubules, many nutrients (amino acids, glucose) and ions (Na^+, K^+, Cl^-, HCO_3^-) are actively reabsorbed back into the bloodstream using ATP as the energy source. Various hormones regulate these reabsorption processes to maintain homeostasis.

This movement of solutes and ions from filtrate into the bloodstream sets up an osmotic gradient that simultaneously drives reabsorption of water from the filtrate into blood. The enormous length of the tubules allows plenty of opportunity to reabsorb water. Thus, as filtrate moves from Bowman's capsule to the collecting tubule, it is progressively concentrated in solutes as a result of the reabsorption of water.

Tubular Secretion

Although urine formation occurs primarily by filtration and reabsorption mechanisms as described above, an auxiliary mechanism called tubular secretion is also involved. Just as certain solutes can travel from the tubular filtrate back into blood, the reverse process can also occur. Cells of the tubular epithelium remove certain molecules and ions (such as H^+ and K^+ ions) from blood and *secrete* these into the filtrate within the tubules. The filtrate is generally more concentrated in these solutes than is plasma (as a result of extensive water reabsorption), so an active transport process has to be in place to move substances from plasma into filtrate against the concentration gradient. Thus, secretion is an active, energy-requiring process that uses protein transporters in tubular epithelium for substances being secreted.

Tubular secretion of H^+ is important for maintaining control of the pH of blood. When pH of blood starts to drop, more hydrogen ions are secreted into urine. If blood should become too alkaline, secretion of H^+ is reduced. Thus, pH of urine can vary between a value as low as 4.5 or as high as 8.5 to maintain a blood pH within its normal limits of 7.3 to 7.4. Normally, urine is more acidic than blood.

The processes of glomerular filtration, tubular reabsorption, and tubular secretion are shown diagrammatically in Figure 12.2.

Rate of Urine Formation

Reabsorption and secretion modify the composition and volume of glomerular filtrate as it travels down the nephron to the collecting tubule. Once these processes are complete, the modified filtrate, now called urine, is transported to the bladder

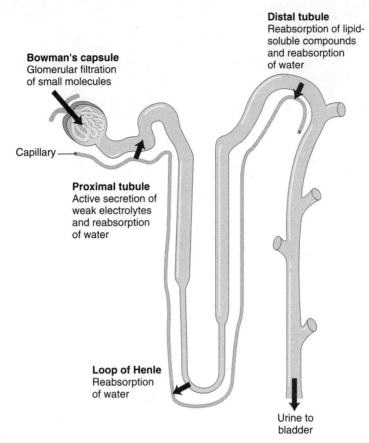

Figure 12.2. Schematic diagram of the processes of glomerular filtration, reabsorption, and secretion in a nephron.

for storage until it can be removed from the body.

The kidneys receive about 1.2 L of blood per minute. About 10% of this is filtered at the glomerulus to form the filtrate, giving a glomerular filtration rate (GFR) of 120 mL/min in an adult with normal renal function. The GFR is, therefore, the volume of blood filtered by the kidneys per minute.

Reabsorption processes leave behind urine that is made up of a small volume of water with a high concentration of urea, unwanted excess salts, and other substances. The rate of urine formation varies between 15 mL/hr and 1500 mL/hr, but is usually around 60 to 120 mL/hr or between 1 to 2 mL/min; this volume goes to the bladder for storage. It is apparent that approximately 99% of water in the filtrate is reabsorbed in the kidneys and returned to blood.

Renal Excretion of Drugs

The kidneys are involved to some extent in excretion of almost every drug or drug metabolite from the body. The processes of filtration, reabsorption, and secretion discussed above determine which and how much drug or metabolite is excreted in urine.

A diagram illustrating the processes involved in renal excretion of drugs is shown in Figure 12.3.

Glomerular Filtration of Drugs

All solutes except proteins and other macromolecules are filtered in the glomerulus

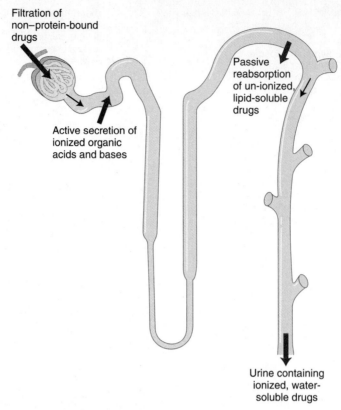

Filtration of
non–protein-bound
drugs

Passive
reabsorption
of un-ionized,
lipid-soluble
drugs

Active secretion of
ionized organic
acids and bases

Urine containing
ionized, water-
soluble drugs

Figure 12.3. Schematic diagram showing the renal excretion of drugs in urine. Active secretion of ionized organic acids and bases occurs primarily in the proximal tubule. Un-ionized and lipid-soluble drugs are passively reabsorbed throughout the tubule.

and appear in the filtrate. Glomerular filtration occurs for all small molecules and ions (molecular weight <5,000) present in plasma. Because filtration is primarily driven by hydrostatic pressure in the glomerulus, the concentration of a drug (or metabolite) in the filtrate will be equal to its concentration in plasma. Protein-bound drugs will not be filtered because they exist as a protein–drug complex. Therefore, more generally, the concentration of a drug or metabolite in the filtrate will be equal to the concentration of its *unbound* or *free* form in plasma.

The GFR of fluid through normal kidneys is about 120 mL/min. We can also define a GFR for each drug, a term that describes the rate at which the particular drug is filtered. GFR of a drug depends on its extent of protein binding, and is given by the equation:

$$GFR_{drug} = f_u \cdot GFR \quad \text{(Eq. 12.1)}$$

where f_u is the fraction of unbound drug in plasma. Highly protein-bound drugs (i.e., those with a low f_u) have a low GFR and are retained in plasma. Conversely, a drug that is not protein-bound will have the same GFR as fluid, 120 mL/min.

Tubular Reabsorption of Drugs

Although the tubular epithelium contains transporters for reabsorption of essential ions and molecules, no special transporters exist for reabsorption of drugs. Thus, the only mechanism available for drug reabsorption from filtrate to blood is passive transcellular diffusion through the epithelial membrane of the tubules. As filtrate travels through the tubules, water reabsorption causes it to become more concentrated in drug, resulting in a higher concentration of drug in filtrate compared with blood. A concentration gradient is set up between filtrate and plasma, allowing drug molecules to diffuse from filtrate back into plasma if their physiochemical properties (such as partition coefficient and pK_a) are appropriate.

Influence of Filtrate pH. Considering that only uncharged, lipophilic molecules can diffuse though the tubular epithelial membrane, reabsorption depends on extent of ionization of a drug in the filtrate—and, therefore, on filtrate pH—and on the partition coefficient of unionized drug. A filtrate pH that favors ionization of a drug will reduce its rate and extent of reabsorption, and vice versa. Because the pH on the two sides (plasma and filtrate) of the tubular epithelial membrane can be (and usually is) different, an *ion-trapping* situation is set up. In alkaline urine, acidic drugs are more ionized and hence are less reabsorbed and more readily excreted, whereas basic drugs are more un-ionized, more reabsorbed, and less readily excreted. The reverse is true in acidic urine.

Ion trapping can be exploited to slow down or speed up excretion of drugs by appropriately altering urine pH. In drug overdose situations, it may be possible to increase excretion of a drug by suitable adjustment of urine pH. Acidifiers such

Methotrexate and Urinary pH

Methotrexate is used in the treatment of several neoplasms such as leukemia, breast cancer, and non-Hodgkin's lymphoma. It is a weak acid with a pK_a of 5.4 and is primarily cleared by the kidneys via glomerular filtration and active secretion. Up to 92% of a single dose is excreted unchanged in the urine within 24 hours after intravenous administration. Methotrexate has poor intrinsic solubility and thus may precipitate in the urine at low pH (below pH 6). A small fraction of the dose is metabolized, mainly to 7-hydroxymethotrexate, which is even more poorly soluble than the parent drug and can also precipitate in the renal tubules. These solubility and precipitation problems are responsible for the risk of nephrotoxicity with methotrexate therapy, especially at high doses. This could lead to renal damage and acute renal failure.

It is very important that patients taking methotrexate are adequately hydrated to prevent high urinary concentrations and precipitation of the drug or the 7-hydroxymethotrexate metabolite in the urine. Additionally, urinary pH should be maintained at 7 or above to further minimize precipitation of methotrexate. Patients are advised to maintain good urine flow by drinking plenty of fluids for 2 days after a high-dose injection (greater than 200 mg), and to keep the urine alkaline by using sodium bicarbonate continuously for at least 24 hours afterward.

Simultaneous administration of other weak organic acids such as salicylates may suppress methotrexate clearance by competition for secretion transporters. Coadministration with other nonsteroidal anti-inflammatory drugs (such as diclofenac, indomethacin, naproxen, or phenylbutazone) can lead to elevated methotrexate plasma levels as a result of its displacement from plasma protein binding sites. These high plasma levels can cause toxicity.

as ammonium chloride and aspirin reduce urine pH, whereas alkalinizers such as calcium carbonate, sodium bicarbonate, and sodium glutamate increase urine pH. Acidic foods (citrus fruits, cranberry juice) and basic foods (milk products) can also change urine pH. An example of altering urine pH in clinical situations is in the case of pentobarbital overdose; renal excretion of pentobarbital (a weak acid) can be increased by alkalinizing urine with sodium bicarbonate injections.

Tubular Secretion of Drugs

Secretion involves transporting drugs from plasma to filtrate against a concentration gradient (from plasma to a more concentrated filtrate) and requires active transporters. Scientists have identified a variety of tubular proteins (primarily located in the epithelium of the proximal tubule) responsible for transport of organic cations, organic anions, neutral and cationic hydrophobic compounds, anionic conjugates, and specific agents such as prostaglandins. These transporters have rather broad substrate specificities; organic anion transporter will bind to and transport many ionized organic acids, and organic cation transporter will do the same for ionized organic bases.

Although transporters bind to only the free form of drug, most protein–drug complexes in blood dissociate rapidly enough to make additional free drug available when some of it has been removed from plasma by secretion. Tubular transporters are so active with some drugs that drug can be completely stripped off plasma proteins in one pass of blood through the kidney. Therefore, plasma protein binding has relatively little influence on rate of tubular secretion.

Because the transporters bind to and secrete only the ionized form of drug, the pH of plasma and its relationship to pK_a of drug are important. A drug that is highly ionized at pH 7.4 will be secreted to a greater extent than a drug only slightly ionized at this pH.

There are two important consequences arising from these active secretion mechanisms.

- Competitive drug interactions: Many drugs share the same secretion transporters, so competition for transporters can occur, leading to desirable or undesirable drug interactions. For example, penicillin and probenecid are both substrates for the organic acid transporter, so probenecid is used clinically to compete with penicillin and reduce its renal excretion. Cimetidine and procainamide are basic drugs that compete with each other for the organic base basic transporter and thus reduce each other's renal excretion.
- Saturable kinetics: The active secretion processes are saturable, so renal excretion can reach a plateau at high doses of a drug. This will lead to a lower excretion rate than expected and, consequently, a higher than anticipated plasma concentration.

Rate of Renal Excretion of Drugs

The rate at which a drug is excreted in urine is the net result of glomerular filtration, reabsorption, and secretion. These processes depend not only on physico-chemical properties of drug but also on the rate of blood flow in the nephron, both in the glomerulus and in tubular capillaries. A more rapid perfusion of the nephron increases the rate of all these processes and usually results in an overall higher drug excretion rate. GFR is a direct measure of perfusion of the kidneys; the greater the blood flow to the kidneys, the higher the GFR.

Secretion and reabsorption of drugs proceed simultaneously in the tubules; secretion increases concentration of drug in the filtrate whereas reabsorption decreases it. Secretion is favored by ionization of drug in the pH 7.4 plasma; reabsorption is favored by lack of ionization of drug in the usually more acidic filtrate.

Thus, the overall rate of drug excretion in urine is governed by a complex relationship between physicochemical properties of drug (pK_a, partition coefficient, and protein binding), pH of plasma and urine, and GFR. In general, the kidneys readily excrete drugs that are water-soluble and ionized in the filtrate, but cannot efficiently excrete drugs that are lipophilic and predominantly unionized in the filtrate.

Renal Clearance

Clearance (CL) is a term that indicates the efficiency with which a drug is removed from plasma. It is defined as the hypothetical volume of plasma from which drug is removed totally and irreversibly per unit time, and has units of volume per time (e.g., mL/min or L/hr). The faster plasma is cleared of drug, the higher the clearance of that drug. The body clears a drug from plasma by two main elimination processes: biotransformation of drug to metabolites or excretion of unchanged drug. Total body clearance is the sum of clearances from all elimination pathways. The concept of clearance is illustrated in Figure 12.4.

Renal clearance (CL_r) is a component of overall drug clearance, and represents the efficiency of removal of unchanged drug in urine by renal excretion. Renal clearance is defined as the volume of plasma that contained the amount of drug appearing in urine per unit time. The rate at which plasma is cleared of drug by the kidneys cannot be directly measured, so an indirect method is used. Renal clearance of a drug can be expressed as:

$$CL_r = \frac{\text{excretion rate in urine}}{\text{plasma concentration}} \quad \text{(Eq. 12.2)}$$

The concentrations of drug in urine and plasma (C_u and C_p, respectively) and volume of urine formation per unit time (V_u) can be measured. From this, CL_r can be calculated using the following equation:

$$CL_r = \frac{C_u \cdot V_u}{C_p} \quad \text{(Eq. 12.3)}$$

Here, ($C_u \times V_u$) represents the excretion rate of drug in urine. Equation 12.3 and the concept of renal clearance can be more clearly understood by considering three illustrative examples.

Renal Clearance of Inulin

Consider a substance such as *inulin,* a carbohydrate found in plants (do not confuse with the hormone *insulin,* which is a protein). Inulin does not bind to plasma proteins and is completely filtered by the kidneys, which means that inulin concentration in the glomerular filtrate is the same as its concentration in plasma. Inulin is not reabsorbed in the

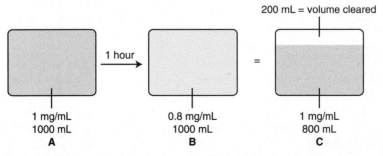

Figure 12.4. A clarification of the concept of clearance. The box (A) represents 1,000 mL of plasma containing 1 mg/mL of a drug. After 1 hour, the plasma concentration of drug drops to 0.8 mg/mL in 1,000 mL as a result of elimination (B). In other words, after 1 hour, only 800 mL of plasma contains the original concentration of drug (1 mg/mL), whereas 200 mL of plasma is completely free of drug, as shown in (C). Thus, the clearance of drug in this example is 200 mL/hr.

tubules (it does not have a high enough partition coefficient) and is not secreted (it is not ionized in plasma).

Therefore, glomerular filtration is the only mechanism contributing to renal excretion of inulin. The renal clearance of inulin should thus be the same as GFR, or approximately 120 mL/min in an adult with normal kidney function. In other words, plasma is cleared of inulin at the same rate that plasma is filtered in the glomerulus. There is no secretion to increase inulin clearance and no reabsorption to decrease clearance. As the filtrate travels down the tubules it becomes concentrated as a result of the reabsorption of water; the final inulin concentration in urine will therefore be significantly higher than in plasma.

If rate of urine formation, V_u, is about 1 to 2 mL/min (the normal range for adults) and CL_r of inulin is 120 mL/min (the normal GFR), then the ratio of concentrations of inulin in urine and plasma can be calculated by rearranging Equation 12.3 as follows:

$$\frac{C_u}{C_p} = \frac{CL_r}{V_u} = \frac{120 \text{ mL/min}}{2 \text{ mL/min}} = 60$$

(Eq. 12.4)

In other words, inulin is about 60 times more concentrated in urine than in plasma.

Conversely, inulin CL_r could be calculated by measuring inulin concentrations in urine and plasma. In fact, renal clearance of *creatinine,* an endogenous substance with properties similar to those of inulin, is often measured to determine an individual's GFR and provide an indication of kidney function.

Creatinine Clearance

Creatinine is a waste product in the blood produced by the normal breakdown of muscle during activity. It is not protein-bound, is freely filtered, is not reabsorbed, and is minimally secreted by the kidneys; thus it is cleared almost exclusively by filtration. Healthy kidneys excrete creatinine in urine and maintain a stable plasma creatinine concentration. Under normal conditions, creatinine excretion is approximately equal to creatinine production, so that the serum creatinine concentration remains fairly constant. When GFR is compromised in renal impairment, creatinine builds up in the serum. The accumulation of creatinine will depend on the degree of loss of glomerular filtration.

Creatinine clearance (CL_{Cr}) is defined as the rate of urinary excretion of creatinine to serum creatinine. In clinical practice, it is determined by collecting urine for 24 hours and taking a blood sample at the midpoint of this time interval. The creatinine concentration is measured in both samples, and equations are used to calculate CL_{Cr} of the patient. A small fraction of creatinine is secreted, and there is some nonrenal elimination as well. As a result, CL_{Cr} values overestimate the actual GFR. A CL_{Cr} significantly lower than 100 mL/min indicates a problem with kidney function.

In patients with reduced muscle mass, CL_{Cr} may appear normal even when kidney function is impaired because both serum creatinine levels and creatinine excretion are lower than normal. Thus, several empirical equations have been developed by clinicians to correct for this by adjusting CL_{Cr} using the patient's age, height, and weight.

Renal Clearance of p-Aminohippuric Acid

Consider a slightly more complex case: a compound not significantly plasma protein-bound, very efficiently secreted by the tubules, but not reabsorbed because of complete ionization in the filtrate. An example is p-*aminohippuric acid* (PAH), a weak acid completely ionized in the filtrate. PAH will be filtered in the glomerulus just like creatinine or inulin. However, as filtrate travels down the tubules, the concentration of PAH will increase not only because of water reabsorption but also because of PAH secretion. In fact, PAH is secreted so efficiently by tubular epithelial transporters that plasma in the tubular capillaries is completely cleared of PAH as it flows through.

Thus, the kidneys remove *all* PAH from plasma in a single pass; blood leaving the kidneys contains virtually no PAH. The CL_r of PAH is, therefore, equal to the rate of plasma flow through the kidneys because that entire volume of plasma has been cleared of drug. The rate of normal renal plasma flow is about 650 mL/min in adults, which represents the highest renal clearance for any substance. Renal clearance of PAH in a patient can give valuable information about kidney function; a PAH clearance much less than 650 mL/min may indicate problems with blood flow in the kidneys.

Renal Clearance of Glucose

Now consider the other extreme—a substance such as glucose that is not protein-bound, but is completely reabsorbed in the tubules (glucose, being an essential nutrient, is reabsorbed by an active transport process). After glomerular filtration, glucose is completely reabsorbed into plasma as the filtrate travels through the tubules. Thus, urine contains no glucose, and CL_r of glucose is zero in healthy adults.

Renal Clearance of Drugs

The three cases discussed above illustrate extreme situations of renal drug excretion and establish minimum and maximum values for renal clearance of drugs. CL_r can range from zero at one extreme to approximately 650 mL/min as the maximum CL_r.

Plasma Protein Binding and Renal Clearance

The examples discussed above (inulin, PAH, and glucose) are compounds not significantly bound to plasma proteins. If a drug is protein-bound, the concentration of drug in the filtrate immediately after glomerular filtration will be less than its concentration in plasma concentration, as we saw in Equation 12.1. The filtrate will then change further in composition owing to reabsorption and secretion processes. Plasma protein binding does not influence overall renal clearance significantly for drugs that are efficiently secreted or reabsorbed. However, for drugs with properties that are less extreme, protein binding will generally decrease CL_r as a result of reduced glomerular filtration.

Excretion Ratio

The excretion ratio (E_{ratio}) of a drug is defined as its renal clearance corrected for plasma protein binding. It is given by:

$$E_{ratio} = \frac{CL_r}{f_u \cdot GFR} = \frac{CL_r}{GFR_{drug}} \quad \text{(Eq. 12.5)}$$

A drug that is protein-bound and cleared by filtration only with no reabsorption or secretion will have an $E_{ratio} = 1$; in other words, its renal clearance, CL_r, equals its GFR. A protein-bound drug with an E_{ratio} greater than 1 indicates secretion is more significant than reabsorption. Conversely, a protein-bound drug with an E_{ratio} less than 1 shows that reabsorption is more significant than secretion. Another way to look at this is by using clearance values.

A drug with CL_r between 0 and 120 mL/min usually indicates reabsorption predominates over secretion, whereas a drug with CL_r between 120 and 650 mL/min usually indicates secretion predominates over reabsorption.

Excretion by the Liver

Although the liver is primarily an organ in which drugs are biotransformed, it also plays a role in drug excretion. Blood supply to the liver comes via the hepatic artery from the systemic circulation and via the portal vein from the intestines. The main functions of the liver are metabolism and energy production.

The liver secretes about 0.5 to 1.0 L per day of a fluid called bile, which is stored in the gallbladder and emptied into the small intestines as needed to aid in digestion of food. The extent of bile production depends on the type of food present, with food high in proteins resulting in greatest bile secretion. At the same time, the liver removes drugs and other substances from the portal and arterial blood for metabolism. These drugs can be secreted into bile in much the same manner as the kidney secretes drugs into urine. This is also an active transport process involving anion and cation transporters in various cells of the liver. Drugs secreted into bile are emptied along with bile into the duodenum, from where they are removed from the body in feces; this elimination pathway is called biliary excretion.

However, many drugs secreted into bile may not be eliminated in feces. If the drug has appropriate physicochemical properties (partition coefficient, pK_a), it can be partially reabsorbed from intestines back into the bloodstream just like an orally administered drug; this process is known as enterohepatic recycling. Such drugs can continue to be secreted in bile and reabsorbed into blood, until some other process eventually eliminates them from the body. Enterohepatic recycling, therefore, increases the persistence of drugs in the body. Biliary excretion represents an important elimination mechanism for drugs extensively ionized in the small intestines (such as weak acids), making reabsorption into blood unlikely. Figure 12.5 illustrates the

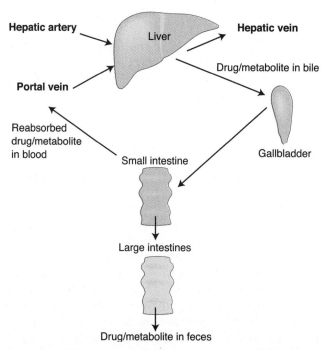

Figure 12.5. The processes of biliary excretion and enterohepatic recycling of drugs and metabolites.

processes of biliary excretion and entero-hepatic recycling of drugs and metabolites. The following is a list of some drugs excreted in the bile:

- Adriamycin
- Vincristine
- Estradiol
- Estriol
- Testosterone
- Digitoxin
- Indomethacin
- Clomiphene

Excretion by Other Organs

Just as drugs are excreted into fluids such as urine in the kidney and bile in the liver, they can be excreted into other fluids as well.

Excretion in Saliva

Several drugs are secreted into saliva made by salivary glands in the mouth. The mechanism for transport of drugs from blood into saliva is passive transcellular diffusion of free (unbound) drug. Salivary secretion is not a significant route of drug excretion because saliva is usually swallowed and enters the gastrointestinal tract. The drug, therefore, can be reabsorbed from the small intestines, resulting in a process of salivary recycling. Drugs that appear in saliva include phenytoin, lithium, digoxin, and salicylates. One application of salivary drug excretion is for routine and noninvasive monitoring of drug levels in patients by measuring concentrations in saliva.

Excretion in Breast Milk

Many drugs pass into the milk of lactating mothers. The primary mechanism of transport is passive diffusion, with some contribution of ion trapping because breast milk has a lower pH (approximately 6.8) compared with blood (7.4).

Thus, weak base drugs tend to be more concentrated in breast milk than in plasma. An illustrative example is erythromycin, which shows concentrations approximately eight times higher in milk than blood. Other examples include heroin, methadone, tetracycline, and diazepam. Some cases of active transport into breast milk have been seen as well. The appearance of high concentrations of drugs in breast milk can have serious consequences for the infant, and nursing mothers are cautioned against the use of drugs during breast-feeding.

Excretion in Sweat

Sweat is a watery fluid produced primarily by glands distributed widely across the skin surface of humans. The primary purpose of sweat production is heat regulation; consequently, the amount of sweat produced is highly dependent on environmental conditions. Several drugs such as amphetamine, cocaine, morphine, and ethanol have been found in sweat. Because the volume of sweat produced is small, excretion in sweat is a possible but not significant mode of drug excretion. However, sweat is being examined as a convenient fluid for detection of illegal drug use.

Excretion in Expired Air

The lung is a major organ of excretion for gaseous and volatile substances, and is a significant route of excretion for volatile drugs such as anesthetics and ethanol. In fact, the Breathalyzer test is based on a measurement of pulmonary excretion of ethanol in expired air. Most organs that excrete drugs eliminate polar compounds more readily than lipophilic compounds. The exception to this premise is the lungs, in which volatility of drug or metabolite is more important than its polarity. Other examples of drugs that appear in expired air are sulfanilamide and sulfapyridine.

KEY CONCEPTS

- Drug excretion is the removal of unchanged drug from plasma.

- The kidney is the main organ for drug excretion, and transfers drug from plasma into urine for elimination.

- Urinary drug (and metabolite) excretion depends on physicochemical properties of the compound, its plasma protein binding, and urine pH.

- Glomerular filtration rate is a measure of kidney function. The GFR of a drug depends on its extent of plasma protein binding.

- Lipophilic, un-ionized compounds can be reabsorbed from the tubules, decreasing their urinary excretion.

- Drugs ionized in plasma are actively secreted into urine; this process is saturable.

- Renal clearance, CL_r, is the efficiency of removal of unchanged drug in urine by the kidneys.

- Drugs are also excreted in bile, and to a lesser extent, in sweat, expired air, saliva, and breast milk. Biliary excretion may result in enterohepatic recycling.

ADDITIONAL READING

1. Shargel L, Yu ABC. Applied Biopharmaceutics and Pharmacokinetics, 4th ed. McGraw-Hill/Appleton & Lange, 1999.

2. Ritschel WA, Kearns GL. Handbook of Basic Pharmacokinetics, 5th ed. American Pharmaceutical Association, 1999.

3. Dipiro JT, Spruill WJ, Blouin RA, Pruemer JM, Hermann J. Concepts in Clinical Pharmacokinetics, 3rd ed. American Hospital Association, 2002.

4. Rowland M, Tozer TN. Clinical Pharmacokinetics: Concepts and Applications, 3rd ed. Lippincott Williams & Wilkins, 1995.

REVIEW QUESTIONS

1. What physicochemical properties favor (1) glomerular filtration, (2) secretion, and (3) reabsorption of drugs in the kidney?

2. Why is secretion the only process that can be competitively inhibited or saturated? What are the consequences of inhibition or saturation?

3. Why can some drugs be excreted in the urine without the need for biotransformation? What types of drugs need to be biotransformed before they can be eliminated?

4. Why does plasma protein binding decrease drug clearance?

5. How can urinary pH be altered to increase the excretion of (1) a weak acid, and (2) a weak base?

6. Why is creatinine clearance a convenient indicator of kidney function?

7. What types of drugs are successfully eliminated in the feces after biliary secretion? What types of drugs undergo enterohepatic recycling?

8. What are the other pathways of drug excretion? Discuss the relative significance of each.

Drug Metabolism

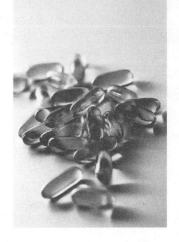

Metabolism or biotransformation is a chemical change in a compound caused by biochemical reactions to give reaction products called *metabolites*. Both terms are found in the literature and are used interchangeably. Do not confuse this type of metabolism with metabolic processes that describe how the body breaks down and uses food.

Biotransformation, along with excretion, is a component of drug elimination. We have seen that polar, water-soluble compounds are readily excreted in urine because of their poor reabsorption from the filtrate in renal tubules. Urinary excretion is also enhanced if the compound is ionized in urine (greater secretion in tubules) and not extensively plasma protein-bound (higher effective glomerular filtration rate [GFR]). Drugs that meet these criteria are excreted largely unchanged in urine. Many drugs, however, are lipophilic and have to be metabolized to some degree before they are excreted.

The primary functions of drug biotransformation reactions are to:

- Make the drug suitable for excretion from the body
- Inactivate the drug to end biological activity

The liver is the primary site of drug bio-transformation. In addition, significant metabolism of some drugs occurs in the gastrointestinal (GI) tract, and to a lesser extent in plasma, lungs, kidney, and skin.

Drugs, Enzymes, and Metabolites

The three major components of a drug bio-transformation reaction are the reactant (drug or *xenobiotic*), product (metabolite), and reaction catalyst (enzyme).

Xenobiotics

When a foreign organism or a macromol-ecule enters the body, our immune system may produce antibodies that interact with and destroy it. However, some foreign molecules called xenobiotics do not trig-ger an antibody response. Instead, the body's numerous enzymes metabolize such foreign molecules and toxins to less-reactive metabolites that can be readily excreted in urine. This method of xenobi-otic detoxification and elimination is very important in handling the variety of for-eign materials to which we are exposed. The body treats drugs as xenobiotics and uses the same enzymes to metabolize and eliminate drugs as quickly as it can.

Metabolites

We have seen that renal excretion is a pri-mary route for removing drugs from the body. The kidney readily excretes polar, water-soluble substances but is much less efficient at excreting lipid-soluble drugs because of their tubular reabsorption. Lipophilic compounds will remain in the body unless they are made polar enough for excretion in urine. Most biotransfor-mation reactions change the chemical structure of drugs to make them polar enough for efficient clearance in urine. Some drugs may already be sufficiently

polar to be excreted unchanged without need for biotransformation. Most drugs, however, are metabolized to some extent before excretion. The role of biotransfor-mation in eliminating a lipophilic drug is shown in Figure 13.1.

Drug metabolites, the products of drug biotransformation reactions, are usually more hydrophilic than the parent drug. Consequently, they are distributed less effectively across capillary endothelia into intracellular water, are less protein-bound, and are less likely to be reabsorbed from the renal tubule. Most metabolites are also less active than the parent drug, so that biotransformation usually results in an end to the drug's biological activity. However, metabolites of a few drugs are pharmacologically active, sometimes even more so than the parent drug. In some cases, the metabolite has a completely dif-ferent biological activity (and toxicity) compared with the parent drug.

Enzymes

Enzymes are biological catalysts involved in many different biochemical pathways. They are cellular proteins that catalyze thermodynamically possible reactions such that the reaction proceeds at a con-trolled rate suitable for the cell's needs. Enzymes change the rate of a reaction without being consumed during the reac-tion, and can speed up reactions by a fac-tor greater than 1,000. In Chapter 6, Drugs and Their Targets, we saw that many cellular enzymes serve as receptors for ligands and drugs. Other enzymes catalyze xenobiotic biotransformation re-actions; these enzymes are found mainly in the liver and to a lesser degree in the intestinal wall, lungs, kidneys, plasma, and skin.

Enzyme Specificity

An important characteristic of enzymes is their degree of *substrate specificity*. Recall that enzyme specificity is the ability of an

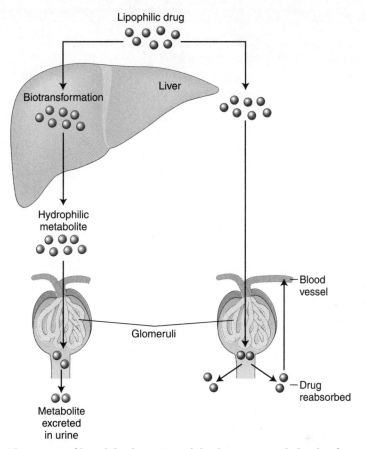

Figure 13.1. Elimination of lipophilic drugs. Lipophilic drugs are metabolized to form relatively more polar metabolites than the parent drug, and these metabolites are thus more easily excreted.

enzyme to bind to substrates with a defined structure while having little or no interaction with other molecules of similar structure. An enzyme binds with substrates of a particular three-dimensional structure because of the conformation of the active site. Enzymes are commonly classified based on the type of reaction catalyzed, as shown in Table 13.1.

Many drug-metabolizing enzymes exhibit broad substrate specificity in that a given enzyme can metabolize a variety of chemically different compounds. Other enzymes show group specificity; that is, a large group of similar compounds (e.g., primary amines) may serve as substrates for the enzyme. The biotransformation of a drug may proceed via more than one reaction, each catalyzed by different enzymes, resulting in several metabolites of the drug.

Because many endogenous substrates are chiral, it follows that stereochemical factors play an important role in the action of enzymes. Some metabolizing enzymes may demonstrate stereospecificity in which one stereoisomer of the drug is metabolized more rapidly than, or to the exclusion of, others.

Kinetics of Drug Metabolism

Enzyme-catalyzed reactions are governed by Michaelis–Menten kinetics, discussed in Chapter 4, Rates of Pharmaceutical Processes. The rate of biotransformation

	TABLE 13.1. Classification of Important Enzymes	
Class	*Reaction catalyzed*	*Names*
Hydrolases	Hydrolysis of substrate	Esterase Peptidase Glycosidase
Ligases	Bond formation	Carboxylase Synthetase
Transferases	Transfer of group between molecules	Aminotransferase Phosphorylase
Lyases	Elimination and addition reactions	Decarboxylase Aldolase
Isomerases	Rearrangement reactions	Racemase *cis-trans* isomerase
Oxidoreductases	Oxidation or reduction	Oxidase Reductase Dehydrogenase

of a substrate by an enzyme is given by the *Michaelis–Menten* equation:

$$V = \frac{V_{max}[S]}{K_m + [S]} \quad \text{(Eq. 13.1)}$$

where [S] is the concentration of the substrate (drug), V_{max} is the maximum rate of metabolism, and K_m is the Michaelis constant. V_{max} depends on the concentration of enzyme available and $1/K_m$ is a measure of the *affinity* between drug (substrate) and enzyme.

The exact concentration of drug at the site of metabolism is not known. However, because blood circulation carries drug to this site, it is reasonable to assume that [S] is equal to drug plasma concentration $[C_p]$, which is readily measured by taking blood samples. In this situation, the Michaelis–Menten equation can be written as:

$$V = \frac{V_{max}[C_p]}{K_m + [C_p]} \quad \text{(Eq. 13.2)}$$

When plasma drug concentration is low, $[C] << K_m$, and Equation 13.2 simplifies to:

$$V = \frac{V_{max}}{K_m}[C_p] = k_m[C_p] \quad \text{(Eq. 13.3)}$$

where k_m is called the *apparent metabolic rate constant* given by V_{max}/K_m. Thus, at low plasma concentrations of drug, the rate of biotransformation is directly proportional to plasma drug concentration and can be described as a first-order process.

If plasma drug concentration is high such that $[C_p] >> K_m$, the rate of biotransformation becomes:

$$V = \frac{V_{max}[C_p]}{[C_p]} = V_{max} \quad \text{(Eq. 13.4)}$$

In other words, the rate reaches the maximum that the amount of enzyme available can handle; the enzyme is *saturated*. The rate of biotransformation is now independent of drug concentration, a characteristic of a zero-order process. This means any additional amount of drug will not be metabolized until some enzyme molecules become available. Such situations could result in accumulation of drug and higher plasma concentrations than expected.

The therapeutic doses of most drugs are such that plasma concentrations remain below saturation levels of the metabolizing enzyme systems. However, saturation of metabolizing enzymes can occur under certain circumstances.

Biotransformation Reactions

Biotransformation pathways are commonly divided into two major groups based on the type of reaction:

- Phase I (*nonsynthetic*) reactions, in which small chemical changes occur in one or more functional groups of drug.
- Phase II (*synthetic* or *conjugation*) reactions, in which a molecule provided by the body is added to the drug.

Phase I reactions introduce or expose a *reactive functional group* on the drug molecule and often precede phase II reactions. Phase I reactions are considered nonsynthetic because only minor changes occur in drug structure. These reactions prepare the drug for subsequent phase II processes in which an endogenous molecule is conjugated with the reactive functional group on the drug.

The main types of phase I reactions are oxidation, reduction, and hydrolysis, which introduce one of the following easily conjugated reactive groups onto the drug:

- hydroxyl (–OH)
- amino (–NH$_2$)
- carboxyl (–COOH)
- sulfhydryl (–SH)

Phase II pathways are called synthetic or conjugation reactions because, commonly, a highly polar molecule or group provided by the body becomes attached or *conjugated* to the reactive group on the drug. The conjugation reaction results in formation of a polar, water-soluble metabolite that can be readily excreted in urine. An illustration of an enzyme catalyzing the reaction between two substrates (one of which could be the drug) is shown in Figure 13.2.

Drugs that already possess one or more reactive groups can be directly metabolized by phase II conjugation without necessity of a phase I process. A drug that does not have a reactive group must first undergo a phase I reaction to unmask or introduce such a group on the molecule. The phase I derivative then undergoes a phase II conjugation to make it suitable for excretion.

A phase I reaction itself may make the drug sufficiently polar to be excreted without subsequent phase II conjugation. In many cases, a drug may experience all the above events, in which case urine will contain some unchanged drug as well as some phase I and phase II metabolites. Figure 13.3 illustrates phase I and phase II reactions and their relationship to excreted metabolites.

Phase I Reactions

A drug may undergo more than one phase I reaction leading to several phase I derivatives. Phase I reactions typically result in a relatively small increase in hydrophilicity of the drug. Although this

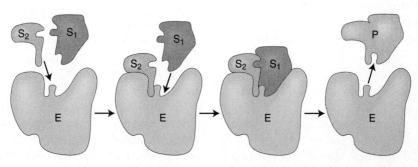

Figure 13.2. An enzyme (E) catalyzing a reaction between two substrates (S$_1$ and S$_2$) to form the product (P).

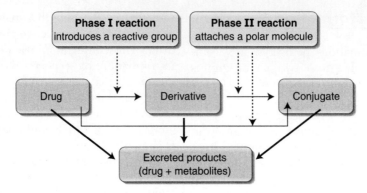

Figure 13.3. Scheme showing the phases of drug biotransformation reactions.

modest structural change usually causes most drugs to lose their intended biological activity, the reaction may activate certain drugs or modify their activity. Drugs that are inactive or have very low activity before biotransformation but are activated after a phase I reaction are called prodrugs. We will discuss prodrugs later in the chapter.

The major types of phase I reactions are:

- Oxidation
- Reduction
- Hydrolysis

Oxidation

Oxidation is the most common type of biotransformation reaction because there are many different ways in which drug molecules can be oxidized, and abundant enzymes to catalyze oxidations. Most oxidations take place in the smooth endoplasmic reticulum (SER) of cells in metabolizing organs such as the liver and intestines.

Microsomal Enzymes. When metabolizing cells are isolated and homogenized during laboratory experiments, the SER becomes fragmented and forms structures called *microsomes*. Although microsomes do not exist in intact cells, enzymes contained in SER are often called microsomal enzymes. These enzymes are capable of metabolizing a wide variety of xenobiotics, particularly lipophilic compounds. Oxidation reactions catalyzed by microsomal enzymes are shown in Figure 13.4.

The Cytochrome P-450 System. Widely distributed microsomal enzymes, specifically a group called the *mixed-function oxidases* (MFOs), catalyze most oxidations. The most important MFO system is the cytochrome P-450 (abbreviated as CYP, CYP450, or P450) superfamily of enzymes, which is subdivided into families and subfamilies based on amino acid sequences. CYP proteins have molecular weights in the range of 45,000 to 60,000.

CYP Nomenclature. Nomenclature of CYP enzymes is based on their amino acid sequence rather than on function. *Families* are CYP enzymes with at least 40% homology in their amino acid sequences and are indicated by Arabic numerals after the CYP root, as in CYP1, CYP2, CYP3, and so forth. Within a family, *subfamilies* have greater than 60% homology in their amino acid sequences and are indicated by a letter after the family designation, e.g., CYP1A, CYP2B, CYP3A, and so on. Arabic numerals are added sequentially when more than one enzyme within a subfamily has been identified, e.g., CYP1A2, CYP2B6, CYP3A4, and so on. These are known as *isoenzymes* or

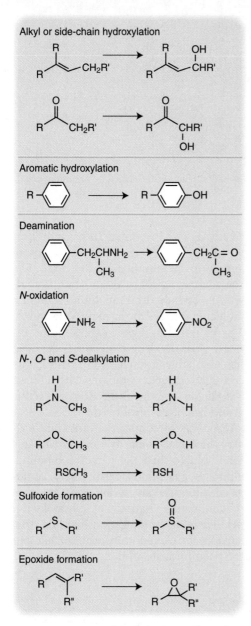

Figure 13.4. Examples of phase I oxidative biotransformation reactions catalyzed by microsomal enzyme systems, particularly cytochrome P-450.

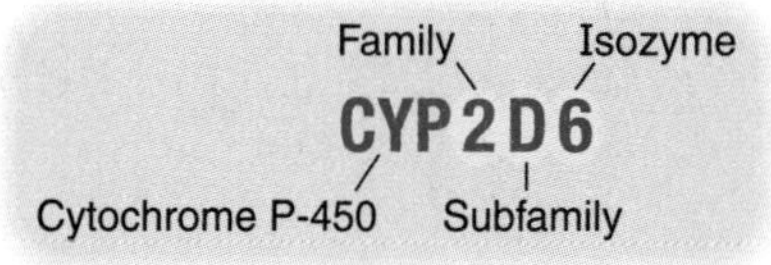

Family   Isozyme

CYP 2 D 6

Cytochrome P-450   Subfamily

Figure 13.5. Nomenclature of cytochrome P-450 (CYP) enzymes.

isozymes. A simple way to understand the nomenclature is shown in Figure 13.5. Genes that code for CYP enzymes are named similarly but are usually designated in italics as in *CYP1A2*, *CYP3A4*, and so forth. To date 12 *CYP* gene families and 50 functional *CYP* genes have been identified in humans.

CYP enzymes have numerous physiological roles, one of them being xenobiotic biotransformation. The majority of drug biotransformation reactions are catalyzed by only three families, CYP1, CYP2, and CYP3. At least 50 different CYP isozymes in these families have been identified, with different specificities for different types of drugs. However, of these, only seven CYP isozymes (CYP1A2, CYP2B6, CYP2C9, CYP2C19, CYP2D6, CYP2E1, and CYP3A4) are known to catalyze the oxidation of more than 90% of drugs.

Nonmicrosomal Enzymes. Nonmicrosomal enzymes present in mitochondrial and soluble fractions of tissues can also catalyze oxidations. These types of reactions are generally dehydrogenations followed by addition of oxygen or water. Oxidation reactions catalyzed by nonmicrosomal enzymes are shown in Figure 13.6.

Reduction

Reduction is a relatively uncommon pathway of drug biotransformation, although it may be important for a few drugs. In general, reduction involves either adding hydrogen, e.g., across a $-CO$ double bond, or removing oxygen and adding hydrogen, e.g., converting $-NO_2$ to $-NH_2$. These reactions introduce hydroxyl and amino groups that are readily susceptible to phase II conjugations.

Reductions occur in the liver and in the lumen of the lower intestines. Anaerobic intestinal bacteria carry out many reductions in the lower intestines, so some drugs may be metabolized even before they can be absorbed. Examples of phase I reductions are shown in Figure 13.7.

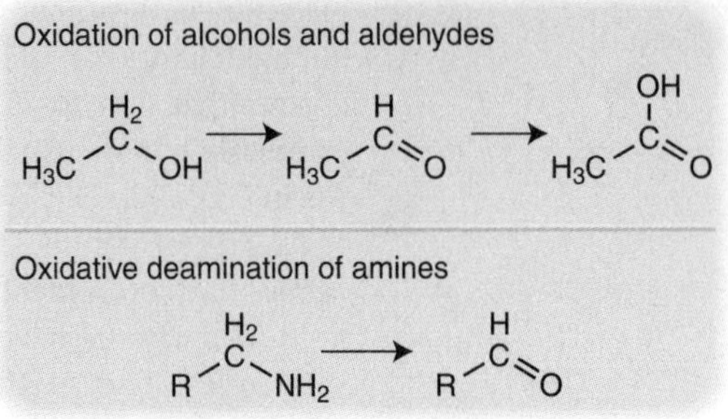

Oxidation of alcohols and aldehydes

Oxidative deamination of amines

Figure 13.6. Examples of phase I oxidative biotransformation reactions catalyzed by nonmicrosomal enzyme systems.

Hydrolysis

Hydrolysis is a common pathway of biotransformation, particularly for esters and some amides. *Esterases* (enzymes that hydrolyze esters) are found in the GI tract, plasma, liver, and many other tissues, and are primarily nonmicrosomal. The hydrolysis of an ester yields an alcohol and a carboxylic acid. *Amidases* (enzymes that hydrolyze amides) are found mainly in the liver and are also nonmicrosomal; hydrolysis of an amide gives an amine and a carboxylic acid. Examples of phase I hydrolysis reactions are shown in Figure 13.8.

Phase II Reactions

Phase II or conjugation reactions involve combination of the drug (or phase I de-

rivative) with a conjugating agent provided by the body. They also require energy to be supplied by the body. The *conjugating agent* is often (but not always) a carbohydrate, an amino acid, or a molecule derived from these substances. The conjugating agent can combine directly with the drug molecule if the drug has a suitable reactive group. If not, the conjugating agent combines with a phase I derivative of the drug after a reactive group has been introduced.

Products of conjugation are almost always biologically inactive and usually less lipid soluble than the parent compound, although exceptions exist. Many conjugated products are weak acids that are predominantly ionized at physiological pH. Therefore, conjugation makes a drug suitable for excretion in urine or bile but too polar for reabsorption.

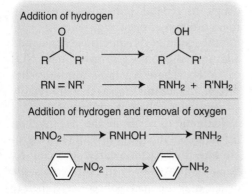

Figure 13.7. Examples of phase I reduction reactions.

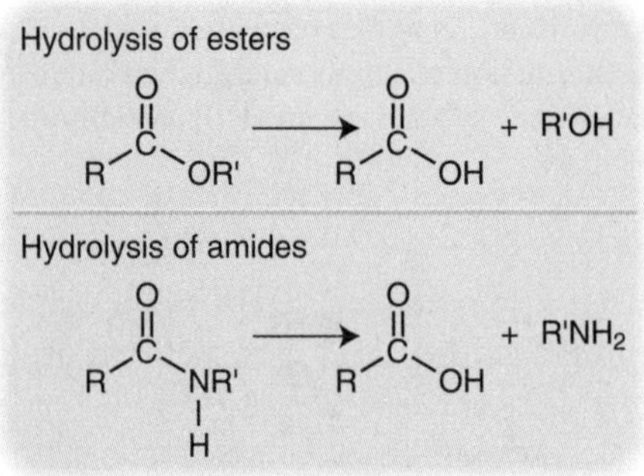

Figure 13.8. Examples of phase I hydrolysis reactions.

CYP3A4

Isozymes of the CYP3A subfamily are the most abundant CYP enzymes in humans. This subfamily comprises two genes expressed in adults, *CYP3A4* and *CYP3A5*, and a third, *CYP3A7*, expressed only during fetal life. Whereas CYP3A5 isozyme plays only a minor role in drug metabolism, CYP3A4 is arguably the single most important drug-metabolizing P450, metabolizing around 60% of current drugs to some extent. CYP3A4 is also the predominant P450 in human liver, where it comprises up to 60% of total P450, and is also the major P450 isozyme expressed in the human intestine. Some drugs metabolized by CYP3A4 are listed below.

CYP3A4 activity varies considerably between individuals and may be increased by a several drugs, including rifampicin, phenobarbital, macrolide antibiotics, and steroids. The repeated observation of wide interindividual variability in CYP3A4 activity has prompted close scrutiny of the *CYP3A4* gene.

Amitriptyline (Elavil)	Benzodiazepines
Alprazolam (Xanax)	Triazolam (Halcion)
Midazolam (Versed)	Calcium blockers
Carbamazepine (Tegretol)	Cisapride (Propulsid)
Dexamethasone (Decadron)	Erythromycin
Ethinyl estradiol (Estraderm, Estrace)	Glyburide (Glynase, Micronase)
	Ketoconazole (Nizoral)
Imipramine (Tofranil)	Nefazodone (Serzone)
Lovastatin (Mevacor)	Astemizole (Hismanal)
Terfenadine (Seldane-D)	Sertraline (Zoloft)
Verapamil (Calan, Isoptin)	Theophylline
Testosterone	Ritonavir (Norvir)
Venlafaxine (Effexor)	Indinavir (Crixivan)
Saquinavir (Invirase)	
Nelfinavir (Viracept)	

Just as a drug may undergo more than one type of phase I reaction, it may also undergo more than one type of phase II reaction. The outcome is an array of metabolites excreted in urine and feces.

There are six types of conjugation reactions important in the biotransformation of drugs:

- Glucuronidation
- Sulfation
- Amino acid conjugation
- Acetylation
- Glutathione conjugation
- Methylation

Glucuronidation

Glucuronidation, also called glucuronide conjugation, is the most common phase II reaction and accounts for most conjugated metabolites seen in the urine. The conjugating agent is *glucuronic acid* in its activated form of *uridine diphosphate glucuronic acid* (UDPGA)(see Figure 13.9).

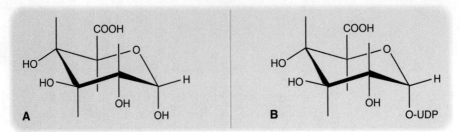

Figure 13.9. **A.** Structure of glucoronic acid (GA). **B.** Structure of uridine diphosphate glucoronic acid (UDPGA).

The drug or phase I derivative reacts with UDPGA by displacing and taking the place of UDP. Glucuronidation is catalyzed by the microsomal enzyme *UDP-glucuronosyltransferase*. The products (called glucuronides) are polar weak acids (as a result of the carboxylic group of GA) that are highly ionized (anionic) at physiological pH and readily excreted in urine and bile.

Glucuronic acid is derived from glucose and is therefore available in ample supply in the body. This is one reason for the predominance of glucuronidation over other conjugation reactions. Another reason is that UDPGA is not selective and can combine with drug molecules containing any reactive group (such as amino, carboxyl, hydroxyl, or sulfhydryl). Figure 13.10 shows examples of common glucuronidation reactions.

Sulfation

Conjugation with a sulfate group is a common phase II pathway for aromatic hydroxy compounds, such as phenols and catechols, and some amines; it occurs to a lesser extent with aliphatic alcohols.

The sulfate group (from sulfur-containing amino acids such as cysteine) combines enzymatically with ATP to convert to its active form, 3'-phosphoadenosine-5'-phosphosulfate (PAPS). PAPS then combines with the drug or its phase I derivative to form the sulfate conjugate (see Figure 13.11).

The reaction is catalyzed by *sulfotransferases* found in the liver, small intestine,

brain, and kidney. The highly ionizable sulfate group makes sulfate conjugates water-soluble and readily cleared in urine and sometimes in bile.

In general, sulfate conjugation occurs less frequently than glucuronidation presumably because of the limited supply of inorganic sulfate and fewer functional groups that can undergo this reaction. The limited supply of sulfate in the body can be exhausted during metabolism.

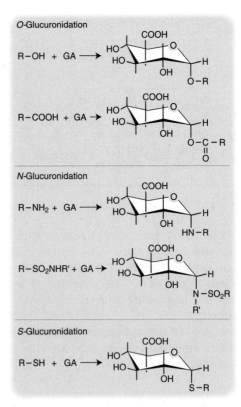

Figure 13.10. Examples of phase II glucuronidation reactions.

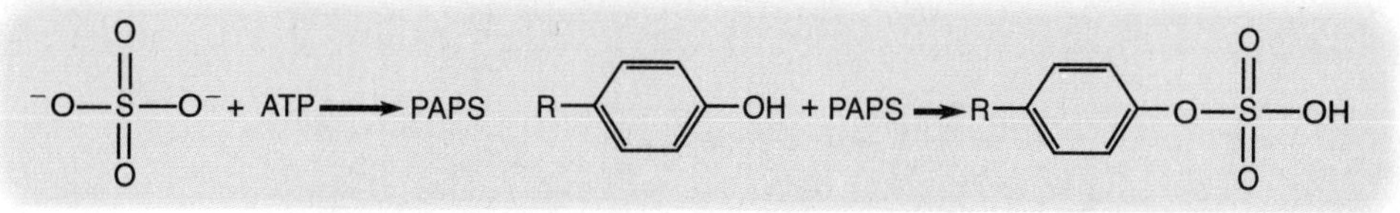

Figure 13.11. The process of sulfate conjugation. PAPS, generated from a sulfur-containing amino acid and ATP, reacts with the drug or a phase I derivative to form the sulfate conjugate.

When sulfate becomes depleted, other conjugation reactions like glucuronidation usually take over.

Amino Acid Conjugation

Many endogenous amino acids (typically glycine and glutamine) can act as conjugating agents, reacting with compounds containing a carboxylic acid group (see Figure 13.12).

The carboxylic acids have to be first activated by combining with ATP, and then converted to form coenzyme A (CoA) thioester derivatives. This step is catalyzed by *acyl CoA synthetases*.

These CoA derivatives are then conjugated with glycine or glutamine, forming a peptide or amide bond between the drug and amino acid. The reaction is catalyzed by N-*acyltransferases* (see Figure 13.13).

Amino acid conjugates are more water-soluble than the original carboxylic acid drug and are readily excreted in urine and bile.

Acetylation

Primary alkyl and aromatic amines can be conjugated with acetic acid to form the corresponding acetyl conjugate. The reaction involves the transfer of an acetyl group (in its activated form, *acetyl coenzyme A*) to the drug, and is catalyzed by *acetyltransferases* (see Figure 13.14).

Acetylation occurs primarily in the liver. Although most conjugation reactions yield soluble metabolites, acetylation often gives conjugated metabolites less water-soluble than the parent because it converts an ionizable amine into a non-ionizable amide. Nevertheless, acetylation

does serve to further deactivate the drug. Because many amine-containing drugs bind to their receptors in cationic conjugate acid form, losing the ability to take on a proton at physiological pH results in a loss of affinity for targets, leading to a loss of biological activity.

Glutathione Conjugation

Glutathione conjugation is a nonspecific reaction involving the combination of an electrophilic compound with the tripeptide glutathione (GSH), found in almost all tissues (see Figure 13.15).

The electrophilic compound combines with the sulfhydryl (−SH) group of GSH to give a thioether conjugate; the reaction is catalyzed by *glutathione S-transferase* in nonmicrosomal fractions of the liver. A wide range of functional groups form thioether conjugates of GSH. Glutathione conjugates are rarely excreted in urine because of their large molecular weight, but may be excreted in bile. They are generally further metabolized to other

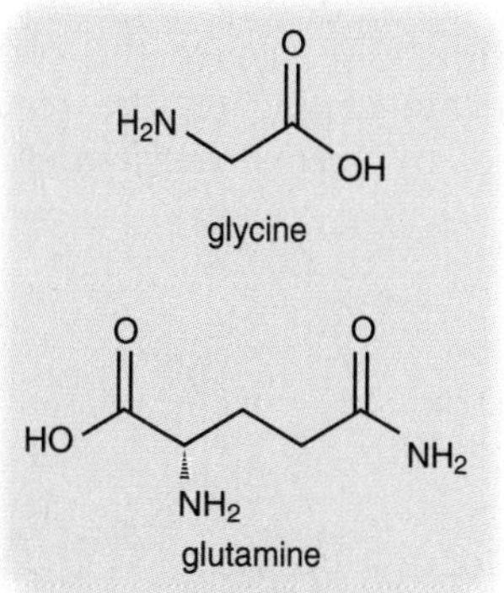

Figure 13.12. Typical amino acids (glycine and glutamine) involved in amino acid conjugation.

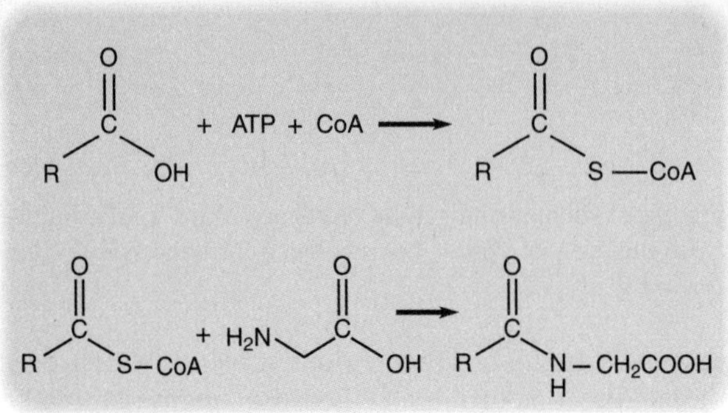

Figure 13.13. The process of amino acid conjugation. A carboxylic acid group on the drug or phase I derivative is first activated to form a CoA thioester, which then conjugates with glycine or glutamine to give the amino acid conjugate.

derivatives. Glutathione stores in cells can become quickly exhausted, leading to accumulation of the starting phase I derivatives in the body.

Methylation

O- and N-methylation (addition of a $-CH_3$ group) is an important biochemical pathway for synthesis and metabolism of endogenous compounds but is of only minor importance in drug biotransformation. Nevertheless, some drugs such as epinephrine and isoproterenol are readily methylated, accounting for their short duration of action (see Figure 13.16).

The methyl group comes from the amino acid methionine, which is first activated to S-adenosylmethionine (SAM). The compound to be metabolized (such as an alcohol, phenol, or amine) combines with SAM to give the corresponding methyl conjugate; the reaction is catalyzed by methyltransferases. Meth-

ylation, like acetylation, results in conjugates less polar than the original compound.

Sites of Biotransformation

Enzymes capable of metabolizing drugs are present in cells of most tissues and organs. However, significant metabolism occurs only in organs that contain high concentrations of enzymes, receive a large fraction of administered drug, and are structurally designed to maximize these reactions.

The liver, because of its structure and location, is the most important organ for drug biotransformation. It has an abundance of microsomal enzymes, particularly the CYP superfamily. We will discuss the liver in detail below, and then follow with a discussion of other metabolizing organs and tissues.

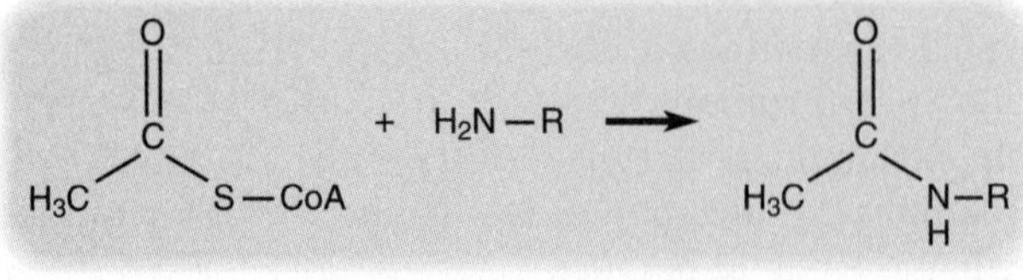

Figure 13.14. The process of acetylation. Acetyl CoA reacts with an amine drug or phase I derivative to give the acetyl conjugate of the drug.

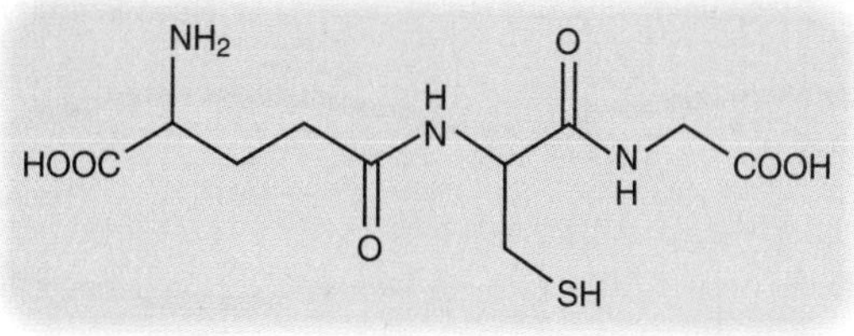

Figure 13.15. Structure of glutathione.

Biotransformation in the Liver

The liver has varied and complex functions involving metabolic and synthetic processes. It also has secretory and excretory functions, such as the production of bile, that provide a pathway for biliary excretion of drugs.

Liver Structure and Function

Blood enters the liver through two major blood vessels—the *hepatic artery* carrying arterial blood and the *portal vein* coming directly from the GI tract. The liver receives approximately 30% of resting cardiac output and is therefore a very vascular organ. The hepatic vascular system is dynamic, meaning it has considerable ability to both store and release blood, and can be thought of as a reservoir within the general circulation. The hepatic artery carries oxygen to the liver and is responsible for about 25% of liver blood supply. The portal vein carries nutrients to the liver and accounts for 75% of blood flow to the liver. Thus, drugs absorbed from the GI tract into the bloodstream have to first pass through the

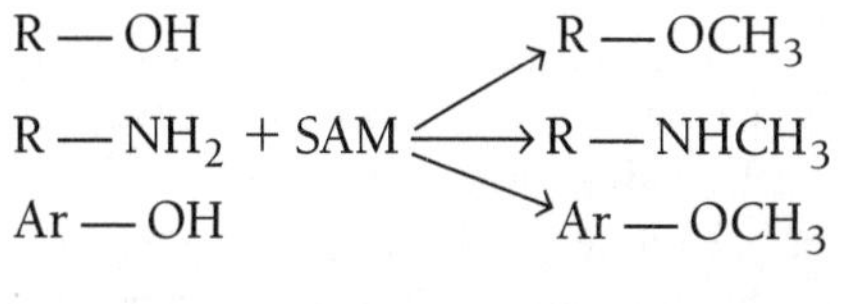

Figure 13.16. The process of methylation. The methyl group comes from activated methionine (SAM), which reacts with the drug or phase I derivative (an alcohol, phenol or amine) to give the corresponding methyl conjugate.

liver before entering the general circulation. Circulation of blood among these organs is illustrated in Figure 13.17.

The functional hepatic unit is the *liver lobule* illustrated in Figure 13.18; a human liver contains about a million such lobules. Each lobule consists of liver cells (hepatocytes) arranged in plates that radiate out from the central vein, which carries blood out of the liver. Liver capillaries called sinusoids containing blood from both the portal vein and hepatic artery separate the plates from one another. The region between the sinusoids and hepatocytes is known as the *space of Disse*. Hepatocytes have *microvilli* that enter the space of Disse, maximizing the surface area of contact between blood and hepatic cells.

The endothelium of liver sinusoids permits free transport of solutes, including proteins and protein-bound substrates, from the sinusoid to the space of Disse. Sinusoidal junctions average 175 nm in diameter and occupy approximately 6 to 8% of the sinusoidal surface area. There is no basal lamina, allowing free passage of macromolecules up to medium-sized chylomicrons. This feature explains why the liver can metabolize a variety of tightly protein-bound xenobiotics.

Thus, drugs and other molecules in the portal and systemic circulations come into close contact with hepatocytes. Lipophilic drugs are readily transported into hepatocytes by transcellular diffusion. Polar or ionized drugs have a more difficult time entering the hepatocyte and may require carrier-mediated processes

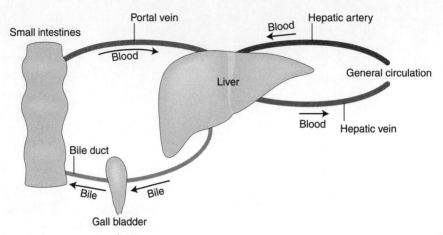

Figure 13.17. Diagram showing movement of blood among the small intestines, liver, and general circulation, and movement of bile from the liver to the small intestines via the gall bladder.

and specific transporters. Several transporters are present in hepatocytes to transport substrates in and allow efflux of other substances, including products of metabolism, out.

A secretory function of hepatocytes is to produce and filter *bile,* a fluid consisting of bile salts, cholesterol, lecithin, and fatty acids. Bile salts are an important component of lipid digestion in the intestines; they help to emulsify fat droplets contained in food to facilitate digestion by intestinal enzymes. Bile also serves an excretory role; bilirubin, an end product of hemoglobin degradation, is actively absorbed from blood by hepatocytes and secreted into canaliculi with bile salts. Drugs and their metabolites may also be excreted in bile.

Blood eventually leaves the liver via the hepatic vein, which empties into the vena cava, carrying drug and its metabolites to the general circulation.

Hepatic Clearance

The concept of clearance can be applied to elimination of a drug by biotransformation in the liver. Hepatic clearance, CL_h, is defined as the volume of plasma flowing through the liver that is completely cleared of drug per unit time. Factors affecting hepatic clearance of a drug are:

- Extraction ratio of the drug
- Blood flow to the liver

Hepatic Extraction Ratio. Consider a drug administered by intravenous injection. As the drug distributes in the systemic circulation and enters the liver via the hepatic artery, a portion of it is removed by metabolism or biliary excretion. Therefore, the drug concentration in blood leaving the liver via the hepatic vein is less than the arterial concentration that entered the liver. The hepatic extraction ratio (ER_h) is defined as the fraction of the drug removed from blood by the liver in one pass:

$$ER_h = \frac{C_a - C_v}{C_a} \quad \text{(Eq. 13.5)}$$

where C_a and C_v are drug concentrations in the hepatic artery and vein, respectively. ER_h values range from 0 to 1.0. An ER_h of 0.2 means 20% of the drug was removed by the liver in one pass. The hepatic extraction ratio depends on the inherent ability of liver enzymes to metabolize drug and is related to V_{max} and K_m of the metabolizing enzymes.

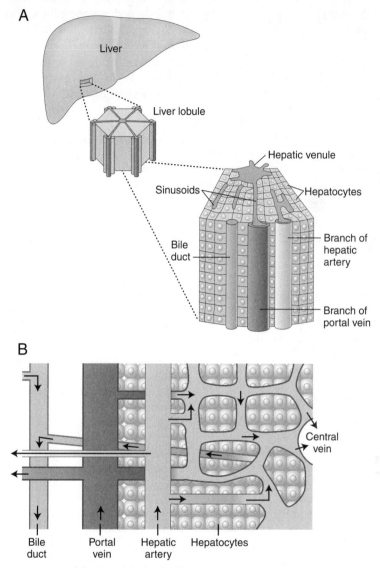

Figure 13.18. Diagram of the liver lobule, the functional unit of the liver (**A**), showing blood flow through sinusoids (**B**).

Liver Blood Flow. It is apparent that drug can be metabolized in the liver only as fast as drug is delivered to the liver by blood. If blood flow to the liver is expressed as Q (mL/min or L/hr), hepatic clearance is given by:

$$CL_h = Q \cdot ER_h \qquad \text{(Eq. 13.6)}$$

For drugs with a high ER_h (>0.7), the liver can remove drug almost as fast as the blood flows through the liver. Thus, changes in liver blood flow can change hepatic clearance of such drugs significantly. If blood flow increases, hepatic clearance increases.

On the other hand, drugs with low ER_h values (<0.2) are less affected by changes in Q than are drugs with high ER_h values. Hepatic clearance of low ER_h drugs depends primarily on efficiency of the enzyme system in catalyzing the biotransformation reaction.

Biotransformation in Other Organs

CYP and other metabolizing enzymes are found in epithelial cells lining the intestinal tract, lung, kidney, brain, skin, and nasal tissue. Significant metabolism of some drugs may occur in one or more of these locations. A clearance and extraction ratio can be defined for each of these sites of biotransformation. Biotransformation in these organs becomes particularly important when drug is administered via the particular organ, such as during nasal, inhalation, or dermal delivery.

Presystemic Biotransformation

The entire dose of a drug administered intravenously enters the systemic circulation. When drugs are given by other routes, however, only a portion of the administered dose may reach the systemic circulation because of biotransformation during absorption and entry into the circulation. This phenomenon, in which a drug is metabolized before it can distribute in the systemic circulation, is called presystemic biotransformation. Epithelial cells of the GI tract and nasal and pulmonary mucosa are capable of metabolizing a wide variety of drugs during absorption. When administered orally, a drug may also undergo significant biotransformation in the liver before entering the systemic circulation.

First-Pass Metabolism

The pattern of blood flow to the liver via the portal vein is such that all orally administered drugs must first pass through the liver after absorption before entering the systemic circulation. If the liver rapidly and efficiently metabolizes the drug during this first passage, then very little drug reaches the general circulation. This phenomenon is called hepatic first-pass me-

tabolism and is significant for drugs with a high hepatic extraction ratio ($E_h > 0.7$). Drugs prone to this effect and with inactive metabolites are usually unsuitable for oral administration and have to be administered by another route.

Gut Wall Metabolism

The intestinal mucosa (*gut wall*) is important in biotransformation of orally administered drugs prone to phase I microsomal oxidation and phase II glucuronidation or sulfation. The highest concentration of intestinal CYP enzymes is found in the duodenum with a gradual decrease further down the intestinal tract. Presystemic metabolism by the intestinal epithelium is often greater than liver metabolism for some drugs and seriously limits the amount of parent drug absorbed into the circulation. For such drugs, oral administration may not be appropriate and an alternative route may be necessary.

Presystemic Metabolism in Other Organs

The lungs have been examined as another tissue in which measurable presystemic metabolism can occur. The lungs are extremely well perfused for purposes of respiration, and blood moves through the lungs rapidly. Thus, even a small amount of metabolic activity in the lungs could play an important role in overall biotransformation of a drug administered by inhalation.

Total Clearance

A drug can be eliminated from the body by excretion of unchanged drug in urine and bile or by biotransformation to metabolites in the liver and in other organs. All these pathways contribute to the total clearance of drug from plasma.

The total clearance is given by the sum of individual clearances:

$$CL_{total} = CL_{renal} + CL_{biliary} + CL_{hepatic} + CL_{other} \quad \text{(Eq. 13.7)}$$

Factors Affecting Biotransformation

Metabolizing enzymes are continually produced and decomposed in the body. The rates of these processes are equal under normal conditions, keeping enzyme concentrations constant. However, changes in enzyme levels can alter the rate of metabolism and consequently result in higher or lower drug plasma concentrations than expected. If left uncorrected, this can lead to increased side effects or failure of therapy. Consider some general situations that alter biotransformation rates of drugs.

Enzyme Inhibition

If a substance interferes with the ability of an enzyme to bind to its substrate, the affinity between the enzyme and substrate decreases, causing an increase in K_m and a consequent decrease in rate of metabolism. The interfering substance is called an **enzyme inhibitor**. Enzyme inhibition is also a mechanism by which some drugs produce their pharmacological effect, as we will see in Chapter 16, Mechanisms of Drug Action. An inhibitor of a metabolic enzyme can be another drug, a drug metabolite, or even a food substance. There are two types of enzyme inhibition: competitive and noncompetitive.

Competitive Inhibition

An enzyme inhibitor is said to be *competitive* if it is:

- also a substrate for the enzyme
- not a substrate for the enzyme, but combines reversibly with the enzyme

Most competitive inhibitors have structures similar to that of the drug whose metabolism they are inhibiting and therefore bind at the same active site of the enzyme. Thus, inhibitor and substrate compete for the same binding site and the same quantity of enzyme. The result is that the concentration of enzyme available for the substrate is decreased, and so is the biotransformation rate of the substrate.

The inhibitor may be a substrate itself, in which case it is metabolized by the enzyme. If the inhibitor is not a substrate for the enzyme, it merely occupies the active site in a reversible fashion. Both processes are reversible because the inhibitor can dissociate from the enzyme.

The degree of competitive inhibition depends on relative affinities of substrate and inhibitor for the active site, and on the relative concentrations of the inhibitor and substrate. If the inhibitor concentration is very large compared with substrate concentration, the inhibitor will occupy almost all the active sites and the substrate will not be metabolized. Conversely, if substrate concentration is made large enough, it will be able to compete with and displace the inhibitor from the active site. Thus, competitive inhibition is less pronounced at high substrate concentrations.

Many drugs biotransformed by the same metabolic enzymes behave as competitive inhibitors of one another. This is a particular problem for drugs oxidized by CYP enzymes because a few isozymes are responsible for biotransformation of many different drugs. Foods and endogenous substrates can also competitively inhibit the biotransformation of drugs.

Noncompetitive Inhibition

Compounds significantly different in structure from the substrate can also act as inhibitors. In this case, the inhibitor binds to the enzyme not at the active site but at another *allosteric* site. This inhibitor–enzyme binding causes a change in conformation of the enzyme active site such that

Prodrugs

A prodrug is a pharmacologically inactive compound that is converted to an active drug by a biotransformation reaction. The prodrug is usually a structural derivative of the active drug, synthesized by modifying a functional group or groups (the *promoiety*) on the drug molecule. A popular approach to prodrug design involves using a hydrolysis reaction to release active drug. In particular, the ester is the most common prodrug form of drugs containing hydroxyl or carboxylic functional groups. Esterases found in almost all tissues make conversion of prodrug to drug very facile. Esters can be synthesized fairly easily with desired degrees of lipophilicity or hydrophilicity, and with controlled rates of the activating hydrolytic reaction.

There are many reasons for which one may wish to administer a prodrug instead of active drug. Some typical situations arise when the drug is too polar for effective oral absorption, or for penetration into the site of action such as the brain. In such cases, a functional group that enhances membrane transport is attached to the drug. After absorption or distribution to the site of action has occurred, the group is metabolically cleaved, releasing active drug. For example, L-dopa is an amino acid prodrug actively transported across the blood–brain barrier and metabolized to dopamine in the brain (see Box Figure 13.1).

Another example is *enalaprilat,* the active drug that is highly ionized in the

Box Figure 13.1. Structures of L-DOPA (prodrug) and dopamine (active drug).

GI tract and poorly absorbed after oral administration. Converting one of the carboxylic groups to an ester (*enalapril*) reduces ionization and improves oral absorption by passive diffusion. An active transport system in the intestines may also be partially responsible for the absorption of the ester prodrug (see Box Figure 13.2).

Other reasons for synthesizing prodrugs are poor stability or poor patient acceptability of the active drug (taste, odor, gastric irritation, pain on injection, and so forth), or a desire to extend the half-life of the drug in the body.

Box Figure 13.2. Structures of enalapril (prodrug) and enalaprilat (active drug).

the substrate can no longer bind to it. This is called noncompetitive inhibition because the substrate cannot compete with and displace inhibitor at any concentration. Noncompetitive inhibition can be reversible, in which inhibitor will dissociate from the enzyme, or irreversible, in which inhibitor will remain bound to the enzyme for the life of the enzyme molecule.

Although inhibition of biotransformation of drugs is generally regarded as undesirable and potentially dangerous, it can sometimes be exploited to improve therapy. If a drug is prone to very rapid metabolism resulting in low plasma levels, metabolism can be intentionally slowed down by simultaneously giving a metabolic inhibitor of the drug.

Enzyme Induction

Some enzymes involved in biotransformation have a unique characteristic; their ability to metabolize drugs can be increased or stimulated by certain substances called enzyme inducers. It is believed inducers increase production rate of the metabolizing enzyme so more enzyme is available for biotransformation.

One type of enzyme induction is *self-induction,* in which a drug stimulates its own metabolism. Continued dosing of a self-inducing drug usually results in progressively decreasing plasma levels, therapeutic activity, and side effects. However, if the metabolites are active or toxic, observed pharmacological activity and side effects may actually increase.

Many drugs, pesticides, herbicides, and food components have been shown to induce their own biotransformation or that of other drugs. The effect of enzyme induction can persist for some time after the inducer is eliminated from the body, because enzyme levels remain high until

TABLE 13.2. Common Substances Involved in Induction of Metabolic Enzymes	
Prescription	*Nonprescription*
Carbamazepine	Chronic cigarette smoking
Dexamethasone	Chronic ethanol use
Isoniazid	Chronic marijuana smoking
Modafinil	St. John's wort
Omeprazole	
Oxcarbazepine	
Phenobarbital	
Phenytoin	
Prednisone	
Primidone	
Rifampin	

the enzyme is decomposed through natural processes. Common agents involved in metabolic enzyme induction are shown in Table 13.2.

Genetic Variability

Genetic factors contribute significantly to interindividual variability in drug metabolism. Genes and gene products regulate all enzymes involved in drug biotransformation. Evolutionary and environmental influences have resulted in significant variations in these genes throughout the population. Mutations in a gene can result in enzyme variants with higher, lower, or no activity compared with the norm, with higher or lower levels of enzymes, or with no enzyme at all in certain individuals. It is not unusual to find a tenfold difference in rates of drug metabolism among patients, solely related to genetic differences. Chapter 20, Pharmacogenomics, will examine genetic variability in all aspects of drug response.

KEY CONCEPTS

- Biotransformation is a necessary first step before excretion of lipophilic drugs.
- Drug metabolism occurs primarily in the liver, but may occur in other tissues. Metabolites are usually more polar than the drug and suitable for excretion in the urine and in other body fluids.
- Phase I reactions convert the drug into a suitable derivative for further conjugation in phase II reactions.

- Most drugs are metabolized by phase I oxidation by a select group of isozymes of the CYP450 superfamily.
- The rate of biotransformation is governed by Michaelis–Menten kinetics, and metabolizing enzymes are subject to saturation, inhibition, and induction.

ADDITIONAL READING

1. Gordon Gibson G, Skett P. Introduction to Drug Metabolism, 3rd ed. Stanley Thornes Pub Ltd, 2001.
2. Ritschel WA, Kearns GL. Handbook of Basic Pharmacokinetics, 5th ed. American Pharmaceutical Association, 1999.
3. Smith DA, van de Waterbeemd H, Walker DK, Mannhold R, Kubinyi H, Timmerman H. Pharmacokinetics and Metabolism in Drug Design. Wiley-VCH, 2000.
4. Rowland M, Tozer TN. Clinical Pharmacokinetics: Concepts and Applications, 3rd ed. Lippincott Williams & Wilkins, 1995.

REVIEW QUESTIONS

1. What physicochemical properties make drugs unsuitable for urinary excretion as unchanged drug? How does biotransformation solve this problem?
2. Why are phase I reactions often necessary before a conjugation reaction can occur? What types of drugs do not require a phase I reaction to precede a phase II reaction?
3. Which is the most common type of phase I reaction? Why?
4. Which enzyme system is most important in drug metabolism? Why?
5. Under what conditions does Michaelis–Menten kinetics approximate a first-order process? A zero-order process? What happens to the rate of metabolism when metabolizing enzymes are saturated?
6. What is meant by hepatic extraction ratio and hepatic clearance?
7. Under what circumstances does first-pass metabolism occur? What is the consequence?
8. What are the other pathways of presystemic metabolism?
9. What is meant by induction and inhibition of drug-metabolizing enzymes? How might this affect plasma concentrations of drugs?

Plasma Concentration–Time Curves

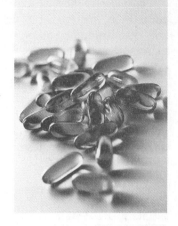

The aim of drug therapy is to reach and maintain the desired concentration of drug at the site of action. The relationship between drug concentration at the receptor and the subsequent pharmacological response is referred to as *pharmacodynamics,* which we will address in greater detail in subsequent chapters. The concentration reaching the receptor depends on a drug's absorption, distribution, metabolism, and excretion (ADME) behavior; differences in ADME are frequently responsible for variability in efficacy and toxicity of the same drug in different individuals.

Drug levels in various tissues, including the site of action, depend on the relative *rates* of ADME processes after administration. Although we have discussed absorption, distribution, excretion, and metabolism pathways separately, it is important to remember that all these processes are proceeding simultaneously after drug administration. Absorption allows the drug to enter the bloodstream, distribution from blood enables it to reach the receptor and other tissues; simultaneously, biotransformation and excretion pathways remove the drug from the bloodstream. The net effect of these dynamic processes determines whether and for how long optimal drug concentration is achieved and maintained in the blood-stream and, therefore, at the site of action.

Pharmacokinetics describes the time course and pattern of drug absorption and disposition; in other words, it is a quantitative description of what the body does to the drug. It describes the temporal (when) and spatial (where) distribution patterns of a drug in the body. Pharmacokinetic information about a drug is important in determining dosage and frequency of dosage for desired therapeutic response.

Blood, Plasma, and Serum

The most direct approach of obtaining pharmacokinetic information is by administering the drug and then measuring drug concentrations in the bloodstream as a function of time. Drug concentration assays often use serum or plasma rather than whole blood. *Plasma* is the clear, yellowish fluid portion of blood in which blood cells are suspended. It differs from *serum* in that plasma contains fibrin and other soluble clotting substances. When whole blood is allowed to clot, serum is the supernatant liquid after centrifugation; if an anticoagulant is added to the blood before centrifugation, plasma is the supernatant.

Drug Concentration in Plasma

Plasma perfuses all tissues and carries drug to various regions of the body. Drug in plasma can exist as either free drug or drug bound to plasma proteins. Partitioning into blood cells or binding to blood cells may also be quite significant for some drugs. Free (unbound) drug can readily leave capillaries in most tissues and equilibrate with interstitial fluid. If physicochemical properties allow, the drug can further distribute into intracellular fluid.

Some tissues and organs in the body are well-perfused, meaning that they have good blood flow; examples are the heart, liver, kidney, and brain. Distribution of drug to well-perfused tissues is rapid, and we can assume that drug in plasma is in dynamic equilibrium with drug in the tissue at all times. This means that the concentrations of free drug in plasma and the tissue are equal. As plasma concentrations decline owing to elimination, tissue concentrations decline as well.

Other tissues, such as muscle and fat, are poorly perfused because they receive blood at a lower rate. Drug distribution to these regions is slower, and distribution equilibrium may not be reached for some time after drug administration. Before distribution equilibrium is established, tissue concentrations in poorly perfused regions will continue to increase despite declining plasma concentrations. Once distribution equilibrium is reached, plasma and tissue concentrations of free drug can be considered equal, and will decline in a parallel manner.

Therefore, changes in drug plasma levels after distribution equilibrium reflect corresponding changes in drug tissue levels in the body. Plasma drug concentrations can be readily measured, giving us a convenient estimate of tissue drug levels and consequently of drug concentration at the receptor.

Pharmacokinetic Compartments

One objective of pharmacokinetic analysis is to use plasma concentrations to develop simple mathematical models that describe drug disposition (distribution and elimination) after administration. For this purpose, the body is divided into a few (usually one to three) imaginary *compartments* that can be viewed as well-stirred, interconnected tanks. Drug is assumed to move between these

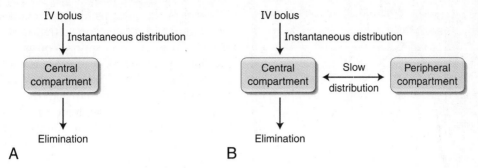

Figure 14.1. Schematic diagram of compartmental modeling. **A.** One-compartment model. **B.** Two-compartment model. Note that elimination occurs out of the central compartment. IV, intravenous.

compartments at defined rates. Tissues into which drug distributes at the same rate are grouped together in the same compartment.

A one-compartment model assumes that the body is composed of a single homogeneous compartment (the *central compartment*) into which drug distributes rapidly and uniformly, for example, a compartment consisting of plasma and well-perfused tissues. A two-compartment model divides the body into a central compartment as before, with a second *peripheral compartment* of poorly perfused tissues. Figure 14.1 shows a schematic diagram of one- and two-compartment models. A more detailed discussion of compartmental pharmacokinetics is beyond the scope of this book.

Plasma Level Curves

The plasma level curve (also called a *plasma level versus time curve* or a *blood level curve*) is a graph depicting drug concentration in plasma as a function of time after dosing. Data for this graph are obtained by administering a known dose of drug to an individual and taking blood samples at various times after administration. The concentration of drug (and sometimes metabolites) in the plasma samples is measured, and results are plotted with time of sampling on the *x*-axis and corresponding plasma concentration on the *y*-axis.

Pharmacokinetic Features of a Plasma Level Curve

The shape of a plasma level curve depends on the route of administration and the rates of ADME processes. Figures 14.2 and 14.3 show typical plasma level curves after administration of a single intravenous (IV) and oral dose of a drug, respectively. We will restrict our discussion to drugs that follow a one-compartment model, i.e., that distribute rapidly into a single central compartment.

Rate of Absorption

The first step after administration of a drug is absorption of drug into the bloodstream.

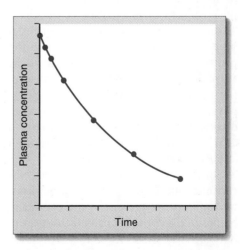

Figure 14.2. Typical plasma level curve after bolus intravenous administration of a drug. Note that the maximum plasma concentration is obtained at time = 0, immediately after dosing.

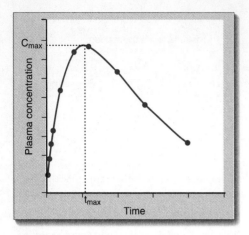

Figure 14.3. A typical plasma level curve obtained after oral dosing of a drug product. The maximum plasma concentration (C_{max}) is reached at a time t_{max} after administration.

Consider a single dose of a drug given orally. After administration, the drug begins to be released from the oral dosage form and starts dissolving in gastrointestinal (GI) fluids. Dissolved drug is available for absorption from the small intestines, most commonly by passive diffusion in accordance with Fick's law. The rate of absorption of dissolved drug depends on its concentration gradient, the properties of the epithelial membrane at the absorption site, and the physicochemical properties of the drug. Absorption is generally a first-order process because the absorption rate depends on the concentration of drug available for absorption. Overall absorption behavior depends on the drug's physicochemical properties and rate of dissolution from the dosage form and is characterized by a first-order absorption rate constant.

Some drugs may be absorbed by carrier-mediated transport if appropriate transporters are present in the cell membranes of the epithelial cells at the absorption site. In such cases, the absorption rate is first-order when drug concentrations are low, but may approach a zero-order process if the transporters become saturated.

As absorption begins, drug enters the circulation and plasma concentration begins to rise. As absorption continues, plasma concentration keeps increasing until it reaches a maximum designated as C_{max}; the time taken to reach C_{max} is called t_{max}. These two parameters provide a measure of the rate of absorption of the drug in the patient; C_{max} is high and t_{max} is short for rapidly and extensively absorbed drugs.

As soon as drug enters the bloodstream, it is distributed rapidly to the central compartment and starts being eliminated by biotransformation and excretion. (If one or more peripheral compartments exist there is further slower distribution into these regions.) Absorption causes plasma concentration of drug to increase, whereas elimination causes it to decrease. The maximum plasma concentration C_{max} is reached when the rate of absorption is equal to the rate of elimination. Absorption predominates before t_{max} when there is a large concentration gradient driving absorption. As drug concentration at the absorption site declines, absorption rate decreases and eventually becomes zero when all available drug has been absorbed. After this time, elimination processes alone determine plasma concentration of drug.

If drug is administered as an IV *bolus* (meaning that the dose is given all at once), the entire dose enters plasma almost instantaneously, and there is no detectable absorption phase. The maximum plasma concentration is attained immediately after administration (at time zero), and plasma concentration then declines as elimination processes begin.

Rate of Distribution

Distribution equilibrium of one-compartment drugs is also achieved immediately after administration of an IV bolus. The large cardiac output moves blood rapidly throughout the body so that distribution to well-perfused tissues is complete almost as soon as drug enters the bloodstream. For example, the initial plasma concentration after an IV bolus dose reflects the drug concentration after distribution equilibrium has been reached. As discussed in Chapter 11, Drug Distribution, the volume of distribution V_d of a drug is given by:

$$V_d = \frac{\text{dose}}{\text{initial plasma concentration}}$$

$$= \frac{X}{C_0} \qquad \text{(Eq. 14.1)}$$

where X is the IV bolus dose of drug in mg and C_0 is the initial (and also the maximum) plasma concentration. Equation 14.1 can be rearranged to give an expression for initial plasma concentration:

$$C_0 = \frac{X}{V_d} \qquad \text{(Eq. 14.2)}$$

Equation 14.2 shows that the initial plasma concentration after IV bolus dosing of a one-compartment drug depends on the dose administered and volume of distribution of the drug; the higher the volume of distribution, the lower the initial plasma concentration. The subsequent decline in concentration is related to elimination processes only.

Distribution equilibrium is reached more slowly for drugs that distribute further to poorly perfused tissues in peripheral compartments. For such multicompartment drugs, the decline in plasma concentration after a single IV dose reflects both distribution and elimination processes.

Rate of Elimination

The elimination behavior of a drug depends on all the factors discussed in Chapter 12, Drug Excretion, and Chapter 13, Drug Metabolism. Elimination begins as soon as drug enters the blood and rapidly distributes to eliminating organs such as the liver and kidney. The drug

may be excreted in its unchanged form in urine or other body fluids, or biotransformed and excreted as metabolites in these fluids. Regardless, plasma concentration of drug decreases progressively with time.

Both biotransformation and excretion are first-order processes (except in a few special cases) in that their rates are proportional to plasma concentration of drug. Because we know that plasma concentration of a drug is related to its volume of distribution, it follows that the rate of elimination is also dependent on V_d. When plasma concentrations are low, the rate of elimination is small. Additionally, the rate of elimination depends on the efficiency of excretion and biotransformation, i.e., on the clearance (CL) of drug by these processes. The total clearance CL of a drug is given by:

$$CL = CL_{\text{renal}} + CL_{\text{biliary}}$$
$$+ CL_{\text{hepatic}} + CL_{\text{other}} \qquad \text{(Eq. 14.3)}$$

Chapter 4, Rates of Pharmaceutical Processes, discussed first-order kinetics principles that can now be applied to the time course of drug concentration in plasma. Consider the IV bolus administration of X milligrams of a one-compartment drug to an individual. The drug distributes rapidly into its volume of distribution, V_d, giving an initial plasma concentration C_0.

Elimination now begins and plasma concentration decreases in a first-order manner; the concentration at any time after dosing is given by:

$$C_t = C_0 e^{-kt} \qquad \text{(Eq. 14.4)}$$

where C_t is plasma concentration at time t after dosing, and k is the first-order elimination rate constant for the drug, with units of $time^{-1}$. The elimination rate constant k can be viewed as the fractional decrease in plasma concentration in a given time interval. For example, $k = 0.05 \text{ hr}^{-1}$

means that plasma concentration decreases by 5% of its value every hour. The elimination rate constant is related to the two fundamental pharmacokinetic parameters of a drug, volume of distribution and total clearance, by the following expression:

$$k = \frac{CL}{V_d} \qquad \text{(Eq. 14.5)}$$

CL and V_d of a drug do not change with dose administered or route of administration.

Plasma Half-Life

Elimination of drug from the bloodstream by biotransformation and excretion is often characterized by a secondary parameter called plasma half-life ($t_{1/2}$ or $t_{0.5}$), defined as the time required for plasma drug concentration to decrease by one half. This definition is similar to one discussed in Chapter 4, Rates of Pharmaceutical Processes, for the half-life of a chemical reaction:

$$t_{1/2} = \frac{0.693}{k} \qquad \text{(Eq. 14.6)}$$

A drug that is rapidly eliminated will have a short $t_{1/2}$ whereas one that is slowly eliminated will have a long $t_{1/2}$. Like the elimination rate constant, the plasma half-life of a drug is a property of the drug and does not usually change with dose or route of administration.

Area Under the Curve

The relative rates of ADME processes are usually in the order distribution > absorption > elimination, giving the typical plasma level curves seen in Figures 14.1 and 14.2. The area under the curve (AUC) is a measure of the total amount of drug in the body after administration. AUC depends on the amount of the administered dose reaching the systemic circulation and the efficiency of drug removal from the body. For a drug administered by IV bolus, AUC is given by:

$$AUC = \frac{X}{CL} \qquad \text{(Eq. 14.7)}$$

Because the entire dose enters the systemic circulation, AUC is proportional to X; as the dose increases so does plasma concentration and, consequently, AUC. In addition, AUC depends on the total clearance of the drug. A drug that is cleared rapidly will give low plasma concentrations and thus have a small AUC.

AUC can also be calculated as the area under the drug plasma concentration–time curve by integrating Equation 14.4 from $t = 0$ to $t = \infty$:

$$AUC = \int_0^\infty C_t dt \qquad \text{(Eq. 14.8)}$$

The units of AUC are concentration $\times$ time (e.g., mg hr L^{-1}).

Because the entire dose enters the systemic circulation after IV administration, this administration route represents the maximum AUC for a given dose of a drug. If the same dose is given orally, the AUC may be less because of incomplete dissolution, incomplete absorption, or presystemic or first-pass metabolism.

Bioavailability

The bioavailability of a drug product is defined as the rate and extent of drug absorption from a dosage form into the systemic circulation. In common usage, bioavailability is often used to describe only extent of absorption.

Absolute Bioavailability. The absolute bioavailability (F) of a drug product is the fraction of the administered dose that reaches the systemic circulation intact after administration. It is generally measured by comparing the AUC of the product with the AUC obtained after giving the *same dose* intravenously. For example, absolute bioavailability of an oral product is given by the following equation:

$$F = \frac{AUC_{oral}}{AUC_{iv}} \qquad \text{(Eq. 14.9)}$$

where AUC_{oral} and AUC_{iv} are the areas under the curve after oral and IV administration of the same dose, respectively. Absolute bioavailability is often represented as a percentage:

$$\%F = \frac{AUC_{oral}}{AUC_{iv}} \times 100 \qquad \text{(Eq. 14.10)}$$

Formulation or toxicity considerations often make it inappropriate to give the same dose of drug orally and IV; usually, a smaller dose is used for IV administration. In this situation, Equation 14.9 must be modified to account for the difference in doses to:

$$F = \frac{AUC_{oral}}{AUC_{iv}} \times \frac{dose_{iv}}{dose_{oral}} \qquad \text{(Eq. 14.11)}$$

For IV administration of drugs, F is equal to 1, or 100%, because the entire dose reaches the systemic circulation. For all other routes, F is less than or equal to 1.

Causes of Poor Bioavailability. It is important to note that bioavailability depends on dissolution of drug from the dosage form (see Chapter 10, Drug Delivery Systems), permeability of dissolved drug through the epithelial membrane at the absorption site (see Chapter 8, Transport Across Biological Barriers), and loss by presystemic metabolism (see Chapter 13, Drug Metabolism).

Bioavailability less than 1 implies that only a portion of the administered dose reaches the systemic circulation. This may be attributable to:

- incomplete release of drug from the dosage form
- poor permeability of drug through tissues at the absorption site
- insufficient time for absorption of all the drug
- instability of the drug at site of administration
- presystemic metabolism, e.g., gut wall metabolism or first-pass effect
- physiological issues pertaining to the patient
- drug interactions

Sources of poor bioavailability are summarized in Figure 14.4.

Drugs that dissolve rapidly from their dosage forms and have good permeability across absorption epithelia tend to be almost completely absorbed. However, absorption of many drugs is not always complete. Low bioavailability is most common with products of poorly water-soluble, low-permeability drugs. Poor permeability could be related to a low partition coefficient, an unsuitable pK_a, or large molecular size. Incomplete release

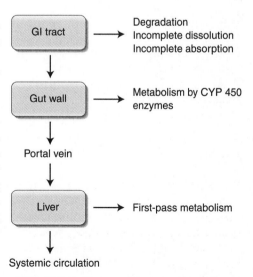

Figure 14.4. Diagram showing sources of poor bioavailability ($F < 1$) after oral dosing.

of drug from a poorly designed dosage form will also prevent a portion of the drug from being available for absorption.

Insufficient time for absorption contributes to low bioavailability of poorly absorbed drugs. For example, orally administered drugs are exposed to the GI tract for about 24 to 48 hours at most, and to the small intestine for about 4 hours. If the drug dissolves slowly or has poor permeability across the intestinal epithelium, this length of time at the absorption site may be insufficient. In such cases, bioavailability tends to be low as well as highly variable.

A drug may be unstable and decompose at the absorption site, reducing the amount of intact drug available for absorption. For example, drugs can hydrolyze at the acidic pH of the stomach or be metabolized by digestive enzymes or intestinal bacteria. Some of the dissolved drug in the GI tract may be unavailable for absorption because of binding or complexation with food or other substances in the GI tract.

Even if a drug is completely absorbed after oral administration, presystemic metabolism (gut-wall metabolism or first-pass effect) will reduce bioavailability.

The patient's health may influence absorptive ability of many tissues. Finally, food and drug interactions may also reduce the amount of a given drug that is absorbed. Thus, the overall bioavailability of a drug from a product depends on a complex set of parameters including properties of the drug, dosage form, and patient.

Effect of Route and Delivery System

The route of administration and delivery system influence the shape of the plasma level curve. We have already noted the differences between plasma level curves

Bioavailability of Digoxin

Digoxin is a drug primarily used to treat congestive heart failure and arrhythmias. It is available in a variety of dosage forms for oral and injectable (intravenous or intramuscular) administration. Oral dosage forms include an elixir, soft-gelatin capsules (sgc), and tablets; bioavailability of digoxin from each of these dosage forms is different and shows considerable interindividual variability. The average bioavailabilities are $F_{tablets} = 0.7$, $F_{elixir} = 0.8$, and $F_{sgc} = 1.0$. The injectable formulations are completely bioavailable ($F = 1$). Thus, clinicians recommend that dosage should be reduced by approximately 20 to 25% when switching a patient from an oral product to an injection.

When digoxin is taken orally with meals, the rate of absorption is slowed but bioavailability is usually unchanged. When taken with meals high in fiber, however, the amount absorbed from an oral dose may be reduced.

In some patients, digoxin in the intestines is degraded to inactive reduction products (e.g., dihydrodigoxin) by colonic bacteria in the gut. Data suggest that 40% or more of the ingested dose will degrade in 10% of patients treated with digoxin tablets. Certain antibiotics that kill intestinal bacteria may actually increase the absorption of digoxin in patients and give higher blood levels and AUC. Drugs that decrease digoxin absorption are antacids, cholestyramine, colestipol, kaolin-pectin, cimetidine, metoclopramide, some chemotherapy drugs, and penicillamine.

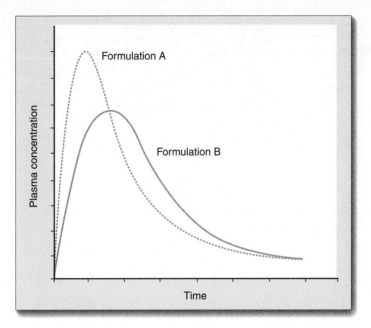

Figure 14.5. Plasma level curves of two oral formulations containing the same dose of a drug. Note that the maximal concentration (C_{max}) and time to reach maximal concentration (t_{max}) of the two curves are different. The area under the curve (AUC) values of the two curves may also be different.

obtained after oral and IV administration. Plasma level curves will be altered when the same dose of drug is given via different routes primarily because of differences in the absorption phase.

Figure 14.5 illustrates the influence of delivery system design on plasma level curves for two tablet formulations, *A* and *B*, containing the same dose of the same drug. The C_{max} and t_{max} values are different for the two formulations, presumably because *A* releases the drug faster than *B*, resulting in a faster absorption rate for *A*. The AUC values of these two formulations are different as well, indicating that formulation *B* has a lower bioavailability than formulation *A*.

Relationship Between Pharmacokinetics and Pharmacodynamics

One goal of pharmacokinetic analysis of a drug is to use the information to quantify clinical pharmacological effects in patients. An assumption made in pharmacokinetic analysis is that tissue drug concentrations (including concentration at the site of action) are related to plasma concentrations; consequently, pharmacological effect can often be correlated to plasma concentration of drug. If such correlations between pharmacokinetics and pharmacodynamics exist, they can help to understand drug action and drug safety, and to establish an optimal dose and dosing schedule for a drug. The relationship between pharmacokinetics and pharmacodynamics is illustrated in Figure 14.6.

Pharmacological Features of a Plasma Level Curve

Plasma concentrations of a systemically acting drug can be related to certain pharmacological parameters as shown in Figure 14.7, and therefore to therapeutic effectiveness of the drug. The minimum effective concentration (MEC) is the lowest plasma concentration needed for therapeutic effect. The minimum toxic concentration (MTC), also called *the maximum safe concentration*, is the plasma concentration above which toxic effects

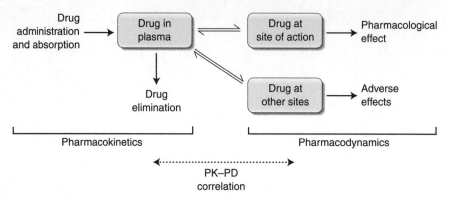

Figure 14.6. Schematic diagram defining the pharmacokinetics (PK) and pharmacodynamics (PD) of a drug, and showing the concept of PK–PD correlation.

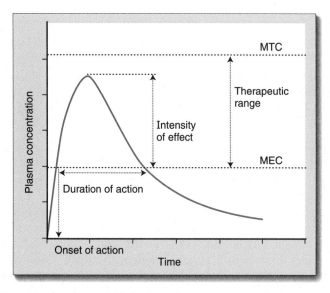

Figure 14.7. Plasma level curve after oral administration showing typical pharmacological features. Onset of action occurs when the plasma level reaches the minimum effective concentration (MEC). The duration of action is the time period for which the plasma level is at or above the MEC. The intensity of effect depends on how high the maximal concentration (C_{max}) is above the MEC. The plasma levels should remain below the minimum toxic concentration (MTC) to minimize adverse reactions.

are seen. Consequently, the aim of drug therapy is to maintain plasma concentration in the range between MEC and MTC; this range is known as the therapeutic range or therapeutic window of a drug. The larger the therapeutic range, the safer the drug is considered to be.

After administration of a single dose of a drug product, therapeutic effect is first seen when plasma concentration reaches the drug's MEC; this is the time required for onset of action. Therapeutic effective-ness lasts as long as plasma concentration remains above MEC; this length of time is the duration of action of the drug product. The intensity of effect often depends on how high the plasma concentration reaches above MEC.

Plasma levels will depend on the dose of drug given. A larger dose will give a higher C_{max} and greater intensity of effect, but perhaps also a higher incidence of side effects. Plasma levels will also depend on the design of the dosage form.

Digoxin Therapy

Digoxin is an old drug that has been used clinically for more than 200 years. The accepted therapeutic range for digoxin is 0.8 to 2.0 μg/L for congestive heart failure and 1.5 to 2.5 μg/L for arrhythmias, although the exact therapeutic range remains controversial. This is partly because there is considerable variation among patients. The problem with the upper concentration limit is that it overlaps with concentrations at which patients may experience toxic effects. Although cardiotoxic effects usually are not seen until the concentration exceeds 2.6 μg/L, noncardiac side effects such as nausea, vomiting, and anorexia may occur at concentrations between 1.3 and 2.6 μg/L. On the other hand, serum digoxin concentrations less than 0.8 μg/L are ineffective in most patients. Thus, digoxin is considered to have a narrow therapeutic range, and plasma concentrations have to be carefully monitored to maintain efficacy and prevent toxicity.

Digoxin is eliminated primarily through renal excretion; about 60 to 80% of administered drug appears as unchanged drug in the urine. Thus, adjustments of dosing need to be made in patients with reduced renal function and a lower creatinine clearance than normal.

The challenging aspects of digoxin therapy are its narrow therapeutic range, the variability in plasma concentrations and bioavailability in patients given the same dose, and the difficulty in measuring clinical efficacy. Digoxin toxicity is a frequently encountered cause of hospitalization. However, interpretation of the serum digoxin concentration must be tailored to the individual because some patients can manifest signs and symptoms of toxicity within the accepted therapeutic range. This has led clinicians to develop nomograms and equations to estimate optimal digoxin dosage based on factors such as age, weight, sex, renal function, disease state, and concurrent drug therapy.

Multiple-Dosing Regimens

We have examined the features of plasma level curves after a single dose. Most clinical applications require achieving and maintaining a therapeutic drug concentration for the duration of therapy. An initial effective concentration can be reached with the appropriate dose; maintaining the concentration in the therapeutic range for an extended period is a challenge. A thorough knowledge of the pharmacokinetics of a drug allows scientists and clinicians to design appropriate multiple-dosing regimens (dose and dosing interval) for each situation. The approach is to administer drug at the same rate that it will be eliminated from the body so that a fairly consistent plasma concentration (**steady state**) in the therapeutic range is achieved.

When a drug is administered on a multiple-dosing regimen, each successive dose is administered before the preceding dose is completely eliminated. The result is accumulation of the drug in the body, yielding a higher maximum plasma drug concentration (C_{max}) with each dose. This accumulation phenomenon, however, does not cause the plasma concentration to rise indefinitely. The C_{max} eventually reaches a plateau at steady state as does the minimum plasma concentration,

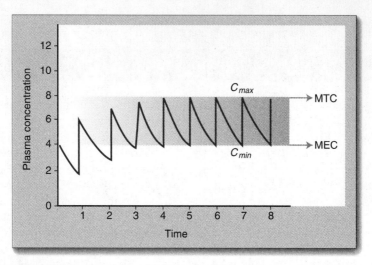

Figure 14.8. Plasma level curve after multiple dosing of a drug showing accumulation of drug and the eventual approach to steady state. In this example, the same dose of drug is given by intravenous bolus at 1-hour dosing intervals. For the first five doses, there is an accumulation of drug with each dose, as seen by the increase in maximal concentration (C_{max}). At steady state, the C_{max} and minimal concentration (C_{min}) remain consistent, within the therapeutic range of the drug.

C_{min}. In designing a dosing regimen then, the objective is to keep C_{min} above the minimum effective concentration (MEC) and the C_{max} below the minimum toxic concentration (MTC) as shown in Figure 14.8. A detailed discussion of multiple dosing is outside the scope of this book.

KEY CONCEPTS

- Compartmental modeling is used in pharmacokinetics to quantitatively describe the disposition and time course of drug in the body.

- The shape of a plasma level curve depends on the relative rates of absorption, distribution, and elimination of the drug.

- The fraction of the dose reaching the systemic circulation (bioavailability) depends on the physicochemical and pharmacokinetic properties of the drug, dosage form properties, and the physiology of the patient.

- For drugs that work systemically, the plasma concentration is usually related to the efficacy and toxicity of the drug.

- A minimum plasma concentration is necessary for efficacy, and too high a plasma concentration can cause toxicity.

- The goal of drug therapy is to maintain plasma concentration in the therapeutic range for the desired time, usually by multiple dosing of drug.

ADDITIONAL READING

1. Shargel L, Yu ABC. Applied Biopharmaceutics and Pharmacokinetics, 4th ed. McGraw-Hill/Appleton & Lange, 1999.

2. Dipiro JT, Spruill WJ, Blouin RA, Pruemer JM, Hermann J. Concepts in Clinical Pharmacokinetics, 3rd ed. American Hospital Association, 2002.

3. Rowland M, Tozer TN. Clinical Pharmacokinetics: Concepts and Applications, 3rd ed. Lippincott Williams & Wilkins, 1995.

4. Levine RR, Walsh CT, Schwartz-Bloom RD. Pharmacology: Drug Actions and Reactions, 6th ed. CRC Press-Parthenon Publishers, 2000.

REVIEW QUESTIONS

1. What is a pharmacokinetic compartmental model? What are the differences between a one- and two-compartment model?

2. What do the parameters C_{max}, t_{max}, elimination rate constant, plasma half-life, and AUC tell you about a drug product? Which of these are independent of the dose and the route of administration?

3. What is meant by the absolute bioavailability of a drug? Why is the absolute bioavailability after IV administration equal to 1?

4. What are the reasons for poor bioavailability of a drug after oral administration? How can a drug that is completely absorbed orally still have a bioavailability of less than 1?

5. Why is it important to measure plasma concentrations of a drug? How are these concentrations related to the efficacy and toxicity of a drug?

6. What is the therapeutic range of a drug? Why is it important to maintain plasma concentrations in the therapeutic range?

Section V • Drug Action

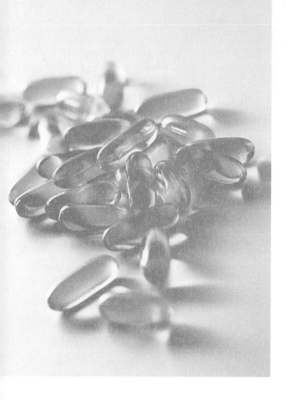

Ligands and Receptors

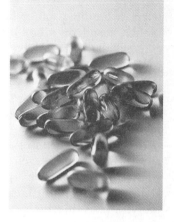

Cells in our body live in association with other cells and must communicate and interact with each other. Cells use chemicals for communication with each other to regulate metabolism, electrical signaling, contraction, growth, ion transport, and other important processes. These chemical messengers, called ligands, are released by one set of cells as needed and bind to their receptors to cause a cellular response. Cellular communication progresses and adjusts normally in a healthy individual to maintain overall well-being. However, one or more cell communication pathways may become impaired with age or disease, and drugs may be needed to restore normal balance between cells.

Chapter 6, Drugs and Their Targets, introduced receptors, ligands, and concepts that underlie receptor–ligand binding. This chapter will describe common types of ligands that carry signals for cellular communication. Further, this chapter will discuss the major types of receptors that serve as important ligand and drug targets and explain further the outcomes of ligand–receptor binding.

In the broadest sense, any interaction of a chemical signal with a biological macromolecule (protein, DNA, RNA) can be considered to be a receptor–ligand interaction if some response occurs after binding. The word "signal" in this context refers to nothing more than molecules (either ligand or drug) present in the extracellular fluid. However, we shall confine our discussion to the interaction of signal molecules with protein receptors, as generally accepted. Many enzymes, such as those with allosteric regulation, can also be considered to be receptors. Sometimes a receptor has enzymatic activity as well.

On binding to the appropriate ligand, the receptor transmits a signal that initiates biochemical changes in the target cell by a wide variety of possible pathways. Cells are exposed to many ligands from their environment, each carrying a chemical message and capable of initiating a different receptor response.

The Signaling Process

Cell signaling is the process by which cells release, transmit, receive, and respond to information from their environment and from each other. This information is carried by endogenous ligands (also called *mediators* or *signaling molecules*) made and released by cells as needed. Human cells can also detect and respond to external signals such as noxious agents, bacteria, viruses, and toxins.

There are three main players involved in the signaling process: the signaling cell, the ligand, and the recipient of the signal, the receptor. The synthesis and release of a ligand by a cell is often itself the result of a ligand–receptor interaction. The binding of the released ligand to a complementary receptor initiates a cascade of biochemical reactions that ultimately result in a physiological action. Only very small amounts of a signal are necessary to mediate body functions, cell–cell communication, and many disease processes.

The overall behavior of a cell depends on the signals it is exposed to in its environment, and each cell responds to signals according to its own specific character. A cell may respond to one set of signals by multiplying, to another set by carrying out a biochemical reaction, and to yet another set by differentiating. Different types of cells require different sets of signals for survival, and the same ligand often has different effects on different cell types.

Many drugs act by competing with or taking the place of an endogenous ligand or by modifying the signaling pathway in some manner. In this way, a drug can make a quantitative change in an existing physiological or biochemical process; however, most drugs do not qualitatively alter the nature of the process. Understanding cell signaling is a first step in understanding drug effects and enables scientists to design better drugs.

The major steps in the signaling process can be described as follows:

1. Signaling cells synthesize the appropriate ligand, usually based on a signal they themselves receive.
2. The cells release ligand molecules, usually into the extracellular fluid.
3. Ligand molecules are transported to target cells in a variety of ways, as we shall see shortly. Depending on its physicochemical properties, the ligand may remain in the extracellular fluid or enter the target cell.
4. Appropriate receptors in the target cells recognize and bind to the ligands with specificity, forming a complex. Receptors may be located either inside the target cells (intracellular receptors) or in the cell membrane (cell-surface receptors).
5. The ligand–receptor complex transforms the signal into an intracellular message and triggers a response in target cells.
6. The ligand is removed, terminating the response.

Endogenous Ligands

A simple classification of ligands secreted by the body is difficult because their chemical structures and physicochemical properties vary considerably. Some ligands are small molecules whereas others are peptides and proteins; some are charged in the physiological pH range whereas others are uncharged; some are hydrophobic whereas others are polar. Furthermore, a given ligand can bind to extracellular, membrane-bound, or intracellular components to initiate signaling cascades that result in different responses depending on the conditions.

One way to group ligands is based on their ability to cross cell membranes. The vast majority of ligands (e.g., peptides) are polar or charged and thus unable to cross the lipid bilayer of the cell membrane. Their receptor proteins must therefore reside in the cell membrane, be able to detect ligand presence in extracellular fluid, and transmit this information into the interior of the cell. These cell-surface receptors serve as conduits for transfer of information from the cell exterior to the cell interior.

Hydrophobic ligands such as steroids, some vitamins, and gases such as nitric oxide can cross the cell membrane by passive diffusion and enter cells. Their target receptors may be on the cell surface but often are located in the cytoplasm or the nucleus. Table 15.1 lists examples of common ligands classified by their hydrophilicity or hydrophobicity. Figure 15.1 illustrates the difference in signaling by hydrophilic and hydrophobic ligands.

Another method of classifying ligands is based on the type of cells that produce them. For example, neurotransmitters are produced by nerve cells and hormones are produced by endocrine glands.

Modes of Cell Signaling

Ligands are synthesized and secreted by many different types of cells and move from signaling cells to target cells in a variety of ways. The major modes of signaling are endocrine signaling by hormones and local signaling by autacoids.

Endocrine Signaling

Glands (extensions of the surface epithelium into underlying connective tissue)

TABLE 15.1. Examples of Various Types of Ligands Grouped by Their Hydrophilicity and Hydrophobicity[a]

Hydrophilic ligands (cell-surface receptors)	Hydrophobic ligands (intracellular receptors)	Hydrophobic ligands (cell-surface receptors)
Small molecule hormones	Steroid hormones	Arachidonic acid derivatives
Peptide hormones	Retinoids	Prostaglandins
Neurotransmitters	Thyroxins	Leukotrienes
Growth factors	Vitamin D	Platelet activating factor
Trophic factors	Cortisol	
Cytokines	Nitric oxide	
Chemokines		
Neuromodulatory peptides		

[a]Hydrophilic ligands cannot cross the cell membrane and can act only on cell surface receptors. Hydrophobic ligands may have intracellular or cell surface receptors.

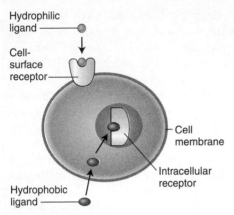

Figure 15.1. Interaction of hydrophilic ligands with cell-surface receptors and hydrophobic ligands with intracellular receptors.

contain cells whose main function is secretion. Glands that maintain contact with the surface by a system of ducts are called *exocrine* or ducted glands, such as the sweat and salivary glands. These glands release their secretions (sweat, tears, mucus, bile) into tubes or ducts that lead to internal or external body surfaces, but are not an important source of signaling molecules.

Many ligands are synthesized and secreted by **endocrine** or ductless glands that have lost their duct system and are isolated in connective tissue; examples are the thyroid and adrenal glands. Endocrine glands have good blood flow, and their secretions, called **hormones**, diffuse into capillaries and are distributed by the bloodstream to target cells. Hormones may have to travel long distances to reach their target cells as illustrated in Figure 15.2, making endocrine signaling a relatively slow process. Thus, hormones are involved in the slow and steady regulation of responses all over the body.

Because most hormones circulate in blood, they come into contact with essentially all cells. However, a given hormone usually affects only its target cells, i.e., those with receptors for the hormone. A few hormones, such as the thyroid hormones, are secreted in a relatively steady amount so that their concentration in the blood remains essentially constant under normal conditions. Other hormones are secreted on a specific cycle. For example, glucocorticoids are secreted on a 24-hour or diurnal rhythm, whereas female sex hormones are secreted on a 4-week cycle. Still other hormones, like insulin, antidiuretic hormone (ADH), epinephrine, and norepinephrine, are secreted on demand, depending on the physiological situation, or as a response to internal or external stimuli.

Types of Hormones. Hormones may be categorized into four structural groups, with members of each group having many properties in common.

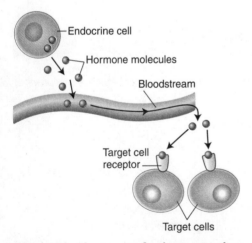

Figure 15.2. The process of endocrine signaling by hormones. Hormones released by the signaling cells enter the bloodstream and travel to the distant target cells. Here they exit the bloodstream and bind to receptors to elicit a response.

- Steroids: Steroids are lipids derived from cholesterol. Examples include the sex hormones, such as testosterone, and adrenal hormones, such as cortisol (Fig. 15.3).
- Modified amino acid derivatives: These comprise catecholamines, histamine, serotonin, and melatonin. Catecholamines (dopamine, norepinephrine, and epinephrine) are derived from tyrosine, serotonin and melatonin are synthesized from tryptophan, and histamine is derived from glutamic acid (Fig. 15.4).

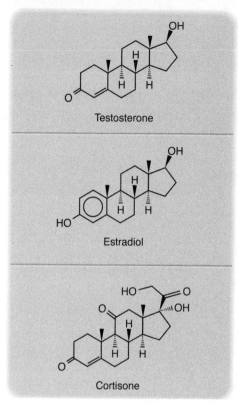

Figure 15.3. Structures of some common steroid hormones.

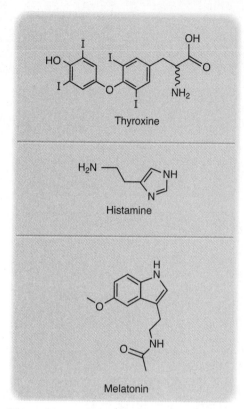

Figure 15.4. Structures of some hormones derived from amino acids.

- Peptides and proteins: Peptide and protein hormones are products of translation and vary considerably in size and posttranslational modifications, ranging from peptides as short as three amino acids to large, multisubunit glycoproteins. Examples are the neuropeptides (vasopressin, oxytocin), pituitary hormones (corticotropin, gonadotropins), and gastrointestinal hormones (insulin) (Fig. 15.5).
- Eicosanoids: This is a large group of molecules derived from polyunsaturated fatty acids, particularly arachidonic acid. The main types of hormones in this class are prostaglandins, prostacyclins, leukotrienes, and thromboxanes (Fig. 15.6).

Despite their molecular diversity, hormones can be categorized into one of two types based on the location of their receptors as either hormones with intracellular receptors or hormones with cell-surface receptors.

Hydrophobic hormones (e.g., the steroids) can cross cell membranes by passive diffusion and carry their signal into the cell. Examples are the sex hormones (androgens, estrogens, and gestagens) and the adrenal hormones (mineralocorticoids and glucocorticoids). Thus, their receptors are usually located in the cell, either in the cytoplasm or the nucleus. Thyroid hormones (e.g., thyroxin, amino acid derivatives) enter the cell by facilitated diffusion and also bind to intracellular receptors. The primary mechanism of action of hormones with intracellular receptors is to modulate gene expression in target cells.

Most polar or charged hormones, such as the protein and peptide hormones, catecholamines, and eicosanoids, cannot cross the cell membrane, and have cell-

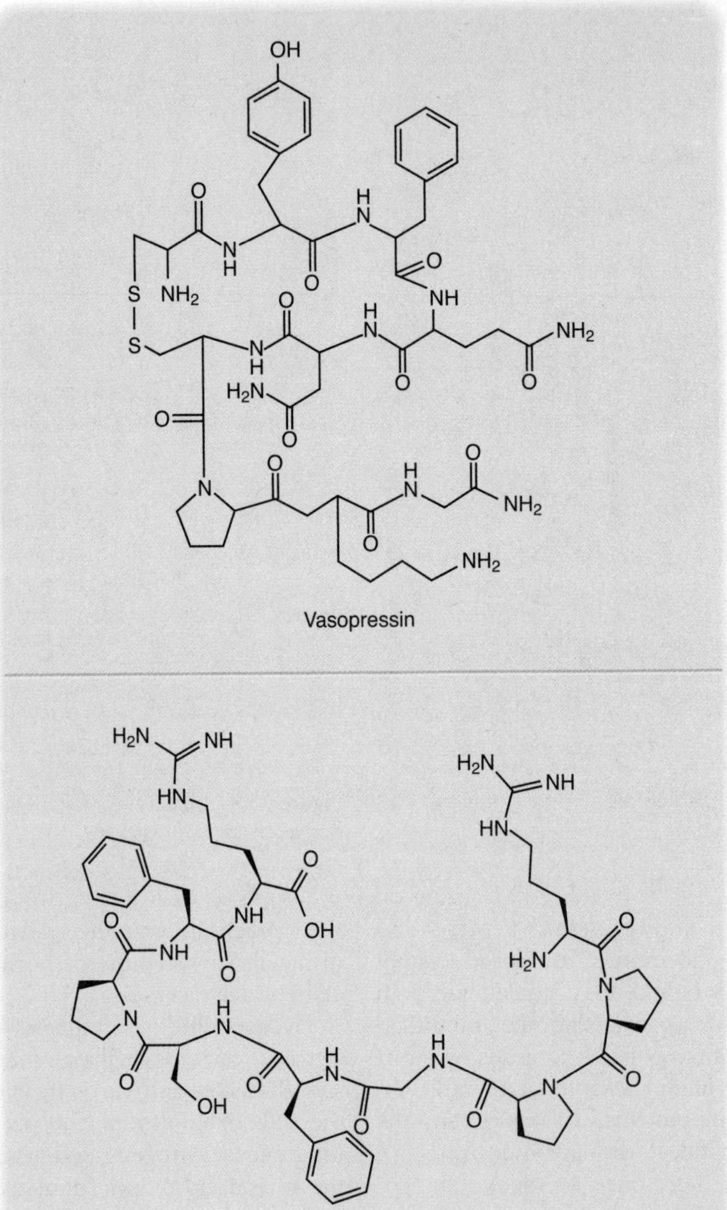

Figure 15.5. Structures of some peptide hormones.

surface receptors. Binding of hormone to its receptor initiates a series of events that leads to generation of so-called *second messengers* within the cell (the hormone is the first messenger) that transmit the signal inside the cell. We shall examine second messengers later in the chapter.

Signaling by hormones decreases and stops as hormones are eliminated from the bloodstream. Elimination takes place by biotransformation in the liver, bloodstream, and other sites. Hormones are also eliminated by excretion in the urine or bile.

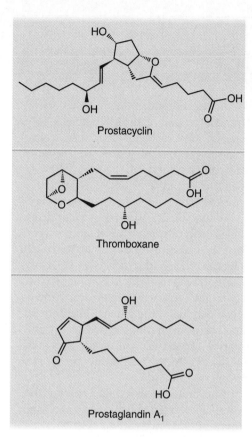

Figure 15.6. Structures of some eicosanoid hormones derived from fatty acids.

Plasma protein binding protects small hormone molecules (such as thyroid hormone) from rapid elimination. Protein binding also serves as a reservoir of hormone, so the concentration of free hormone in plasma is kept small and fairly stable.

Mechanisms of Hormone Action. Hormones exert their action by one of two fundamental mechanisms: activation of enzymes or modulation of gene expression.

Most enzymes shuttle between catalytically active and inactive conformational states. Many hormones affect their target cells by inducing such transitions, usually causing an activation of one or more enzymes. Because enzymes are catalytic and often serve to activate additional enzymes, a small change induced by

hormone–receptor binding can lead to widespread consequences within the cell.

In particular, hormones induce their biochemical changes in the cell through changes in the amount of phosphate bound to proteins. Approximately one third of the proteins present in a typical human cell may be phosphorylated (covalently bound to phosphate) at one time or another. Protein phosphorylation and dephosphorylation are controlled by two enzymes: *protein kinases* that put phosphate on a protein and *phosphatases* that remove phosphate attached to a protein. Phosphorylation can increase or decrease the biological activity of an enzyme, help move proteins between subcellular compartments, and allow interactions between proteins to occur, as well as label proteins for degradation. The variety of responses to phosphorylation is immense, and many human diseases are associated with the abnormal phosphorylation of cellular proteins.

The binding of hormones to their receptors on the surface of a cell often results in the activation of kinases and phosphatases, as illustrated in Figure 15.7. Once activated, cellular phosphorylation patterns will begin to change, with many proteins being phosphorylated or dephosphorylated. The final result will be various changes in cellular behavior.

The other major mode of action of hormones is stimulating transcription of a group of genes. This can alter a cell's phenotype by leading to synthesis of new proteins. Similarly, if transcription of a group of previously active genes is shut off, the corresponding proteins will soon disappear from the cell. When the hormone binds to its intracellular receptor, a conformational change in the receptor results in receptor activation. The major consequence of activation is that the receptor becomes capable of binding to DNA, and transcription from genes to which the receptor is bound is affected. Most commonly, receptor binding stimulates transcription, and the hormone–receptor complex functions as a transcription factor.

Antagonistic Hormone Pairs

Many hormones work in antagonistic hormone pairs with exactly opposite roles. When a body function exceeds its homeostatic level, one hormone can be released to bring the level down to normal; when that same body function falls below the homeostatic level, a completely different hormone might be released to bring the function up to normal. An example is the hormone pair of insulin and glucagon, both of which regulate blood glucose levels. Both hormones are secreted by the islets of Langerhans, a special group of cells in the pancreas; insulin is secreted by the beta cells of the islets, and glucagon by the alpha cells of the islets. Both cell types release their hormones simultaneously at a basal level. Insulin and glucagon are critical participants in glucose homeostasis and serve as acute regulators of blood glucose concentration.

When blood glucose levels rise above normal, such as after a meal, there is a rapid increase in insulin production by the beta cells. Insulin lowers blood glucose levels by mediating glucose uptake into skeletal muscle, liver, and adipose cells. When insulin binds to its receptor on the membrane of these cells, glucose transporters are activated, allowing increased uptake of glucose. Insulin increases the use of glucose by muscle cells and its storage in the liver as glycogen and in adipose tissue as fat. This causes blood glucose levels to drop.

When blood glucose levels drop below the normal level, insulin secretion is markedly reduced to its basal level. Additionally, the alpha cells release glucagon, which stimulates the liver and muscles to break down glycogen, releasing glucose and reversing the drop in blood glucose concentration. Moreover, glucagon activates pathways in which amino acids are converted into glucose.

The brain in particular has an absolute dependence on glucose as a fuel because neurons cannot use alternative energy sources like fatty acids to any significant extent. When blood levels of glucose begin to fall below the normal range, it is critical to release additional glucose into blood. In this manner, insulin and glucagon act together to balance each other and maintain homeostasis. Type 1 diabetes is a potentially fatal disease in which insulin secretion fails.

Local Signaling

In addition to true endocrine glands and cells, there are other types of ductless glands and cells that secrete molecules for local signaling. In fact, almost every cell is capable of secreting a variety of ligands that help to maintain homeostasis. Ligands responsible for local effects are referred to as autacoids or local hormones.

Types of Autacoids. Classification of autacoids is difficult because this group encompasses a wide variety of structurally diverse compounds. In fact, many ligands can function as both endocrine and local signaling molecules; the main differences lie in the speed and selectivity with which the molecules are delivered to their targets. Thus, although the traditional definition of hormones describes them as being secreted into blood and af-

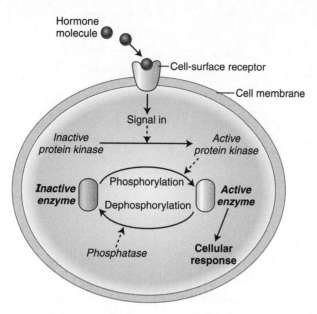

Figure 15.7. Activation and deactivation of an enzyme mediated by hormones. The binding of a hormone to its cell-surface receptor sends a signal that is transmitted into the cell interior. The signal activates a protein kinase that results in phosphorylation of another enzyme, eventually resulting in a cellular response. The active enzyme is deactivated by a phosphatase, and awaits another signal.

fecting cells at distant sites, many hormones also affect neighboring cells or even have effects on the same cells that secreted them. Figure 15.8 shows structures of some common autacoids.

Collectively, autacoids have three features in common: they do not need to be transported by the bloodstream, they exert effects near the site where they are synthesized and secreted, and the effects are typically of short duration. Most autacoids are secreted on demand at transiently high concentrations and then rapidly degraded, so their actions are local and short-lived. Even if not quickly degraded, they become diluted as they diffuse away from the site of secretion, so concentrations rapidly become low enough to be ineffective.

Autacoids are necessary for communication between cells during defense and repair processes and are involved in helping the body deal with some sort of insult or injury. They mediate the interactions between cells by either attracting or activating cells, or both.

Local signaling by autacoids can be classified, according to the way in which the target cell receives the signal, as paracrine, autocrine, or juxtacrine.

Paracrine Signaling. Paracrine signals are those that influence neighboring cells. A signaling cell releases ligands into the extracellular fluid, which diffuse to neighboring cells, bind to specific cell surface receptors, and transmit a signal into the cell. This is illustrated in Figure 15.9. An example of paracrine ligands is a group of related compounds called growth factors that stimulate neighboring cells to divide and grow.

A special type of paracrine signaling is neuronal signaling used by neurons; the ligands are called neurotransmitters. An electrical impulse triggers the release of the neurotransmitter from the neuron. The initial electrical message is sent over the length of the axon, but the neurotransmitter itself travels only the short distance of the gap, or synapse, between the signaling neuron and the target cell; an illustration is shown in Figure 15.10.

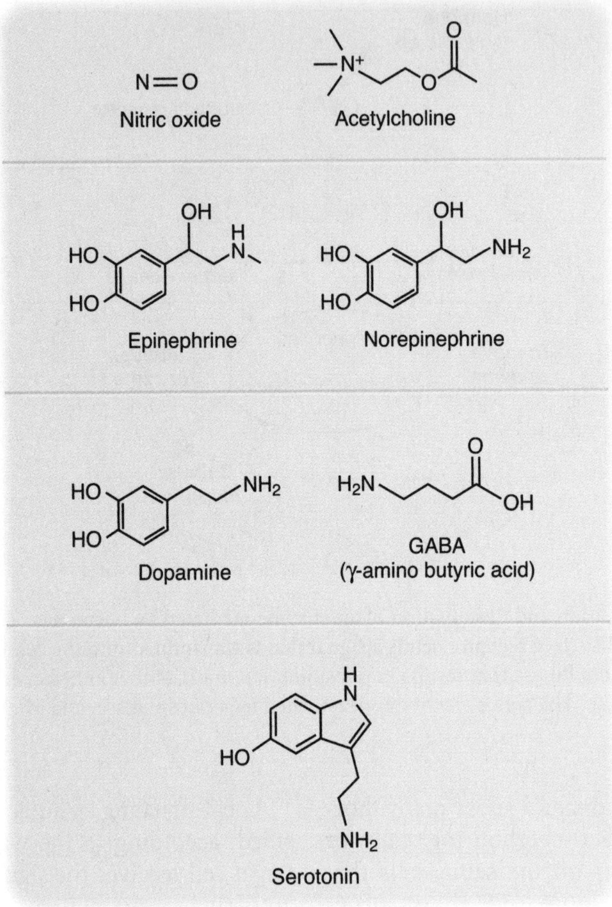

Figure 15.8. Structures of some common small-molecule autacoids.

Neuronal signaling, like all local signaling, is fast, and neurotransmitters are responsible for rapid transfer of information and quick responses at discrete sites. Several drugs act by either mimicking or blocking actions of neurotransmitters at specific locations in the body.

Autocrine Signaling. Autocrine signaling is a variation of paracrine signaling and occurs when cells respond to substances they themselves secrete, i.e., the signaling cell is also the target cell. If there is only one cell involved, the signal is weak, but a strong signal can be obtained if a group of identical cells are involved. Autocrine signaling is a mechanism to encourage a group of cells to adopt a similar behavior—a group of identical cells signal to themselves and each other to reinforce developmental decisions and create identical groups of cells. Autocrine signaling is illustrated in Figure 15.11.

Juxtacrine Signaling. Juxtacrine signaling, often called contact-dependent signaling, requires direct contact between the signaling cell and the target cell. The ligands are not released into the extracellular fluid but are directly transferred between the signaling and target cells, as shown in Figure 15.12. In one type of juxtacrine signaling, the ligand remains attached to the cell membrane of the signaling cell, and the signal is transmitted only when the target cell comes in direct contact with the attached ligand. Another type of juxtacrine signaling involves direct transfer of

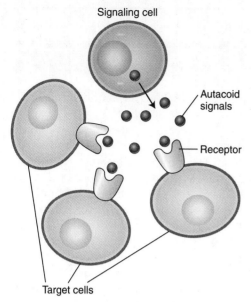

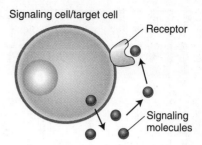

Figure 15.11. Autocrine signaling. The signaling cell is also the target cell.

Figure 15.9. Schematic showing the process of paracrine signaling. The ligands are released by the signaling cells and bind to specific receptors on the target cells.

signaling molecules from one cell to another through gap junctions between adjacent cells. Recall that gap junctions are communicating junctions that allow small molecules and ions to pass directly from the cytoplasm of one cell to another. An example of juxtacrine signaling is electrical transduction from cardiac cell to cardiac cell via the gap junction.

Signal Transduction

We have seen that hydrophobic ligands and those capable of facilitated diffusion can enter the target cell and directly bind

to an intracellular receptor to cause an intracellular response. However, when a ligand binds to a cell-surface receptor, the signal needs to be relayed inside the cell to initiate an intracellular effect.

Signal transduction refers to the processes by which an extracellular ligand–receptor interaction causes an intracellular change without the ligand entering the cell. In other words, it is the translation of an extracellular signal into changes in cell behavior. Additional cellular molecules often become involved in transmitting the message to its ultimate destination in the cell.

The ligand is considered the *first messenger*, carrying a signal from the signaling cell to the target cell-surface receptor. Once the initial ligand–receptor binding has occurred, other compounds called second messengers play an important role in transmitting the signal to specific intracellular sites in the cytoplasm or nucleus. Second messengers are short-lived molecules that mediate the transduction of the extracellular signals, and are usually generated strictly in response to a

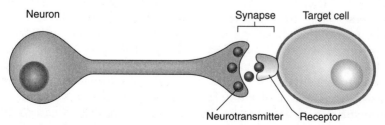

Figure 15.10. Neuronal or synaptic signaling, a special type of paracrine signaling. The signaling cell is the neuron, and the target cell may be another neuron or some other type of cell. The ligands are called neurotransmitters. The space over which the neurotransmitters travel between two neurons is the synapse.

The Insulin Receptor

Like receptors for other protein hormones, the receptor for insulin is embedded in the cell membrane of target cells (hepatocytes and myocytes). The insulin receptor is a tyrosine kinase–linked transmembrane glycoprotein with a dimeric structure capable of binding two insulin molecules at any given moment. It is composed of two α subunits and two β subunits linked by disulfide bonds. The α chains are entirely extracellular and contain the insulin binding domains. The linked β chains penetrate through the cell membrane into the cell and contain ATP-binding and tyrosine kinase domains.

The receptor functions as an enzyme that transfers phosphate groups from ATP to tyrosine residues on intracellular target proteins. Binding of insulin to the α subunits is the initial step in a signal transduction pathway that mediates glucose uptake and metabolism. The binding causes the β subunits to phosphorylate themselves (autophosphorylation), activating the catalytic activity of the receptor. The activated receptor then phosphorylates a number of intracellular proteins, which in turn alters their activity and generates the biological response.

Signal transduction by the insulin receptor is not limited to its activation at the cell surface. The activated ligand–receptor complex initially present at the cell surface can be internalized into the cell by endocytosis, forming vesicles or *endosomes*. Endocytosis of activated receptors concentrates receptors within endosomes and also allows the insulin receptor tyrosine kinase to phosphorylate substrates that are further inside the cell.

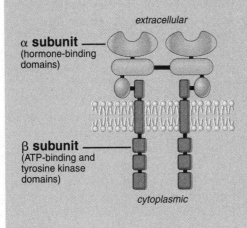

extracellular

α **subunit**
(hormone-binding domains)

β **subunit**
(ATP-binding and tyrosine kinase domains)

cytoplasmic

specific ligand–receptor interaction. Particularly important second messengers in a variety of signaling pathways include cyclic AMP (cAMP), calcium ions, inositol 1,4,5-trisphosphate (IP$_3$), and diacylglycerol (DAG).

The signal transduction pathway is nonlinear such that one molecule of an agonist can produce a large signal. As an illustration, consider one molecule of an agonist activating one receptor. This activates 10 adenylyl cylases, generating 100 molecules of cAMP, which activate 1,000 protein kinases, which phosphorylate 10,000 calcium channels, which allow 100,000 units of calcium to enter the cell. which finally causes 1 million units of contraction.

Protein phosphorylation is a common means of information transfer and many second messengers elicit responses by activating protein kinases. The use of common second messengers in multiple signaling pathways creates both opportunities and potential problems. Input from several signaling pathways, often

A
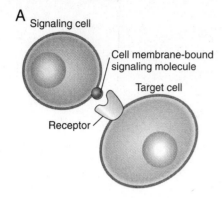

called *crosstalk*, may affect the concentrations of common second messengers. Crosstalk permits more finely tuned regulation of cell activity than would the action of individual independent pathways. However, inappropriate crosstalk can cause the signal carried by second messengers to be misinterpreted. An overview of the signal transduction process is illustrated in Figure 15.13.

After a signaling process has been initiated and the information has been transduced to affect other cellular processes, these processes must be terminated. Without such termination, cells lose their responsiveness to new signals. Moreover, signaling processes that fail to be terminated properly may lead to uncontrolled cell growth and the possibility of cancer. Protein phosphatases are one mechanism for the termination of a signaling process; the role of protein phosphorylation and dephosphorylation is shown in Figure 15.14.

B
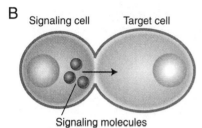

Figure 15.12. Juxtacrine signaling. **A.** Membrane-bound signal. **B.** Signal transmission through gap junctions.

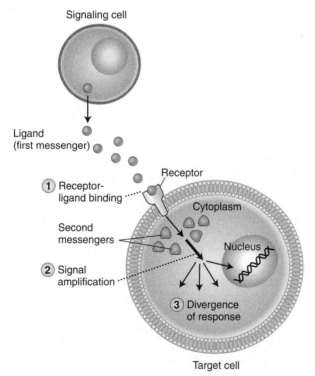

Figure 15.13. Representation of the signal-transduction process. The signaling cell releases a ligand that binds to a surface receptor on the target cell. This binding initiates signal transduction, which may involve second (intracellular) messengers. The outcome is some sort of cellular response in the target cell.

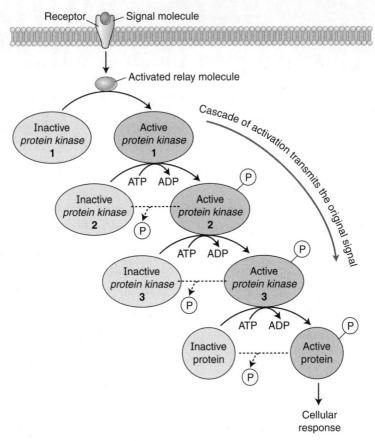

Figure 15.14. A more detailed depiction of the phosphorylation–dephosphorylation cascade that is often seen in signal transduction.

Signal transduction has several important features:

- The signal can undergo **amplification**, a process by which a small amount of ligand can create a large cellular response.
- The signaling pathway can diverge such that several processes in the cell can be influenced at the same time.
- Transmission of the signal can be altered according to the needs of the cell, by variation in the nature and amounts of the second messengers.
- The time course of the response can be controlled.

Several such counterbalanced signal transduction pathways control most cellular functions. Interfering with any step in the signal transduction cascade can be potentially harmful, but may be a useful approach in the treatment of disease.

Consequences of Ligand Signaling

A ligand may act at many different cellular sites—the cell membrane, cytoplasm, or nucleus—and at several different receptors. For example, dopamine activates dopamine receptors as well as adrenergic receptors. It is amazing that a few types of endogenous signaling ligands (neurotransmitters, hormones, and autacoids) are involved in controlling and regulating a vast variety of physiological functions.

Although a ligand may be able to reach many cells, only target cells with a specific receptor for these ligands will respond to the signal. Whether a cell responds to the signal and the manner in which it responds are dictated by what types of receptors the cell expresses and by the kind of signal transduction machinery available for responding to the signal. Variation in receptor type helps segregate the "signal" from the "noise" for various cells.

Different cells can therefore respond differently to the same signaling molecule. In other words, each cell is programmed to respond in a specific way to a signal. Additionally, the response depends on the number and type of other signals being simultaneously received by the cell. Thus, a single response may be dependent on the presence (or absence) of several different ligands. The response of the target cell may be fast (on the order of seconds) or slow (on the order of minutes or hours).

Target cell responses to receptor–ligand interactions may include:

- Alteration in the metabolism of the cell
- Modification in the electrical charge across the cell membrane
- Readjustment of the cytoskeleton
- Secretion of substances
- Cell death
- Activation of DNA to produce cellular proteins

Some common types of cell responses to a signal are illustrated in Figure 15.15.

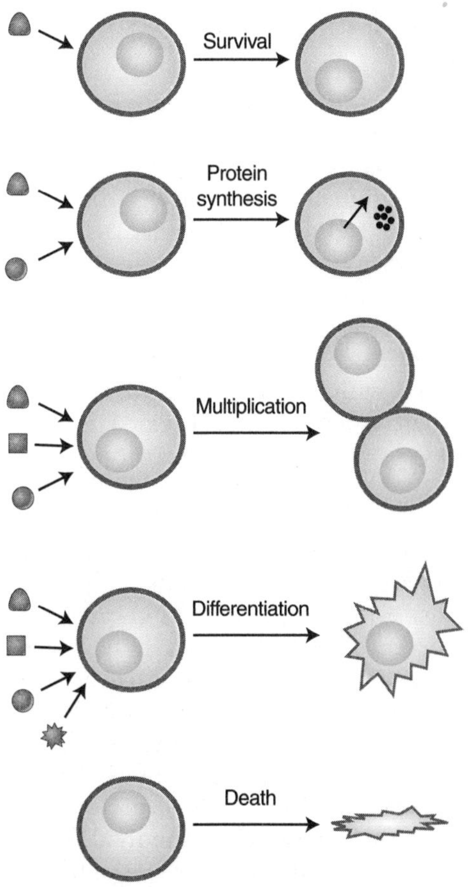

Receptors

As we have seen, a receptor is a cellular protein that binds specifically to a ligand and responds to it, passing a signal along. A cell has numerous different receptors that can respond to various combinations of signal molecules.

Ligand–Receptor Interactions

Recall that the interaction between a receptor (R) and a ligand (L) to produce an effect can be expressed as a two-step process.

$$L + R \rightleftharpoons LR \qquad \text{(Eq. 15.1)}$$

$$LR \rightarrow \rightarrow effect \qquad \text{(Eq. 15.2)}$$

The ligand–receptor complex (LR) is formed in the first step (Eq. 15.1). In the second step, the complex becomes the stimulus for a series of events that lead to the ultimate effect. A ligand that produces a response in the second step (Eq. 15.2) is an *agonist*. A ligand that merely forms a complex but does not produce a subsequent response is an *antagonist*.

Figure 15.15. Examples of different types of responses that result after cell signaling. Each response is a consequence of a different number and type of signals.

A very specific ligand structure is needed for a complex to form because receptor proteins are highly *stereoselective*. The ligand has to exhibit *stereocomplementarity* with the binding site of the receptor. Therefore, a receptor has two functions:

- detect a ligand and complex with it (*recognition*)
- conduct and translate a signal after binding to an agonist (*signal transduction*) to produce the desired effect

Once a ligand binds to a receptor-binding site, we say that the site is *occupied*. The number of receptors available in a particular tissue is usually limited, so that the receptors can be *saturated* if sufficient ligand is available and all the binding sites become occupied.

Noncatalytic and Catalytic Receptors

Many receptors are *noncatalytic*, meaning that ligand–receptor binding is reversible (as shown in Eq. 15.1) and the ligand dissociates intact from the receptor after the effect in Equation 15.2.

Ligands also bind to catalytic *enzymes* either in the cell or on the cell membrane; the ligand in this case is called a *substrate*. Enzymes interact with their substrates to form complexes, but unlike receptors, the enzyme catalytically transforms the substrate into chemically different products that are then released. The process can be viewed as follows:

$$S + E \rightleftharpoons ES \rightarrow product + E \quad (Eq. 15.3)$$

where E is the enzyme and S is the substrate. Therefore, the two major characteristics of enzyme receptors are their ability to recognize a substrate (just like noncatalytic receptors) and their ability to catalyze a reaction of it.

Recent evidence suggests that some noncatalytic receptors have the potential to be active even in the absence of an ag-

onist ligand. Such receptors are referred to as **constitutively active receptors**. Their agonist-independent activity emphasizes the intrinsic regulatory activity of a receptor, i.e., the receptor (not the ligand) contains the information to modulate cell function. Many ligands inhibit this constitutive activity *after* binding to the receptor. These ligands act as **inverse agonists**, displaying negative intrinsic activity. The discovery has led to the concept of inverse agonism, which has emerged as an essential principle of receptor regulation.

Receptor Subtypes

Each agonist ligand has receptors in many different parts of the body and can stimulate a wide range of effects depending on where in the body the ligand–receptor interaction occurs. In fact, a ligand can bind with many slightly different versions of its receptor, each with a unique function, in various locations. Thus, ligands can be thought of as master keys that can fit several different locks or **receptor subtypes** to open different doors (effect).

For example, norepinephrine can interact with α- and β-*adrenoreceptors*, which are further subdivided into α_1 and α_2 and β_1 and β_2 receptors. These receptor subtypes are found in different target organs: for example, the heart contains β_1 receptors whereas β_2 receptors are found in the bronchial smooth muscle. Each receptor subtype has a different function, and the release of norepinephrine locally at each of these sites produces a different physiological effect. Another example is acetylcholine binding to *cholinergic* receptors that can be either *muscarinic* or *nicotinic*; each of these is subdivided into many different subtypes with distinct functions.

The existence of receptor subtypes allows our bodies to use just one ligand for a variety of actions by releasing it in different locations. This phenomenon also allows scientists to design drugs that bind to only one receptor subtype of a ligand. In this way, drugs can be made very selective. Conversely, a drug that can bind to many subtypes of a receptor can cause unwanted side effects.

Receptor Structure and Classification

One way of classifying receptors is by the ligand that binds to them. In fact, many receptors are named after their signaling ligands, such as steroid, insulin, or acetylcholine (ACh) receptors.

A more useful approach to receptor classification is by their structure, function, or signal transduction pathway. On this basis, we can construct five broad categories of receptors:

Cell-surface receptors:

- Ion-channel receptors
- G protein–coupled receptors
- Enzymatic receptors

Intracellular receptors:

- Transcriptional regulation receptors
- Intracellular enzymes

Let us briefly consider each one of these structural classes and see how they work.

Cell-Surface Receptors

The primary mechanism through which a cell senses extracellular stimuli is through cell-surface receptors.

Ion-Channel Receptors. Although the cell membrane is lipidlike, we have seen that it contains proteins that form ion channels through which small ions (e.g., Na^+, K^+, Ca^{2+}, and Cl^-) can enter and leave the cell. The conformation and structure of the channel protein make it selective for transport of a particular ion. Conformational changes in these receptor proteins can open or close these channels, regulating ion movement in and out of a cell.

Many ion channels are opened and closed by the binding of certain neurotransmitters with **ligand-gated ion-channel** receptors. These receptors are integral glycoproteins that traverse through the cell membrane and can exist in one of three states: resting (or closed), open, or desensitized. On binding with a ligand, the closed receptors rapidly change conformation to open the ion channel in a process known as *gating*. Dissociation of the ligand–receptor complex closes the ion channel. However, after prolonged exposure to the ligand, the receptors can become desensitized.

The signal ligands for these ion channels are neurotransmitters. Examples are the nicotinic ACh receptors (where the ligand is acetylcholine, which regulates the Na^+/K^+ channel) in skeletal muscle, and GABA receptors (where the ligand is γ-aminobutyric acid) in the brain. A schematic representation of a ligand-gated ion-channel receptor is shown in Figure 15.16. Signaling by ligand-gated ion channels is very fast—on the order of milliseconds—which is very important for the rapid transfer of information across synapses.

Another type of ion channel is called a **voltage-dependent ion channel**. These channels can be opened or closed by generating a voltage difference across the membrane. Such a voltage can be created as a result of a differential distribution of ions on the two sides of the membrane, resulting in a conformational change of the receptor protein and an opening and closing of the channel. There is no ligand directly involved in the transport of ions by voltage-dependent receptors.

G Protein–Coupled Receptors. The G protein–coupled receptors (GPCRs) are a superfamily of related cell-surface receptors vital for normal cellular health. GPCRs are important as targets for drug design and therapy; it is estimated that

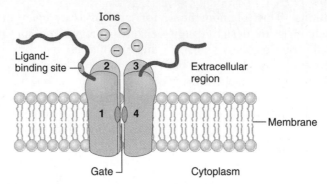

Figure 15.16. Schematic representation of a ligand-gated ion-channel receptor. The receptor is a transmembrane protein (shown here with four transmembrane segments labeled 1–4). The extracellular part of the protein contains the ligand-binding site. Ligand–receptor binding causes a change in the conformation of the receptor. This opens the gate, creating a pore through which ions can diffuse into the cell.

more than half of all the drugs on the market today target GPCRs.

The common structural feature of this class of receptors is a single polypeptide chain that has seven *trans-membrane domains*, i.e., it traverses the lipid bilayer seven times. The term *G protein* in the name occurs because the signal-transduction mechanism in this class of receptors works through small intracellular proteins called *G proteins*, short for *guanine nucleotide-binding proteins*, a family of proteins involved in second messenger cascades. Their name is derived from their signaling mechanism, which uses the exchange of guanine diphosphate (GDP) for guanine triphosphate (GTP) as a molecular "switch" to allow or inhibit biochemical reactions inside the cell.

GPCRs bind to a wide spectrum of extracellular ligands, including hormones, neurotransmitters, and autacoids. Each ligand has a different mode and site of binding on the seven-transmembrane protein, resulting in a different biochemical outcome. Many of the GPCRs act through second messengers.

After a ligand binds to the active site on the cell surface, the receptor undergoes a conformational change that alters the intracellular portion of the receptor,

allowing it to further bind to the G protein in the cell. A G protein is made up of α, β, and γ subunits. Binding of the G protein with the ligand–receptor complex causes the G protein to break up into two active components—an α subunit and a β–γ complex—both of which can regulate the activity of target proteins in the cell membrane. Once the activated α-subunit has propagated its signal to its target protein, it reassociates with the β–γ complex and the signal is shut off. This "on–off" mechanism is a crucial component of controlling many signaling pathways. The receptor stays active while the signal ligand is bound to it, and can therefore catalyze the activation of many molecules of G protein in this way.

Figure 15.17 shows the structure and signal-transduction mechanism of GPCRs. Examples of this class of receptors are acetylcholine muscarinic, α- and β-adrenergic, dopamine, serotonin, and histamine receptors.

Enzymatic Receptors. This simple class of receptors has an extracellular portion that binds to the ligand, a single linear hydrophobic region that traverses the membrane lipid bilayer, and an intracellular portion that is located in the cytoplasm. This intracellular region may

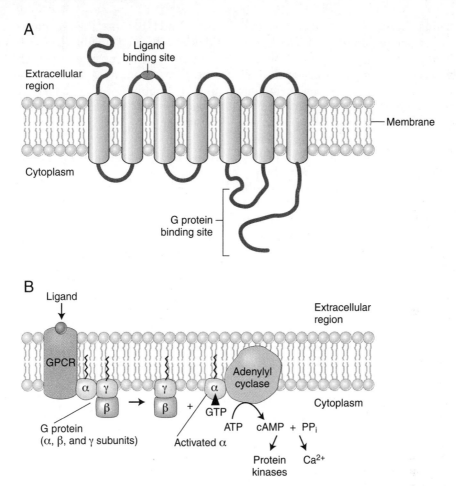

Figure 15.17. A. The structure of G protein–coupled receptors shows the seven-transmembrane (7TM) protein receptor with its seven transmembrane domains, and the binding sites for ligand and G protein. **B.** The signal transduction pathway after activation of a G protein–coupled receptor (GPCR) by a ligand.

have intrinsic enzyme activity that is triggered on binding to a ligand, i.e., the receptor is itself an enzyme. Note that ligand–receptor binding in this case is reversible because the signaling ligand is not the substrate. The substrate is located inside the cell and is transformed to a product on receptor activation by the ligand.

The best understood family of enzymatic receptors is the **protein kinase receptor** family, in which the enzyme activated is a protein kinase. For example, *tyrosine kinases* selectively attach a phos-phate group to the amino acid tyrosine in a protein, and *serine/threonine* kinases to serine and threonine residues. Enzymatic receptors with intrinsic protein kinase activity bind to and mediate actions of most growth factors (epidermal growth factor, nerve growth factor, platelet-derived growth factor [PDGF], and so forth) and are of great interest for their role in cancer.

Alternatively, the receptor may be an **enzyme-linked receptor**; when activated by a ligand these receptors bind to and activate enzymes nearby. Here, too, the signaling ligand is not the substrate. Ligand–receptor binding initiates a cascade of protein phosphorylations that result in the ultimate effect inside the cell. This class of single transmembrane (1TM) receptors is further classified according to the intracellular enzyme system that is activated after ligand binding.

Figure 15.18 illustrates an enzyme-linked receptor showing the single transmembrane protein, the extracellular ligand–binding site, and the intracellular site associated with enzyme activity. For example, the cytokine receptor is a tyrosine kinase–linked receptor. Cytokine receptors must first be activated by their signaling ligands (cytokines, interferons, and human growth factor [HGF]), and then bind to cytoplasmic tyrosine kinases before they are able to phosphorylate their target proteins. Therefore, protein kinases are involved in the process of signal transduction in these pathways as well, as they were with GPCRs.

Intracellular Receptors

Many intracellular proteins act as receptors for signaling ligands and other compounds. Because the receptor is inside the cell, the signaling ligand has to cross the cell membrane, reach the receptor, and bind to it. Thus, the ligands must be lipophilic (like the steroid hormones) so that they can cross the cell membrane.

Transcriptional Regulation Receptors. The transcriptional regulation receptors, also known as *nuclear receptors*, constitute most of the intracellular receptor class. Transcriptional regulation receptors usually trigger an effect when the ligand–receptor complex travels from the cytoplasm into the nucleus, initiating transcription of RNA. They are further subdivided as:

- steroid receptors (e.g., receptors for corticosteroids, sex steroids, and mineralocorticoids)
- nonsteroid receptors (e.g., receptors for thyroid hormones, retinoic acid, and vitamin D)

The process by which a hormone binds to its intracellular receptor and triggers a response is illustrated in Figure 15.19. The hormone crosses the cell membrane

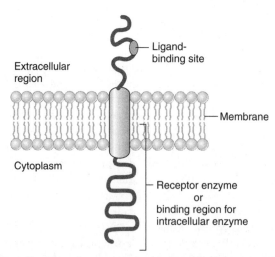

Figure 15.18. Schematic depiction of an enzymatic receptor showing the single transmembrane protein, the extracellular ligand-binding site, and the intracellular site associated with enzyme activity.

Gleevec

Disrupting messages between cells with specificity and limited side effects has become a new model for anticancer drug discovery. The success of signal-transduction inhibitors, such as Gleevec (imatinib mesylate) in first treating chronic myelogenous leukemia (CML) and then gastrointestinal stromal tumors (GISTs) has bolstered this approach to new drug discovery. Imatinib is an inhibitor of the receptor tyrosine kinases for PDGF and stem cell factor (SCF), and inhibits PDGF- and SCF-mediated cellular events.

In healthy individuals, normal receptors on stem cells respond to growth factor signals to produce new blood cells. The receptor can be turned on and off as necessary to produce the number of blood cells the body needs.

Patients with CML have a genetic defect that results in abnormal receptors that have constitutive activity and cannot be turned off, resulting in uncontrolled growth of white blood cells. The receptor needs energy provided by ATP to carry out its kinase activity and propagate signals necessary for cellular proliferation. Imatinib fits into and inhibits the ATP-binding site on the receptor; without ATP, the receptor cannot carry out its kinase activity. Thus, imatinib is a tyrosine kinase inhibitor that prevents the constitutive cell growth signal in the abnormal, cancerous cells.

Tyrosine kinase inhibition reduces the ability of the kinase to transfer phosphate groups from ATP and phosphorylate tyrosine residues on substrate proteins, which in turn prevents the transduction of energy signals necessary for cellular proliferation. Thus, the specific signal-transduction pathway abnormally activated in the leukemic transformation process (and in PDGF-mediated pathways) is inactivated by imatinib.

Imatinib is indicated for the treatment of newly diagnosed adult patients with Philadelphia chromosome–positive CML. It is also now indicated for the treatment of patients with malignant GISTs.

---

by passive diffusion and binds to its receptor in the cytoplasm, thus activating the receptor. The receptor has a hormone-binding site (selective for a given hormone), a DNA-binding site, and a third site whose exact function is unknown. The hormone–receptor complex then travels to the nucleus, where it binds to DNA and initiates transcription of mRNA. The mRNA leaves the nucleus and serves as a template for synthesis of specific proteins within the cytoplasm. This process takes time, and there is generally a lag time—up to several hours—between initial ligand–receptor binding and production of proteins. For this reason, the effect produced by hormones that act at nuclear receptors can persist long after the initial signaling event.

Figure 15.20 shows an overview of signaling by agonist binding to various types of receptors.

Intracellular Enzymes. Enzymes catalyze most cellular processes and reactions. Each cell requires more than 500 different enzymes to carry out all its functions, and the types and concentrations of

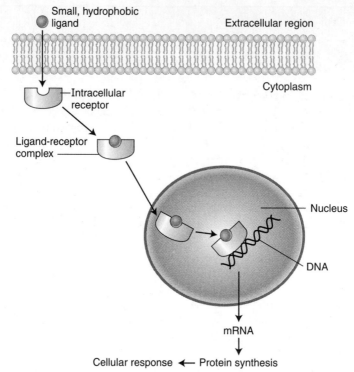

Figure 15.19. Mechanism of action of a typical intracellular hormone receptor. The receptor is located in the cytoplasm of the cell. The hormone (ligand) has to cross the lipid bilayer and enter the cell to bind to the receptor.

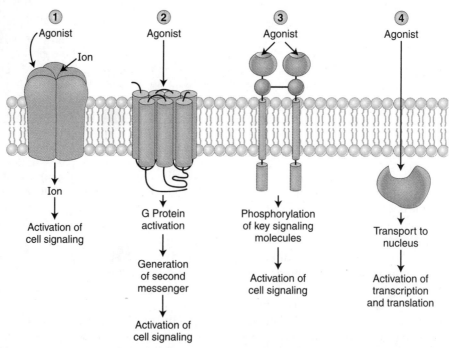

Figure 15.20. Summary of signaling by agonist–receptor binding at (1) ligand-gated ion channels, (2) G protein–coupled receptors, (3) enzyme-linked receptors, and (4) intracellular receptors.

these enzymes vary according to the needs of the cell. Enzymes may be membrane-bound as we have seen already, or may be contained in the cytosol or in various intracellular structures. Many intracellular enzymes are involved in signal transduction cascades as discussed earlier with the protein kinases, and serve as intracellular receptors.

One of the functions of enzymes is to catalyze synthesis or break down of signaling molecules according to the needs of the cell. For example, acetylcholinesterase breaks down the neurotransmitter acetylcholine, whereas dopa decarboxylase converts L-dopa to its active form dopamine.

Modulation of Ligand–Receptor Interactions

Ligand–receptor interactions are the body's way of maintaining homeostasis and defending or repairing itself. Receptors and ligands respond to external perturbations and appropriately adjust physiological processes to maintain normal functioning of our body. Therefore, the nature and extent of these interactions need to be modulated or controlled according to the situation. The body achieves this modulation by controlling or altering several parameters. When one of these modulation mechanisms does not work optimally, the result could be a disorder or disease.

Concentration of Ligand

The concentration of ligand will in part determine how much of the ligand–receptor complex is formed and therefore the strength of the signal. Ligand concentration is controlled by:

- increasing or decreasing ligand synthesis
- increasing or decreasing ligand release

- altering the destruction or removal of ligand from the receptor site

Receptor Density

Receptors also have the capacity to adapt to the changing environment to maintain homeostasis; this ability is known as receptor dynamism. The primary manifestation of this response is a constant fluctuation in receptor density or the number of receptors at a particular site. Receptor density is not fixed but is dynamic, controlled by opposing rates of receptor synthesis and receptor degeneration. The body can modify these rates by:

- Increasing the number of receptors when there is a shortage of ligand, known as receptor up-regulation
- Decreasing the number of receptors when there is an abundance of ligand, known as receptor down-regulation

Allosteric Modulation

Allosteric effects occur when the binding properties of a protein for a ligand change as a consequence of a second molecule binding to the protein; we have discussed this in an earlier chapter. The modulating molecule and ligand bind to different sites on the protein or even to different subunits; the modulator binding location is called the *allosteric* site. The structures of the ligand and modulating molecule can be very different because they bind to different sites. Binding of the modulator to the receptor alters the conformation of the receptor active site and either increases or decreases its affinity for the primary ligand. Thus, the presence and concentration of the modulating molecule can control ligand–receptor interactions, and the presence of an allosteric modulator provides one more means of controlling cell signaling.

Allosteric effects are important in the regulation of enzymatic reactions. Cells use allosteric activators (which enhance activity) and allosteric inhibitors (which reduce activity) to control enzyme reactions. Noncatalytic receptors can also be allosterically modulated. For example, the activation of ligand-gated ion channels is allosterically modulated by compounds such as anesthetics, barbiturates, neurosteroids, neurotoxins, and alcohol.

KEY CONCEPTS

- Cellular communication is carried out by the appropriate release and binding of ligands to their receptors.
- Hydrophilic ligands bind to cell-surface receptors, whereas hydrophobic ligands can bind to intracellular receptors after crossing the cell membrane.
- Hormones are ligands made in endocrine glands and carried by the bloodstream to their target receptors; they act by activating enzymes or modulating gene expression.
- Ductless glands and other cells secrete autacoids for local signaling; many ligands can function as both hormones and local signals.
- Paracrine signals influence neighboring cells; autocrine signaling occurs when cells respond to substances they themselves secrete; and juxtacrine signals are those passed between two cells in contact.
- Signal transduction is the translation of an extracellular signal into changes in cell behavior by a cascade of several second messenger systems.
- Receptors may be noncatalytic (act by binding reversibly to agonists), catalytic (act by catalyzing a reaction), or constitutively active (act in the absence of an agonist).
- Cell-surface receptors (e.g., ion-channel receptors, G protein–coupled receptors, and enzyme-associated receptors) bind to ligands on the cell membrane, whereas intracellular receptors (e.g., transcriptional regulator receptors and enzymes) require the ligand to enter the cell.
- Receptors of the G protein–coupled cell-surface receptor superfamily are targets for almost half of marketed drugs.
- Ligand–receptor interactions are modulated by changes in ligand or receptor concentration or by allosteric effects.

ADDITIONAL READING

1. Foreman JC, Johansen T (eds). Textbook of Receptor Pharmacology, 2nd ed. CRC Press, 2002.

2. Gomperts BD, Kramer IM, Tatham PER. Signal Transduction. Academic Press, 2002.

3. Helmreich EJM. The Biochemistry of Cell Signaling. Oxford University Press, 2001.

4. Krauss G. Biochemistry of Signal Transduction. John Wiley, New York, 2000.

REVIEW QUESTIONS

1. What are the steps involved in cellular communication?

2. Describe the types of hormones secreted by endocrine glands and tissues.

3. Explain the process of endocrine signaling by hormones. What are the key features of endocrine signaling?

4. What are the similarities and differences between endocrine and local signaling by ligands?

5. List the features and differences between paracrine, autocrine, and juxtacrine signaling.

6. Explain the process of signal transduction. Why is transduction essential for polar signaling ligands?

7. What is the role of second messengers in the transduction process? How is a signal altered according to the needs of the cell?

8. Explain how one type of signaling ligand can cause different effects in different locations in the body.

9. What are receptors? Distinguish between catalytic, noncatalytic, and constitutive receptors.

10. List and briefly describe the types of cell-surface and intracellular receptors.

11. Elaborate on the mechanisms by which the body modulates and controls ligand–receptor interactions.

Mechanisms of Drug Action

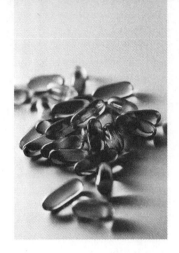

It is widely accepted that the cellular targets of most drugs used for medical treatment are proteins and associated macromolecules, and that most drugs produce their effect by binding to these specific receptors in the body. These concepts were introduced in Chapter 6, Drugs and Their Targets. Drugs usually work by competing with or taking the place of an endogenous ligand or by altering the ligand–receptor interaction in some way. Therefore, a drug generally makes a *quantitative* change in an existing physiological or biochemical process but does not *qualitatively* alter the nature of the process or create a new process.

Importance of Drug Structure

By binding to a receptor, drugs either enhance or inhibit receptor activity. A drug can take the place of an endogenous ligand if drug structure is similar enough to the ligand it is designed to replace. Remember that most receptors are stereoselective so that stereochemistry of drug and ligand has to be similar, and the drug and receptor have to exhibit *stereocomplementarity*. Many drugs of diverse structures are able to bind to the receptor's active site provided that the structure of the pharmacophore can be recognized by the receptor.

The interaction of receptors with a ligand or drug involves the types of reversible molecular bonds we have already discussed. Most interactions involve several kinds of forces simultaneously. Ionic bonds, the most long-range of these forces, are important for the primary phase of attraction between the receptor with ligand or drug. The ionization state of the drug and of the acidic and basic groups of the receptor's active site is important in determining the initial attraction between them. At physiological pH, even mildly acidic groups such as carboxylic acid groups will be entirely in their anionic form, whereas phenolic groups may be partially ionized. Basic groups such as amino groups will be either partially or completely protonated to their cationic form. The pharmacological activity of many drugs can often be correlated with the fraction ionized at the receptor site. However, complete ionization is not desirable if the drug has to cross cell membranes (i.e., has intracellular receptors) to exert its action. Thus, the pK_a of a drug needs to be such that an appropriate balance between the ionized and un-ionized forms exists at physiological pH.

Ionic bonds alone are not sufficient to hold the drug in contact with the receptor long enough, or in the proper orientation, to produce an effect. Hydrogen bonds, hydrophobic forces, and van der Waal's interactions come into play after the initial ionic attraction. They serve to orient the drug appropriately and then to fine tune the fit between receptor and drug.

Drug Action at Noncatalytic Receptors

The discussion in this section applies to *noncatalytic receptors* (including *constitutively active receptors*); we will examine the interaction of drugs with catalytic receptors (enzymes) later in the chapter. A drug with an appropriate pharmacophore can replace the corresponding endogenous ligand and interact with the receptor. In most situations, the ligand L is still available to bind to the receptor, and there is competition between ligand and drug for available receptors. The amount of drug–receptor complex formed versus the amount of ligand–receptor complex formed depends on the concentrations of ligand and drug and their relative affinities for the receptor.

Theory of Drug Action

Chapter 6, Drugs and Their Targets, examined some simple approaches to understanding receptor binding to an endogenous ligand or drug. We now expand on these concepts to account for the varied behavior seen when a drug binds to a receptor.

One theoretical model of drug action is the two-state model, illustrated in Figure 16.1. This model was originally developed to explain constitutive activity of G protein–coupled receptors (GPCRs), but can be used as a general approach to understand drug action at any receptor. The model assumes that the receptor exists in two conformations that are in equilibrium—an inactive form (the R state) and an active form (the R* state). Receptors in the R* conformation can give rise to a response with a magnitude dependent on the fraction of receptors in the R* conformation (i.e., the R/R* ratio). Most receptors exist in the inactive R conformation when not bound to a drug or an endogenous ligand, with only a small fraction in the active R* conformation. Exceptions are the constitutive receptors (discussed in the previous chapter), which have a significant fraction of receptors in the R* state even in the absence of ligand.

For a drug to influence the function of a receptor it first has to have an affinity for and be able to bind to the receptor.

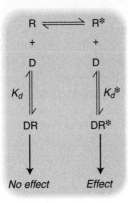

Figure 16.1. A schematic representation of the two-state receptor model. R is the receptor in the inactive state, R* is the receptor in the active state, D is the drug, and DR and DR* are the respective drug–receptor complexes. R, R*, DR, and DR* are in constant equilibrium. K_d and K_d^* are equilibrium constants defined for the dissociation of the drug–receptor complex, and are inversely related to affinities of the drug for the receptor in its inactive and active states, respectively.

Drugs with receptor affinity may bind selectively to either R or R* states, or with equal affinity to both R and R*. Drug–receptor binding can therefore influence receptor function in different ways. In general, a drug can enhance, diminish, or block the transmission of a signal when it binds to a receptor.

Agonists and Antagonists

An agonist is an endogenous ligand or drug that can interact with the active receptor state and stimulate an effect or response characteristic of that receptor. Endogenous ligands and agonist drugs preferentially bind to R* to form the active DR* complex as follows:

$$D + R^* \rightleftharpoons DR^* \xrightarrow{\text{stimulus}} \text{effect}$$

$$\text{(Eq. 16.1)}$$

The equilibrium constant (*affinity*) of this interaction is given by:

$$K^* = \frac{[DR^*]}{[D][R^*]} \quad \text{(Eq. 16.2)}$$

For mathematical convenience, we define a dissociation constant of the drug–receptor complex, K_d^*:

$$K_d^* = \frac{1}{K^*} = \frac{[D][R^*]}{[DR^*]} \quad \text{(Eq. 16.3)}$$

A drug with a large K_d^* has a low affinity for the receptor, and vice versa. The preferential formation of the DR* complex over a DR complex drives the equilibrium between R and R* toward more R*. This increases the proportion of receptors available for signaling and eventually increases pharmacological response.

The selectivity of agonists for R or R* may vary. An agonist drug with great selectivity for R* over R will behave as a **full agonist** and will therefore enhance or augment the response of the endogenous ligand. An agonist with only a small selectivity for R* over R will behave as a **partial agonist** and will not show the extent of response of a full agonist. In some situations, partial agonists may actually block (antagonize) the effects of a full agonist drug or the endogenous agonist ligand. For example, pindolol is a partial agonist at β-adrenergic receptors; it may act as an agonist if no full agonist is present, or as an antagonist if a full agonist, such as isoproterenol, is present.

Some drugs preferentially bind to R over R* to form the inactive DR complex. This binding drives the equilibrium between R and R* toward R, decreasing the proportion of receptors in the R* state available for signaling by the endogenous ligand.

$$R + D \rightleftharpoons DR \xrightarrow{\text{no stimulus}} \text{no effect}$$

$$\text{(Eq. 16.4)}$$

The treatment of the equilibrium constant for binding (affinity; K) and the dissociation constant of the complex (K_d) are analogous to that discussed above for agonist binding to the active receptor state, so that:

$$K_d = \frac{1}{K} = \frac{[D][R]}{[DR]} \quad \text{(Eq. 16.5)}$$

If there is a significant level of constitutive receptor activity, these drugs, known as inverse agonists, will decrease receptor signaling and thereby decrease response. If there is no significant constitutive receptor activity, these drugs will compete with and act as competitive antagonists of the endogenous ligand. Thus, an antagonist drug will reduce or prevent the response of the natural ligand; for this reason, antagonists are often called *receptor blockers*.

Drugs that do not differentiate between R and R*, binding with equal affinity to both conformations, are known as neutral competitive antagonists. They do not alter receptor activity on their own, but can compete with agonists and inverse agonists for receptor binding, thereby competitively antagonizing the responses elicited by agonists and inverse agonists. The clinical significance of the differentiation between neutral competitive antagonists and inverse agonists is not always clear. Figure 16.2 shows a schematic representation of how the two-state receptor model relates to the action of drugs.

In general, there is structural similarity between a series of agonists because they have to bind to the same active receptor conformation and stimulate the same response as the ligand. However, there may be less similarity between the structures of ligands and their antagonists. Antagonists are often more bulky than agonists for two reasons: to prevent receptors from acquiring active conformations, and to increase the number of attractive binding forces with the receptor and compensate for an imperfectly matched structure. Figures 16.3 and 16.4 illustrate these structural concepts with examples of endogenous ligands and their agonists and antagonists. Examples

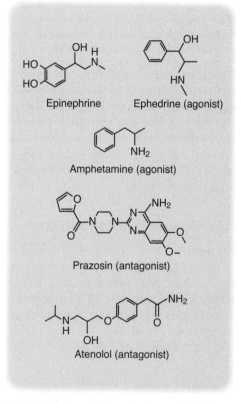

Figure 16.3. Examples of agonists and antagonists of epinephrine. Note structural similarities between epinephrine and its agonists, and the dissimilarities between epinephrine and its antagonists. Ephedrine and amphetamine are stimulants, whereas prazosin and atenolol are antihypertensives and are used to treat high blood pressure.

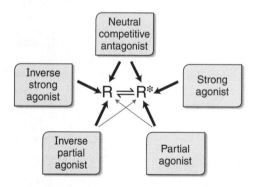

Figure 16.2. The two-state receptor model and its relationship to the mechanism of action of drugs. The heavy arrows indicate a strong affinity between drug and receptor (either in its active or inactive conformation), whereas the light arrows indicate a weak affinity.

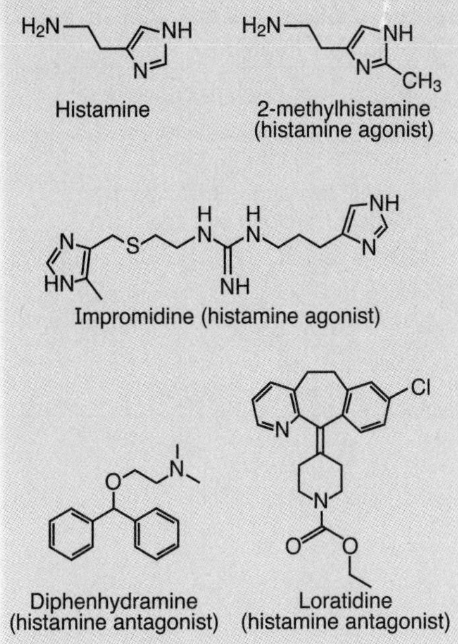

Figure 16.4. Examples of agonists and antagonists of histamine. Note the structural similarities between histamine and its agonists, and the dissimilarities between histamine and its antagonists. Histamine agonists do not have a clinical role, but are used in research. Diphenhydramine and loratidine are antihistamines and are used clinically to treat allergies.

of agonist and antagonist drugs are given in Tables 16.1 and 16.2, respectively.

Allosteric Drugs

The interaction of an agonist drug with its receptor often results in a continuous stimulation of potentially all receptor molecules in the body, which is not necessarily desirable. Similarly, the interaction of an antagonist drug with a receptor may lead to a prolonged blockade of receptor function, which also may be problematic.

There are, however, novel ways to intercede in receptor function that allow for a more controlled and selective "tuning" action of a drug on the receptor. Allosteric modulation has long been recognized as a general and widespread mechanism for control of protein function. Allosteric modulators bind to regulatory sites distinct from the receptor's active site, resulting in conformational changes (such as R to R* or vice versa) that influence ligand binding and protein function profoundly. This concept has been studied intensively and is now considered a classic mechanism to control protein behavior. For example, allosteric enzymes contain regions separate from the substrate-binding site to which small, regulatory molecules (*effectors*) may bind and thereby affect the catalytic activity.

This concept underlies the mechanism of action of allosteric modulators, drugs that bind at an allosteric site and thereby modify the binding of the endogenous ligand at the primary binding site (Fig. 16.5). Examples of an allosteric protein that is an important drug target is HIV reverse transcriptase, which coverts viral DNA to RNA, and is a key target for antiretroviral drugs such as nevirapine.

TABLE 16.1. Examples of Agonist Drugs, Their Receptor Targets, and Conditions That They Treat		
Receptor	*Drug*	*Condition Treated*
α adrenoceptor	Oxymetazoline[a]	Nasal congestion
Opioid receptor	Meperidine, morphine	Analgesia
Glucocorticoid nuclear receptor	Dexamethasone	Inflammation
GABA$_A$ chloride ion channel	Alprazolam	Anxiety
Potassium ion channel	Minoxidil	Hair regrowth

[a]Partial agonist.
GABA, γ-aminobutyric acid.

TABLE 16.2. Examples of Antagonist and Inverse Agonist Drugs, Their Receptor Targets, and Conditions That They Treat		
Receptor	Antagonist Drug	Condition Treated
Calcium ion channel	Diltiazem	Angina, high blood pressure
Angiotensin receptor	Losartan	High blood pressure, heart failure, chronic renal insufficiency
β-adrenoceptor receptor	Propranolol	Angina, myocardial infarction, heart failure, high blood pressure
Mineralocorticoid nuclear receptor	Spironolactone	Edema caused by liver cirrhosis and heart failure
Estrogen nuclear receptor	Tamoxifen	Prevention and treatment of breast cancer
Serotonin transporter	Fluoxetine	Depression
Histamine H_2 receptor	Cimetidine,[a] ranitidine[a]	Gastric acidity

[a]Inverse agonist.

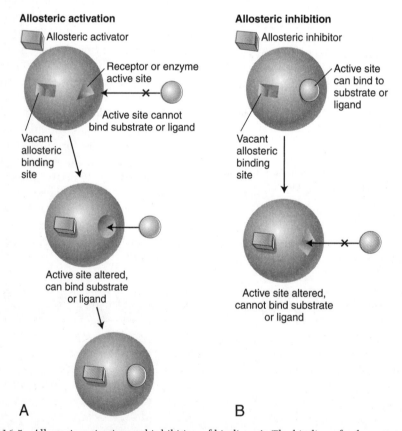

Figure 16.5. Allosteric activation and inhibition of binding. **A.** The binding of a drug at an allosteric site enhances the ability of the ligand or substrate to bind. **B.** The allosteric drug inhibits binding of the ligand or substrate.

Allosteric activators or *enhancers* are drugs that enhance agonist affinity of the ligand while having no effect on their own. *Allosteric antagonists* or *inhibitors* reduce agonist affinity. *Neutral allosteric drugs* bind to an allosteric site without affecting the binding or function of the endogenous ligand but can still block the action of other allosteric modulators that act via the same allosteric site.

Quantitation of Drug–Receptor Interactions

One of the major difficulties in measuring drug–receptor interactions is that the structure, characteristics, and concentrations of many receptors are still unknown. Various empirical parameters and approaches are currently used to describe the interaction between drugs and receptors. These parameters have evolved over several decades, and each gives us different pieces of information. Modeling the actions of drugs and receptors in the ways outlined below is a powerful tool, and allows the actions of drugs to be better understood, analyzed, and described. Let us consider some of the more useful concepts.

Affinity

The first and most obvious concept is that the intensity of drug effect is directly proportional to the concentration of the drug–receptor complex. The most direct measure of this is the *affinity* of the drug for the receptor in the formation of the drug–receptor complex.

The receptor concentration is usually constant at a given time, so that the concentration of the complex depends primarily on the concentration of drug and on the affinity of drug for the receptor. Complex formation is greater when drug concentrations are large and when K_d^* (for agonists) and K_d (for antagonists) are small. In other words, the greater the drug concentration and affinity, the greater the number of receptors occupied by drug.

Occupation Theory

The concept of drug occupancy of receptors led to the occupation theory, which states that the magnitude of pharmacological effect is directly related to the fraction of *occupied receptors*. The implications of this are that maximum drug effect occurs from the occupation of all possible receptors, 50% maximal effect results from occupation of 50% of the receptors, and so on. From this, we can derive an equation (note similarity to the Michaelis–Menten equation) to relate the drug–receptor interaction to pharmacological effect:

$$E = E_{max} \frac{[D]}{K_D + [D]} \quad \text{(Eq. 16.6)}$$

where E is the pharmacological effect, E_{max} is the maximum pharmacological effect, [D] is the concentration of the drug, and K_D is now defined for an equilibrium representing total receptors (R + R*). The K_D value is very often used as a parameter to compare the potency of different drugs that work at the same receptor.

Equation 16.6 implies that at high drug concentrations, [D] is much greater than K_D, and therefore E is essentially equal to E_{max}, i.e., that all drugs produce maximum effect when all available receptors are fully occupied. However, this is not always the case. We have already seen in the previous chapter that the relationship between receptor binding and response is complex. Agonist–receptor binding is only the first step in a series of biochemical events that ultimately produce pharmacological effect. A deficiency of the occupation theory is that it does not provide any information about the ability of the drug to produce a response after binding to the receptor. In particular, it cannot distinguish between full agonists, partial agonists, and antagonists, all of which can occupy receptors fully.

Two concepts—intrinsic activity and efficacy—were introduced to address shortcomings of the occupation theory.

Intrinsic Activity

It was postulated that two factors govern the effect of a drug: affinity and intrinsic activity. Affinity is a measure of drug–receptor binding as discussed above. Intrinsic activity (denoted by α) describes the ability of the drug to evoke a maximal effect after receptor binding. Therefore, both agonists and antagonists have affinity for their receptors, but agonists also have intrinsic activity.

A full agonist, which by definition gives a maximum response when all receptors are occupied (because it binds preferentially to the R* form), is assigned an α value of 1. Partial agonists elicit less than maximal response even when all receptors are occupied (because they bind to both R and R* receptor forms), and have α values less than 1. Antagonists, which have no intrinsic activity (because they bind preferentially to the R form), have an α value of 0.

It is proposed that drug effect is related to intrinsic activity and the concentration of the drug–receptor complex as follows:

$$E = \alpha [DR] \qquad \text{(Eq. 16.7)}$$

We can also say that:

$$E = E_{max} \frac{[DR]}{[R_t]} \qquad \text{(Eq. 16.8)}$$

where $[R_t]$ is the total concentration of receptors.

Equation 16.8 indicates a linear relationship between drug effect E and *fractional receptor occupancy* $[DR]/[R_t]$, until $[DR]/[R_t] = 1$. This suggests that a full agonist ($\alpha = 1$) will exhibit maximal effect when all the receptors are occupied ($[DR] = [R_t]$). A partial agonist ($0 < \alpha < 1$) will not show maximum effect even when all the receptors are occupied.

The assumption so far has been that maximum effect requires the complete occupation of receptors. This is not always the case. There are situations when two full agonists ($\alpha = 1$) can elicit a maximum response ($E = E_{max}$) while occupying different fractions of the available receptors. This is thought to occur because the two agonists activate the receptors to different extents. Such a nonlinear relationship between drug effect and receptor occupancy cannot be explained by this approach.

Efficacy

It was postulated that occupancy of receptors by an agonist first produces a stimulus, S, in the tissue, and this stimulus eventually produces the effect E. The efficacy e of an agonist is a measure of how strongly it stimulates the receptor; an agonist with a higher efficacy has the ability to produce a stronger stimulus. In molecular terms, the stimulus is a measure of the degree to which the agonist–receptor complex can assume its active conformation (DR*). Note that in this context, the term *efficacy* has a different meaning than in clinical pharmacology, in which efficacy refers to how effectively the drug treats the disease or symptoms.

The concept of efficacy explains the apparent ability of agonists to give maximum effect while occupying different fractions of receptors. Different agonists may produce stimuli of different strengths even when they occupy the same fraction of receptors, resulting in different degrees of effect E. Conversely, two drugs can produce the same effect while occupying different fractions of receptors.

Expressing the concept of efficacy mathematically, we can write that the effect of an agonist is a function of the stimulus produced after drug–receptor binding:

$$E = f(S) \qquad \text{(Eq. 16.9)}$$

where f is the function that converts receptor stimulus into response, E is the effect as before, and S is the stimulus. The strength of the stimulus depends on the efficacy e of the drug and on the receptor occupancy, as follows:

$$S = e \frac{[DR]}{[R_t]} \qquad \text{(Eq. 16.10)}$$

The definition of efficacy says that maximum effect can be observed when only a fraction of the receptors are occupied, provided the drug–receptor complex produces a strong enough stimulus. Thus, a highly efficacious drug can stimulate a maximum response while occupying only a small fraction of the receptors. Conversely, a drug with low efficacy may show a submaximal response even at 100% receptor occupancy because of a small stimulus.

Efficacy (e) and intrinsic activity (α) describe two approaches of explaining how a drug modulates pharmacological effect. Although these are two different concepts, they are often used interchangeably in the literature.

Spare Receptors

The above approaches show that drug effect depends on the total number of occupied receptors. However, maximum effect is frequently seen before the drug occupies all available receptors. The excess receptor sites beyond that required for a maximum response are called **spare receptors**, or the *receptor reserve*, i.e., it is the fraction of receptors that are unoccupied by an agonist when the maximal agonist response is obtained.

We can understand this using G protein–coupled receptors as an example. One agonist-occupied GPCR can activate many G proteins. At a certain degree of receptor occupation all available G proteins in the cell are activated, and a further increase in the occupancy of GPCRs will not lead to a subsequent increase in G protein activation and pharmacological effect.

Thus, the spare receptor theory is a hypothesis to explain the particularly high efficiency of some receptor-modulated signaling pathways. The assumption is that spare receptors increase *sensitivity* to a drug, i.e., if a response is produced by occupancy of a certain number of receptors, increasing the number of available receptors allows the same response with a lower concentration of drug. This can be understood by referring to Equation 16.1; a higher concentration of receptors (and, therefore, R*) means that a lower concentration of D can give the same concentration of complex DR*.

Mechanisms of Antagonism

So far, we have mainly dealt with agonist drugs. However, receptor antagonists are very important in drug therapy. Antagonists are compounds that reduce or prevent the effect of agonists. They can be classified as:

- competitive antagonists
- noncompetitive antagonists
- functional antagonists
- chemical antagonists

Competitive Antagonists

Competitive antagonists are compounds that have an affinity for and bind to the same receptor as the agonist. However, the antagonist does not have intrinsic activity and cannot generate a stimulus that leads to the desired effect. The classic explanation of competitive antagonists is that they are "silent" ligands, i.e., agonists and antagonists bind to exactly the same active site of the receptor, but whereas agonists stimulate a response, antagonists do not. According to the two-state receptor model, the lack of intrinsic activity of antagonists is a result of the antagonist binding to the inactive R form of the receptor to form the inactive DR complex. This alters the equilibrium between R and R*, shifting it such that a smaller fraction of receptors is present in the active form.

Regardless of the explanation, an important characteristic of competitive antagonism is that the antagonist and agonist compete with each other for the same receptor depending on their relative concentrations and affinities. Antagonism can always be reversed by increased concentrations of the agonist; conversely, increasing concentrations of the antagonist drug relative to ligand will favor drug binding with the receptor.

The mechanism of action of an agonist and a competitive antagonist is illustrated in Figure 16.6.

Noncompetitive Antagonists

A noncompetitive antagonist can reduce or prevent the activity of an agonist in one of several ways. The antagonist may bind to an allosteric site on the same receptor, changing the conformation of the receptor site and thus interfering with the binding of the agonist. This type of noncompetitive antagonism is called allosteric antagonism, discussed earlier in this chapter. Another way that a noncompetitive antagonist may exert its effect is by interfering with events (such as signal

Competitive Histamine Receptor Antagonists

The signaling ligand histamine is produced by and released from mast cells of the peritoneal cavity and connective tissues. It binds to histamine receptors, of which there are three subtypes, the H_1, H_2, and H_3 receptors. H_1 receptors are found in the smooth muscle of the intestines, bronchi, and blood vessels, H_2 receptors are found in gastric parietal cells and in the vascular and central nervous systems (CNS), and H_3 receptors are found in brain and in the periphery. Anaphylaxis and allergic responses as a result of antibody–antigen interactions are two important responses mediated in part by histamine. Major effects of histamine include arteriolar dilation and increased capillary permeability, decrease in heart rate (H_2), bronchoconstriction (H_1), and gastric acid secretion (H_2). H_3 receptors regulate histamine release.

Many antihistamine drugs such as diphenhydramine, chlorpheniramine, and tripelennamine are competitive H_1 antagonists and are effective in the treatment of allergies. The sedative side effects associated with H_1 antago-

nists may be caused by a blockade of central H_1 receptors involved in wakefulness and attention. Scientists have designed newer H_1 antagonists with reduced transport into the CNS (across the blood–brain barrier), thereby limiting unwanted side effects such as drowsiness. Terfenadine was one of these early H_1 antagonists with reduced CNS penetration, but was problematic because it produced cardiac arrhythmias. Astemizole is an effective H_1 antagonist with low CNS activity.

H_2 antagonist drugs such as cimetidine, famotidine, nizatidine, and ranitidine work by competitive antagonism of H_2 receptor sites on parietal cells. Basal and nocturnal gastric acid secretion is reduced, and these drugs are therefore clinically useful in treating duodenal ulcers. Antihistamines that are used to treat allergies have no beneficial effect on duodenal ulcers, and vice versa.

H_3 antagonists have also been developed with a potential application of enhancing alertness by elevating histamine release in the CNS.

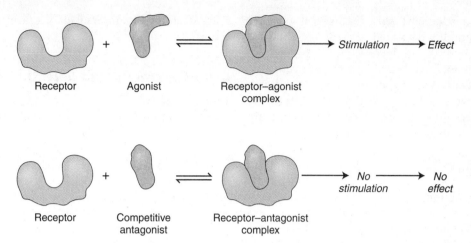

Figure 16.6. Schematic diagram of mechanisms of action of agonists and competitive antagonists. Note that the conformation of the receptor can be altered when it binds with an agonist.

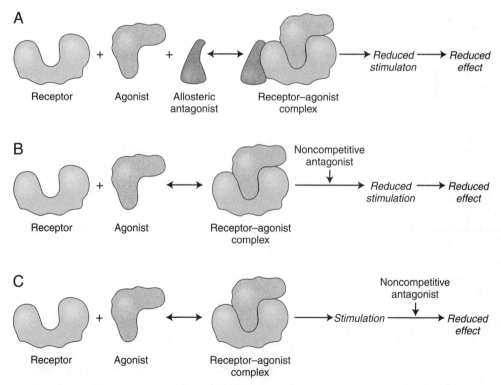

Figure 16.7. Mechanisms of noncompetitive and functional antagonism in drug–receptor interactions. Allosteric antagonist (**A**), antagonist inhibiting signal transduction by agonist (**B**), and antagonist acting at another receptor but converging on the signaling pathway to antagonize the effect (**C**). All result in a reduced or no effect in the presence of agonist.

transduction) after the agonist–receptor complex is formed, thereby reducing the stimulus and decreasing effect. For noncompetitive antagonism, increasing the agonist concentration does not result in a reversal of the effects of the antagonist. The mechanisms of noncompetitive antagonism are illustrated in Figure 16.7.

Functional Antagonists

Functional antagonists are actually agonists that produce an effect that opposes that of another agonist. Usually, a functional antagonist interacts with a different receptor on the same tissue or cell system, or has opposing effects on an intracellular second messenger, thus converging on the signaling pathway to antagonize the effect.

One type of functional antagonism is *physiological antagonism*, in which the action of one agonist exerts an effect opposite to that of the original agonist, usually through a different receptor (e.g., muscarinic agonist inhibition of adrenoceptor-stimulated adenylyl cyclase activity in the heart). Another type is *indirect antagonism*, in which the antagonist competes for the binding site of a second messenger that links agonist binding to the observed effect (e.g., adrenoceptor antagonist blockade of the actions of tyramine, or protein kinase A inhibitors blocking adrenoceptor agonists).

Chemical Antagonists

A **chemical antagonist** reacts with the agonist chemically to change its structure so that it cannot complex with the receptor, making it inactive. These types of antagonists actually decrease the concentration of the agonist at the receptor site, and are useful in treating overdose and poisoning. An example is protamine sulfate, a chemical antagonist of the anticoagulant drug warfarin. Too much warfarin can cause excessive bleeding and hemorrhage. Protamine sulfate (protamine being a weak base) forms a stable inactive complex with warfarin (a weak acid), resulting in reversal of warfarin's action.

Drug Specificity and Selectivity

The **specificity** of a drug is its ability to exert its action by a single mechanism. A drug can have specificity even if it produces a variety of effects if all the effects are caused by a single mechanism of action. For example, atropine has specificity because its only mode of action is as an antagonist at acetylcholine (ACh) receptors. Because ACh receptors with different physiological functions are found all over the body, atropine has a variety of pharmacologic effects.

In contrast, the **selectivity** of a drug is its ability to preferentially produce one pharmacological effect over other effects. Thus, atropine is not selective because it binds relatively equally to all ACh receptors, resulting in a variety of effects. Selectivity is usually related to a drug's ability to stimulate one subtype of a receptor more strongly than other subtypes so the drug is active at lower concentrations at one site compared with another. Selectivity in drug action is desirable because it serves to reduce side effects.

Do not confuse these definitions of drug specificity and selectivity with specificity and selectivity of ligand–protein binding that we saw in Chapter 6, Drugs and Their Targets. Although the concepts behind the definitions are similar, the terms are used differently in different contexts.

Stereoselectivity in Drug Action

We have seen in Chapter 6, Drugs and Their Targets, that the stereochemistry of a molecule has profound consequences on its ability to bind to the active site of proteins. This is particularly true in drug–receptor interactions, where several scenarios are possible with a chiral drug:

- *Enantiomer 1 is active; enantiomer 2 has the same activity:* There is little difference in anticonvulsant activity of the enantiomers of various barbiturates, or anticoagulant activity of the enantiomers of warfarin.

- *Enantiomer 1 is active; enantiomer 2 is inactive:* In –profen nonsteroidal anti-inflammatories (e.g., ibuprofen, ketoprofen, and flurbiprofen), only the (S)-enantiomer has the desired activity.
- *Enantiomer 1 is an agonist; enantiomer 2 is an antagonist of the same receptor:* In dihydropyridines and dihydropyrimidones, the (R) enantiomers have the desired calcium channel antagonism, whereas the (S) enantiomers are calcium channel agonists.
- *Enantiomer 1 is active; enantiomer 2 has a separate, desirable activity:* In β-blockers, the (+) enantiomers block β-adrenergic receptors whereas the (–) enantiomers have beneficial effects on blood lipids.
- *Enantiomer 1 is active; enantiomer 2 is toxic:* Both enantiomers of bupivacaine have the same local anesthetic activity, but the (R) enantiomer is cardiotoxic.

The development of a single enantiomer rather than a racemate is the goal of drug research and development to enhance the efficacy and safety of many racemic drugs. Technology is now available to synthesize single enantiomers in a pure form on a large scale, and most new chiral drugs in development are being designed as single isomers. However, it is sometimes difficult to design a synthetic pathway to produce a single enantiomer; in such cases, the drug is first made as a racemate and then separated into enantiomers. One approach to avoiding the complication introduced by chiral drugs is to specifically design *achiral* drugs, compounds that do not have asymmetric centers. However, this may result in absence of selectivity and the possibility of unwanted toxicity.

Receptor Regulation by Drugs

In Chapter 15, Ligands and Receptors, we learned that when receptors are exposed to a persistent concentration of a ligand, the tissue adjusts by decreasing the number of receptors by *receptor down-regulation*. The same phenomenon can occur with drugs. For example, continuous administration of an agonist drug can result in the development of tolerance, so that the usual dose of drug produces a progressively smaller effect and larger doses are needed to achieve the same effect.

In contrast, if there is a decrease in ligand stimulation of receptors, the body compensates by increasing receptor density; this is known as *receptor up-regulation*. This can occur after continuous treatment with an antagonist that blocks receptors from being stimulated by their ligands. The homeostatic response by the body is an increased rate of receptor synthesis. A *rebound effect* is often seen on abruptly discontinuing the antagonist because of the large number of receptors now available to bind to endogenous ligands or other agonists.

Interaction of Drugs With Enzymes

Enzymes are a special type of receptor because they catalytically change a substrate into a product by enhancing a chemical reaction. Cells in our bodies require hundreds of enzymes to carry out their normal functions, and malfunctions in these processes can lead to illness. Similarly, infectious bacteria require enzymes to survive and multiply. Many diseases and illnesses are treated by specifically interfering with the action of certain human or bacterial enzymes. Although enzyme activation could be exploited therapeutically, most effects are produced by enzyme inhibition.

Enzyme Inhibitors

An enzyme inhibitor is a compound that can bind to the enzyme and decrease or abolish its catalytic activity. Most inhibitors work either by decreasing the affinity of the enzyme for its natural substrate, by decreasing the amount of enzyme available for catalysis, or by a combination of both these effects.

The first enzyme inhibitor drugs developed were antibacterial agents and antitumor agents whose goal was to inhibit cellular replication by blocking enzymes in pathways essential for cell growth. Drugs like 5-fluorouracil (5FU) and 6-mercaptopurine (6MP) block enzymes involved in synthesis of pyrimidine and purine nucleotides, respectively, which are essential for DNA and RNA synthesis.

A large number of current drugs exert their action by inhibiting a target human enzyme. This becomes a useful approach to new drug design when the natural substrate of the enzyme is a beneficial substance that is depleted in a certain disease, or when the products of an enzymatic reaction are harmful.

Assume that a disease is a result of a deficiency of a certain compound, and that this compound is a substrate for the target enzyme. Using a drug that inhibits the target enzyme will slow or prevent the degradation of the substrate, thereby increasing its concentration and treating the disease. An example is seizures that arise from low levels of γ-aminobutyric acid (GABA) in the brain. Inhibition of GABA transferase, an enzyme that degrades GABA, is the mechanism of action of some anticonvulsant drugs.

Conversely, if an excess of a certain compound leads to disease, then inhibiting an enzyme that catalyzes its synthesis will be a useful approach. For example, angiotensin-converting enzyme (ACE) is an important target for antihypertensive drugs. Angiotensin I is converted by ACE to angiotensin II, which is responsible for increases in blood pressure. Inhibiting ACE and thus lowering the concentration of angiotensin II reduces blood pressure. ACE inhibitors such as captopril, enalapril, and lisinopril are very effective antihypertensive drugs.

Enzyme inhibitors can be classified as reversible or irreversible.

Reversible Enzyme Inhibitors

Most inhibitors are **reversible enzyme inhibitors**, meaning that noncovalent interactions are involved in inhibitor–enzyme complex formation, and that the complex can subsequently dissociate. Reversible enzyme inhibitors can be further classified as *competitive* or *noncompetitive* depending on their mechanism of binding to the enzyme.

Competitive Enzyme Inhibitors. Competitive inhibitors bind at the same enzyme active site as the natural substrate. The inhibitor and substrate can therefore displace each other from the binding site depending on their relative affinities and concentrations. Such inhibitors are highly specific for a particular enzyme and have a structure similar to either the substrate or product of the target enzyme. Most enzyme inhibitor drugs are *competitive and reversible*.

Binding of an enzyme E to its substrate S and reversible competitive inhibitor I can be represented by the following set of equations:

$$E + S \xrightleftharpoons{K} ES \rightarrow product$$
$$E + I \xrightleftharpoons{K} EI \rightarrow no\,product$$

(Eq. 16.11)

The free enzyme is capable of reacting with the substrate to give an ES complex, or with the inhibitor to give an EI complex. The ES complex can continue on to form the desired product whereas the EI complex cannot.

Recall that the rate of an enzymatic reaction for converting a substrate to product is mathematically described by the Michaelis–Menten equation:

$$V = \frac{V_{max}\,[S]}{K_m + [S]} \quad \text{(Eq. 16.12)}$$

and that the affinity, K, of the enzyme for the substrate is given by:

$$K = \frac{1}{K_m} = \frac{[ES]}{[E][S]} \quad \text{(Eq. 16.13)}$$

The presence of a competitive inhibitor blocks the active site on some enzyme molecules and therefore decreases the concentration of the [ES] complex. This lowers the apparent affinity of the enzyme for substrate, increasing K_m. V_{max} can still be attained, although a higher concentration of substrate will be needed to achieve this.

Generally, a competitive inhibitor merely binds at the enzyme's active site without further reaction. However, in some cases, the competitive inhibitor may be an alternative substrate for the enzyme and is converted to alternative products after binding to the enzyme.

A reversible inhibitor, whether competitive or noncompetitive, is effective only as long as its concentration at the site of action remains high enough to prevent the enzyme–substrate complex from forming. Thus, additional doses of the inhibitor are necessary to maintain the pharmacological effect.

The sulfonamides, a class of antibacterial drugs, are good examples of competitive enzyme inhibitors. Sulfonamides specifi-cally inhibit the enzyme dihydropteroate synthetase, which is responsible for biosynthesis of tetrahydrofolate, a compound necessary for the replication of bacteria. Thus, sulfonamides are bacteriostatic and are used to treat bacterial infections.

Another example is the group of statin drugs (lovastatin, mevastatin, and simvastatin) that are competitive inhibitors of the enzyme 3-hydroxy-3-methylglutaryl coenzyme A (HMG-CoA) reductase, one of the enzymes that catalyze cholesterol biosynthesis. Inhibition of this enzyme results in a decrease in cholesterol biosynthesis in the body and lowers plasma cholesterol levels.

Noncompetitive Enzyme Inhibitors. Noncompetitive enzyme inhibitors usually bind at an allosteric site on the enzyme, different from the active site where the substrate binds. These inhibitors are generally structurally unrelated to the substrate, but their binding results in a conformational change in the active site so that it can no longer bind effectively with the substrate to convert it to the product. The substrate and inhibitor are capable of binding to the enzyme at the same time to create a ternary complex, but this complex is inactive. This is illustrated in Figure 16.8.

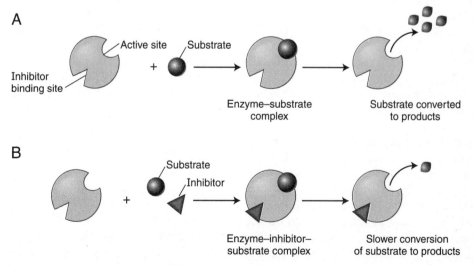

Figure 16.8. Diagram illustrating the effect of a noncompetitive enzyme inhibitor on the rate of an enzymatic reaction. **A.** Reaction without inhibitor. **B.** Reaction with inhibitor.

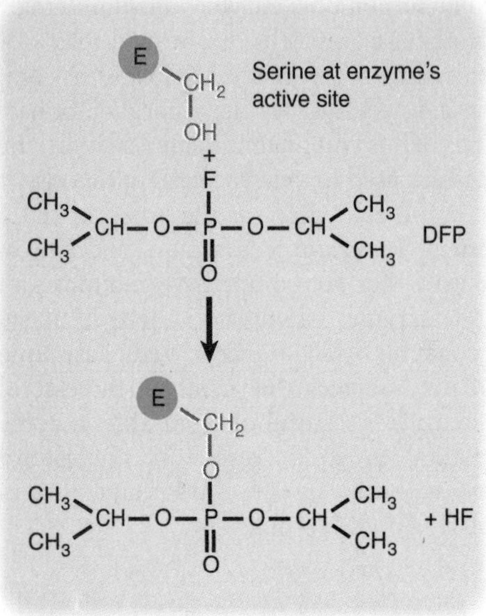

Figure 16.9. Example of covalent bond formation between an enzyme and an irreversible inhibitor. The reaction shown is of the competitive irreversible inhibitor, diisopropyl fluorophosphate (DFP), which can react with serine groups at the active site of an enzyme to form a covalent adduct.

Noncompetitive inhibition can be represented by the following set of equations:

$$
\begin{aligned}
E + I &\rightleftharpoons EI \\
EI + S &\rightleftharpoons EIS \rightarrow no\,product \\
E + S &\rightleftharpoons ES \rightarrow product \\
ES + I &\rightleftharpoons EIS \rightarrow no\,product
\end{aligned}
\qquad (Eq.\ 16.14)
$$

Notice that the enzyme–inhibitor–substrate (EIS) complex can be produced by two routes, but the final result is the same—an inactive complex and no product formation.

The rate of enzyme catalysis is decreased because the catalytic site is influenced by the inhibitor. V_{max} is thus reduced, but because the binding site is not affected, K_m remains unchanged. Because binding occurs at different sites on the enzyme, an excess of substrate cannot displace noncompetitive inhibitors, and thus substrate concentration does not influence the degree of inhibition.

Irreversible Enzyme Inhibitors

Most interactions between an enzyme and substrate are reversible in that the enzyme remains unchanged after the reaction and is available to bind to more substrate molecules. If the interaction of an inhibitor with the enzyme is of a covalent nature, the compound is called an irreversible enzyme inhibitor or enzyme inactivator; an example of this is shown in Figure 16.9. Irreversible inhibitors can sustain their action for a long time because they do not dissociate from the enzyme. However, this does not mean that additional doses of inhibitor are not needed. As the enzyme loses activity, the body synthesizes more enzyme molecules, requiring more inhibitor to sustain the action. New enzyme synthesis can take hours or days, so that the effect of such an inhibitor is of long duration.

Many poisons are harmful to cells because they are potent irreversible inhibitors and denature the enzyme. Examples are heavy metals (mercury, lead, and arsenic) and cyanide.

Many drugs also work by irreversible enzyme inhibition. A familiar example is aspirin's irreversible inhibition of the enzyme prostaglandin synthetase. Antimicrobial drugs such as antibiotics are irreversible enzyme inhibitors as well; for example, penicillins bind to and inactivate the bacterial enzyme transpeptidase, an essential enzyme in bacterial growth. Other irreversible inhibitors such as the nitrogen mustards are used in anticancer therapy.

Selectivity of Enzyme Inhibition

Selectivity in enzyme inhibition is desirable so that beneficial effects are not accompanied by unwanted side effects. As scientists continue to learn more about enzyme activity and structure, the design of more specific inhibitors becomes possible. Both reversible and

Monoamine Oxidase Inhibitors

Neurotransmitters (serotonin, dopamine, and norepinephrine) are monoamines. When released into the synaptic space, neurotransmitters are either reabsorbed or destroyed by monoamine oxidase (MAO) in the synaptic cleft. There are two isoforms of MAO: MAO-A preferentially deaminates serotonin, melatonin, and noradrenaline. MAO-B preferentially deaminates phenylethylamine and trace amines. Dopamine is equally deaminated by both isoforms.

Clinical depression may be related to decreases in concentration of the neurotransmitters. Thus, drug discovery has focused on drugs that can either block the reuptake of neurotransmitters (e.g., cyclic antidepressants and newer selective serotonin reuptake inhibitors) or interfere with the breakdown of the monoamines in the synaptic cleft (monoamine oxidase inhibitors or MAOIs).

MAOIs are one of the oldest classes of antidepressants and are typically used when other antidepressants have not been effective. Irreversible MAOI drugs currently available in the United States include phenelzine sulfate, tranylcypromine sulfate, isocarboxazid, and selegiline (specific for MAO-B). These inhibit the enzyme and increase the synaptic concentrations of the signaling amines. Unfortunately these drugs caused severe cardiovascular side effects in certain patients, resulting in death. These patients had eaten foods high in tyramine (such as cheese, wine, and beer) just before their deaths. Further investigation revealed that tyramine triggers the release of norepinephrine and thus raises blood pressure. Normally, the excess norepinephrine is degraded by MAO, keeping blood pressure under control. However, in patients taking an MAOI, MAO activity is lowered and the norepinephrine cannot be broken down rapidly enough to prevent a hypertensive crisis. Thus, these drugs are to be taken with strict dietary control.

Reversible inhibitors of MAO are available in Europe. Herbal substances, such as St. John's wort, which may have MAOI-like activity, are also frequently used for self-treatment of depression.

---

irreversible enzyme inhibitors can be made selective.

Similarities Between Receptors and Enzymes

Whether a drug works by binding to a cellular receptor or an enzyme, there are many similarities in the principles of binding and processes that affect the function of the protein. These similarities are summarized in Table 16.3.

Non–Receptor-Based Drug Action

Not all drugs act on discrete receptors or at active sites of specific enzymes in the body. Some drugs act extracellularly, and their actions are aimed at noncellular constituents of the body. Still other drugs may act at cellular sites or at membranes, but their actions are primarily the result of their physicochemical properties rather than a specific interaction with a receptor or enzyme. These types of drugs are said to

Nonsteroidal Anti-Inflammatory Drugs

A good example of improving selectivity is seen in the class of drugs called nonsteroidal anti-inflammatory drugs (NSAIDs). These drugs were known to be effective analgesics before the discovery that they worked by inhibiting cyclooxygenase (COX), a component of the enzyme prostaglandin synthetase involved in the production of prostaglandins. These ligands cause the pain and swelling of arthritis inflammation.

However, all NSAIDs also caused disruption of the gastric mucosa, resulting in severe gastric side effects and bleeding. Scientists later discovered that there are two forms of COX: COX-1, which is primarily responsible for unwanted gastric effects, kidney function, and platelet aggregation, and

COX-2, which is responsible for fever, pain, and swelling. These enzymes are about 60% homologous.

Older NSAIDs (aspirin, ibuprofen, and naproxen) inhibited both COX-1 and COX-2 and therefore had serious side effects such as gastric bleeding, and kidney and liver toxicity. Selective COX-2 inhibitors such as celecoxib (Celebrex) and rofecoxib (Vioxx) were then found by selective screening. These drugs are effective COX-2 inhibitors without anti-COX-1 activity. New data indicate an increased risk of major fatal and nonfatal heart attacks in clinical trial participants taking COX-2 inhibitors. Rofecoxib has been withdrawn from the market, and celecoxib is to be used with utmost caution.

work by *nonspecific* mechanisms of action. There are several examples that fit into this category. Gastrointestinal drugs, such as antacids, laxatives, and cathartics, have nonspecific actions in the gastrointestinal tract. Blood plasma substitutes are macro-molecules used in cases of blood loss. Various agents applied to the skin such as sunscreens also fall into this group.

The activity of many nonspecific drugs is related to their lipophilicity. For example, inhalation anesthetics with a

---

TABLE 16.3. Comparison of Terms and Events in Enzymatic and Receptor Processes

Event	Enzyme	Receptor
Compound bound at active site	Endogenous substrate, drug	Endogenous ligand, drug
Complex	ES or ED	RL or DR
Number of binding sites	One or more sites	One or more sites
Binding affinity	K_m	K_d
Molecules that also bind to protein	Inhibitors, activators	Agonists, antagonists
Regulation	Allosteric activation or inhibition	Allosteric activation or inhibition
Outcome	Product formed	Response

ED, enzyme–drug; ES, enzyme–substrate; K_m, Michaelis constant; K_d, dissociation constant; DR, drug–receptor; RL, receptor–ligand.

variety of chemical structures (nitrous oxide and various organic volatile substances like chloroform and ether) all produce similar actions on the brain by forming a monomolecular layer on membranes and altering membrane transport. Chemical disinfectants and germicides act by nonspecifically destroying living membranes and tissue. These actions are irreversible, and the functional integrity of the cells is permanently destroyed. In all these cases, activity can be correlated with the partition coefficient of the drug.

KEY CONCEPTS

- Drugs either enhance the natural activity of a ligand (agonists) or reduce it (antagonists, inhibitors). A few drugs work by nonspecific mechanisms that do not require binding to a receptor or enzyme.

- Agonists interact with the active receptor state to stimulate an effect characteristic of that receptor. Full agonists have a greater selectivity for the active receptor form, whereas partial agonists have a smaller selectivity for the active receptor and show a lesser effect than a full agonist.

- Competitive antagonists compete with agonists for the same receptor depending on their relative concentrations and affinities; competitive antagonism can be reversed by excess agonist.

- Noncompetitive antagonists reduce the effect of an agonist by binding at an allosteric site or by interfering in signal transduction. This antagonism cannot be reversed by excess agonist.

- Specificity of a drug is its ability to exert its action by a single mechanism, whereas selectivity describes a drug's ability to produce only one pharmacological effect.

- The intensity of a drug effect can be characterized by several factors such as affinity, intrinsic activity, and efficacy. Each measures, in different ways, how a drug modulates pharmacological effect.

- Enzyme inhibitors decrease the target enzyme's activity either by reducing the affinity of the enzyme for its natural substrate or by reducing the amount of enzyme available for catalysis, or a combination of both.

- Competitive enzyme inhibitors bind at the same enzyme active site as the natural substrate; this inhibition can be reversed by excess substrate. Noncompetitive enzyme inhibitors bind at an allosteric site on the enzyme; this inhibition cannot be reversed by excess substrate. Irreversible enzyme inhibitors generally work by binding covalently to and inactivating the enzyme.

ADDITIONAL READING

1. Katzung BG (ed). Basic and Clinical Pharmacology, 8th ed. McGraw-Hill/Appleton & Lange, 2000.

2. Mutschler E, Derendorf H. Drug Actions: Basic Principles and Therapeutic Aspects. CRC Press, 1995.

3. Brunton L, Lazo J, Parker K (eds). Goodman & Gilman's The Pharmacological Basis of Therapeutics, 11th ed. McGraw-Hill Professional, 2005.

4. Mycek MJ, Harvey RA, Champe PC. Lippincott's Illustrated Reviews: Pharmacology, 2nd ed. Lippincott Williams & Wilkins, 2000.

REVIEW QUESTIONS

1. How do agonists, antagonists, partial agonists, and inverse agonists differ in their interactions with receptors?
2. Explain the occupation theory of receptors. What are its deficiencies? How are these addressed by the concepts of intrinsic activity?
3. Describe how the concepts of stimulus and efficacy explain the ability of drugs to give maximum effect while occupying different fractions of receptors.
4. How do competitive and noncompetitive antagonists work? What are the differences in their mechanisms?
5. What is drug selectivity and why is it important in the action of drugs?
6. How can drug administration cause up-regulation or down-regulation of receptors? What are the consequences?
7. Explain how enzyme inhibitors work as drugs.
8. Distinguish between the mechanisms of binding and action of competitive, noncompetitive, and irreversible enzyme inhibitors.
9. Elaborate on nonspecific mechanisms of drug action.

Dose–Response Relationships

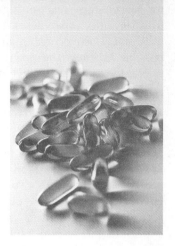

We now understand the mechanisms by which drugs work at the molecular level in the body. This mechanistic knowledge must be translated into practical concepts for effective drug therapy. In particular, clinicians should be able to compare various drugs in terms of their effectiveness, selectivity, and safety, and to understand how these parameters are related to the dose of drug. It is also important to know how to adjust the drug dose in a particular patient to achieve efficacy without toxicity. Understanding the relationship of response to dose is one of the most challenging tasks in new drug development.

In Chapter 16, Mechanisms of Drug Action, we learned that most drugs work by binding to receptors or enzymes, and that the response is related to the concentration of drug available at the active site of the target protein. Let us proceed from there to understand the relationship of drug dose to response.

Concentration–Response Relationships

Using the concepts discussed earlier, we can describe a concentration–effect relationship for the interaction of an agonist and antagonist (or inhibitor) with a receptor. Most of these relationships are derived from *in vitro* experiments on enzymes, cells, and isolated organs, in which it is possible to know the precise concentration of the drug at the active site.

Agonists and Substrates

Figure 17.1 shows a *concentration–effect* or *concentration–response* curve for a full and partial agonist acting at a receptor. The data to construct such a curve are obtained by placing known concentrations of drug in the *in vitro* experimental system (such as a cell, tissue, or isolated organ system) and then measuring the response of the system to the drug. Concentration–response curves are usually governed by the following equation, which was introduced in Chapter 16, Mechanisms of Drug Action:

$$\frac{E}{E_{max}} = \frac{\alpha}{[R_t]}[DR] \qquad \text{(Eq. 17.1)}$$

A plot of E/E_{max} (either as a fraction or as a percentage) on the y axis versus the $[DR]$ on the x axis should give a straight line with a slope equal to $\alpha/[R_t]$.

Although there is no direct way of measuring the concentration of the complex $[DR]$, the *total* concentration of drug $[D_t]$ used in the experiment is known. When $[D_t]$ is small (low drug concentrations), almost all the drug is involved in complex formation, so $[DR]$ is essentially equal to $[D_t]$. This approximation modifies Equation 17.1 to:

$$\frac{E}{E_{max}} = \frac{\alpha}{[R_t]}[D_t] \qquad \text{(Eq. 17.2)}$$

Equation 17.2 shows a linear relationship between E/E_{max} and total drug concentration $[D_t]$; the slope of the line is $\alpha/[R_t]$.

When $[D_t]$ is sufficiently large (i.e., high drug concentrations), all the receptors are occupied (saturated), and maximum pharmacological response (E/E_{max} = 1 or 100%) will be obtained if the drug is a full agonist (α =1). Any further

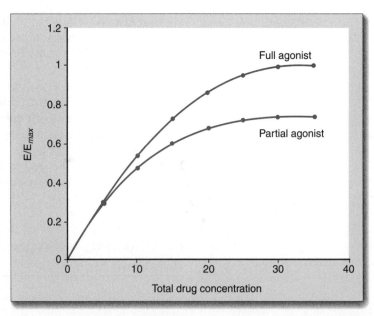

Figure 17.1. A typical concentration–response curve showing the relationship between total drug concentration and the fractional response (E/E_{max}) for a full and partial agonist at a receptor site.

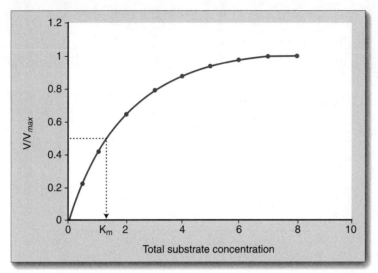

Figure 17.2. A typical concentration–response curve showing the relationship between total substrate concentration and the fractional response (V/V_{max}). The Michaelis constant (K_m) is the substrate concentration at which the rate of the reaction is 50%.

increase in concentration will not give any greater effect; the biological response has reached a plateau. Thus, we obtain a hyperbolic graph when we plot relative response E/E_{max} versus total drug concentration $[D_t]$. For partial agonists ($0 < \alpha < 1$), the receptors will also become saturated at high concentrations, and the response will reach a plateau, but E/E_{max} will be less than 1 at the plateau.

Notice that the concentration to response relationship is not proportional, i.e., the concentration needed for 100% response is not double the concentration for 50% response, but is much larger. Initially, small changes in concentration produce a large change in response. As the response approaches maximum, large changes in concentration are needed to make small changes in response.

Note also the similarity of Figure 17.1 to Figure 17.2, which shows the catalytic response of an enzyme–substrate interaction. Thus, our discussion above about agonists applies to substrates of enzymes as well.

Concentration–response curves are better and more commonly represented with the *logarithm* of the drug concentra-

tion on the x axis, because this allows a broader range of agonist concentrations to be shown. When plotted in this manner, as in Figure 17.3 for an agonist, a sigmoid or S-shaped log concentration–response curve with a center of symmetry at 50% response is obtained. This midpoint represents the concentration that gives 50% of the maximum response and is called the EC_{50}. Another advantage of using a logarithmic concentration scale is that the curve is essentially linear around the EC_{50} (between about 20 and 80% maximal response), making mathematical analysis easier. Therefore, at intermediate agonist concentrations there is a linear relationship between relative response and log concentration. The slope is the highest in this region of the curve, and small changes in agonist concentration can produce large changes in response.

The same type of sigmoid curve is obtained for enzyme–substrate systems; here, V/V_{max} is plotted against the logarithm of the substrate concentration. The midpoint concentration of this curve, representing 50% maximum response, is K_m.

The concentrations of endogenous ligands in the body usually lie near the

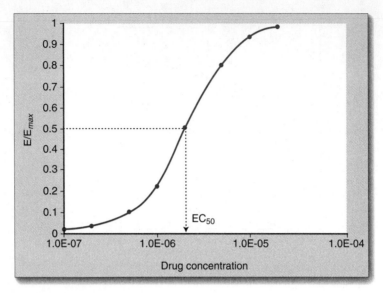

Figure 17.3. A typical logarithmic concentration–response curve for a full agonist. Note the logarithmic *x* axis and the characteristic sigmoid shape of the curve. The EC_{50} is the drug concentration that gives 50% maximal response ($E/E_{max} = 0.5$). Also note the linearity of the curve between approximately 20 and 80% maximal response.

EC_{50} or K_m of the drug–protein interaction, i.e., in the linear portion of the concentration–response curve. By making small changes in ligand concentration, the body can precisely control cellular behavior.

Antagonists and Inhibitors

In Chapter 16, Mechanisms of Drug Action, we discussed the mechanism of action of antagonists and inhibitors. Antagonists are drugs that reduce or prevent the effect of agonists at a receptor. Enzyme inhibitors are drugs that prevent or decrease the rate of the reaction converting substrates to products. *Competitive* antagonists or inhibitors have an affinity for and bind to the same site on the target protein as the agonist (substrate). The endogenous ligand and drug compete for the same active site, and can displace each other from the site depending on their relative concentrations and affinities. On the other hand, *noncompetitive* antagonists or inhibitors usually bind to an allosteric site on the target protein.

Competitive Binding

Figure 17.4 shows the concentration–effect curve for an agonist (or substrate) in the absence and presence of two different concentrations of a competitive antagonist (or inhibitor). To produce an effect, the agonist has to first replace the antagonist at the binding sites. Therefore, higher concentrations of agonist are needed to produce the same degree of effect when an antagonist is present. Furthermore, even higher concentrations of agonist are needed to produce the maximum effect. The result is that the concentration–response curve for the agonist is shifted to the right, i.e., to higher agonist concentrations. This is a parallel shift in curves so that the slopes of the linear portions of the curves remain the same.

Because competition between agonist and antagonist depends on their relative concentrations and affinities for the receptor, the shift to the right is greater for an antagonist present at a higher concentration, or with a greater affinity. The

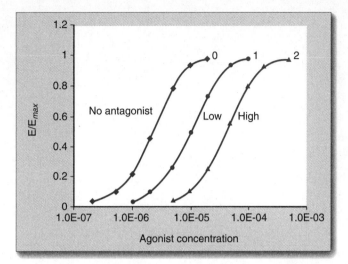

Figure 17.4. Concentration–response curve for a full agonist in the absence and presence of a competitive antagonist. Curve 0 shows the relationship when no antagonist is present. Curves 1 and 2 show the shift in the relationship in the presence of low and high concentrations of the competitive antagonist respectively.

extent of this shift is a useful way of comparing antagonists and is best expressed as a *concentration ratio*. This is the factor by which the agonist concentration must be increased to restore the original response in the presence of an antagonist. This also illustrates the concept that the effect of a competitive antagonist can be reversed by high agonist concentrations.

The same discussion holds true for enzyme substrates and their competitive inhibitors.

Noncompetitive Binding

Figure 17.5 shows concentration–response curves for an agonist in the absence and presence of different concentrations of a noncompetitive antagonist. As with competitive antagonism, the curves are shifted to the right in this case. However, the slope of the linear portion and the maximum effect are both reduced. High concentrations of antagonist may completely prevent effect, even if agonist–receptor binding takes place. Unlike

competitive antagonism, the effect of a noncompetitive antagonist cannot be reversed by high agonist concentrations. Again, the same discussion applies to enzyme substrates and their noncompetitive inhibitors.

Competitive–Noncompetitive Binding

Some antagonists demonstrate both competitive and noncompetitive properties. These drugs are competitive at low concentrations, but noncompetitive at high concentrations. Therefore, at low concentrations, these drugs cause a parallel shift of the agonist curve, and at high concentrations they decrease the slope and maximum effect. Figure 17.6 shows this graphically.

Similarly some enzyme inhibitors show both competitive and noncompetitive behavior and are often called mixed inhibitors, changing both K_m and V_{max} of the enzyme–substrate reaction. The concentration–effect curves in this case are similar to those shown in Figure 17.6.

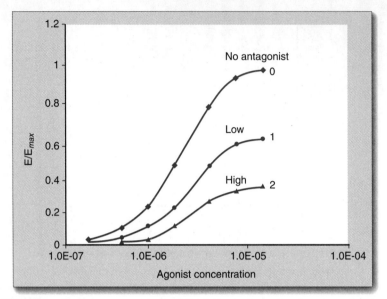

Figure 17.5. Concentration–response curve for a full agonist in the absence and presence of a noncompetitive antagonist. Curve 0 shows the profile when no antagonist is present. Curves 1 and 2 show the shift in the curve in the presence of low and high concentrations of the noncompetitive antagonist respectively.

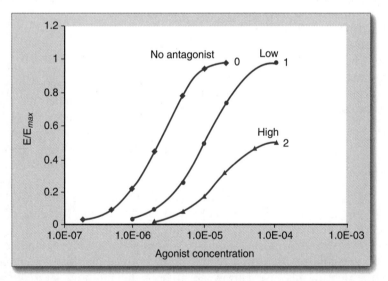

Figure 17.6. Concentration–response curve for a full agonist in the absence and presence of a competitive-noncompetitive antagonist. Curve 0 shows the profile when no antagonist is present. Curves 1 and 2 show the shift in the curve in the presence of low and high concentrations of the antagonist respectively.

Dose–Response Relationships

When dealing with animals or humans, the exact concentration of drug at the receptor is not known. However, this concentration is related to the dose of drug administered; the higher the dose, the greater the concentration at the receptor. Therefore, if the drug dose is known and the pharmacological response can be measured, a *dose–response* or *dose–effect relationship* can be established. Dose–response relationships are a common way to portray data in both experimental and clinical sciences.

From discussions in earlier chapters we know that drug dose is only one of the factors that determine concentration of drug at the receptor active site, and subsequent pharmacological response. The drug's absorption, distribution, metabolism, and excretion (ADME) behavior is also important; ADME determines drug plasma concentration, which in turn affects concentration at the receptor (site of action) and in other tissues. Thus, the same dose of drug administered by a different route, or by different formulations with the same route, can give varying pharmacological responses.

In Chapter 14, Plasma Concentration–Time Curves, we examined the relationship between plasma concentration and response. In most situations, a higher dose of drug gives a proportionately higher plasma concentration (up to a limit), all other conditions being the same. It is in this context that one should understand the discussion of dose–response relationships.

A dose–response curve (DRC) is usually constructed using the *logarithm* of the dose on the *x* axis. The *y* axis shows the response, presented either as intensity of effect in a graded dose–response curve, or as frequency of effect in a quantal dose–response curve.

Graded Dose–Response Curves

A graded dose–response curve is useful in representing the dose–effect relationship in an individual. The assumptions are that the response varies continuously with dose and that a higher dose gives a greater response. An example is shown in Figure 17.7; note that the graded DRC is sigmoid with a center of symmetry at 50% response. The threshold dose is defined as the lowest dose that produces a measurable response. The slope of the curve near its center of symmetry also has significance; a steep slope shows that a small increase in dose produces a large increase in response.

Potency and Efficacy

The potency of a drug is the dose needed to produce a certain defined response in an individual. It is a useful parameter that allows comparisons of different drugs that act at the same target site. The smaller the dose required to produce the defined effect, the more potent the drug; conversely, the more potent the drug, the less of it is required to produce a given effect. Potency is related to the affinity of a drug for the receptor; the higher the affinity, the more potent the drug.

Potency also depends on how much of the dose reaches the receptor after administration. The fraction of the dose that arrives at the receptor site depends on the drug's ADME behavior. Thus, a drug with the best activity *in vitro* may not be the most potent because less of it may reach the receptor site. Moreover, differences in ADME are often responsible for variability in potency of the same drug in different individuals.

Efficacy, on the other hand, is a measure of the maximum response a drug can produce regardless of the dose, and is often related to the intrinsic activity of the drug; drugs with high intrinsic activity usually give a greater maximal efficacy.

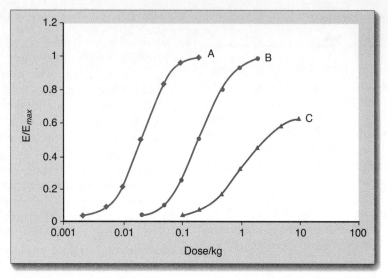

Figure 17.7. A typical graded dose–response curve for three drugs (*A, B,* and *C*) acting at the same receptor. The dose is in arbitrary units. Note the logarithmic *x* axis, and the sigmoid shape of the curve. Drug *A* is 10 times more potent than drug *B*. Drug *C* is less potent than drug *A* or *B*. Both drug *A* and drug *B* reach the same maximal effect and have the same efficacy, whereas the efficacy of drug *C* is lower than that of drug *A* or *B*.

This parameter is also useful in comparing two drugs with the same action.

The potency of agonists can be compared by their position on the *x* axis, and their efficacy can be determined from the maximum response exhibited, by the position on the *y* axis. For example, Figure 17.7 shows that:

- drug A has a higher potency than drugs B or C
- drug B has the same maximal effect as drug A but is less potent
- drug C will never achieve the efficacy of drug A, even at high doses

Potency is useful in determining drug doses when changing from one drug to another, but does not provide any information about effectiveness or safety. Thus, the most potent drug may not necessarily be the best drug. Potency is clinically important only when drugs are very potent (difficult to administer safely) or very weak (difficult to administer conveniently). Efficacy is more important than potency for therapy because it focuses on the effectiveness of a drug rather than on the size of the dose.

Quantal Dose–Response Curves

Not all patients respond to a drug in the same way or to the same extent. Very few individuals show the desired effect at low doses, whereas almost all show the desired effect at very high doses. This illustrates the problem of *biological variability* when dealing with individuals. The variability may be the result of differences in receptors or in the amount of drug reaching the receptor site, or some other reason. We shall discuss the various factors responsible for this behavior in Chapter 18, Therapeutic Variability.

To measure this variability in individual dose–response, the DRC can be constructed to show the *frequency* of a certain response (e.g., the number of individuals exhibiting a defined response to a minimum dose) on the *y* axis. This is useful when studying the effect of a drug on a patient population rather than in an individual patient. For such analysis, the

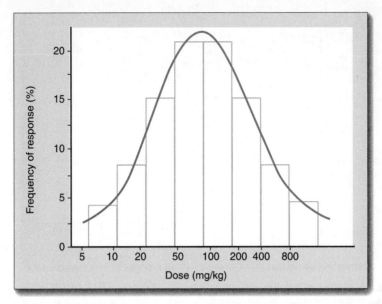

Figure 17.8. A quantal dose–response curve showing the frequency of response (number of patients responding) as a function of the minimum dose administered.

response needs to be well defined, both qualitatively and quantitatively. This is because the measurement of response is *quantal,* not continuously variable; the patient either shows the defined response or does not.

To obtain these data, the population is given increasing drug doses until virtually all patients respond. In essence, one is finding the individual threshold dose for the group. The graphs are usually bell-shaped, following a gaussian or normal distribution as shown in Figure 17.8. This type of curve, called a quantal dose–response curve, is useful in describing the DRC in a group of subjects.

Another way of showing quantal dose–response is to plot the data as the *cumulative* frequency responding to a certain dose, illustrated in Figure 17.9. As the dose is increased more individuals exhibit the defined effect; all individuals show the response at the highest dose. Notice that we again have a sigmoid curve with a center of symmetry at 50% response. The dose at the center of symmetry of a cumulative quantal DRC is called the ED_{50} or the *median effective dose.* The ED_{50} is defined as the dose that produces the desired effect in half of the individuals studied.

One way to compare the potency of two drugs that produce the same response is to compare their ED_{50} values; the lower the value, the more potent the drug. Similarly, we can define ED_{95} as the dose at which 95% of individuals show an effect, and so on.

Drug Selectivity

The *selectivity* of a drug has been discussed in Chapter 16, Mechanisms of Drug Action; it is the ability of a drug to produce one effect (usually the desired effect) at much lower doses than other effects (such as side effects). The DRCs of all the effects of a drug will give a measure of its selectivity; the more widely spaced the DRCs, the more selective the drug.

Dose-Related Toxicity

An ideal drug would produce a therapeutically useful response without

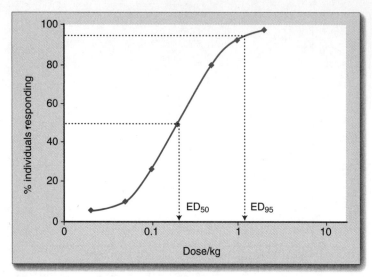

Figure 17.9. A typical quantal dose–response curve with dose per kilogram (dose has arbitrary units) on the logarithmic *x* axis and the cumulative percentage of individuals responding on the *y* axis. The ED_{50} and ED_{95} are the doses at which 50 and 95% of individuals, respectively, show the defined response.

causing any undesirable effects. Unfortunately, every drug produces unwanted side effects at a large enough dose. Side effects are pharmacological effects observed in addition to the primary drug action and vary greatly with the drug, the dose, and the patient. Sometimes these effects cause serious problems (*toxicity*), whereas in other cases they may be relatively harmless. In a few situations, a drug's side effect may even be desirable. Undesirable side effects are known as adverse drug reactions (ADRs).

Most common types of ADRs are related to the dose of the drug and are the result of one or more of the known pharmacological effects of the drug; these account for about 80% of ADRs seen in practice. Dose-related ADRs are frequently predictable and can be avoided. Examples are drowsiness after taking antihistamines or an elevated heart rate after using β-agonists. Other types of side effects are not related to the dose or even directly to the drug's biological action. These are generally called "*idiosyncratic*

reactions" or *allergic* effects. We will discuss this type of side effect in Chapter 18, Therapeutic Variability.

Just as we can construct quantal DRCs for the beneficial effects of a drug, we can also construct similar curves for the dose-dependent ADRs of drugs.

Therapeutic Index

The ultimate adverse side effect of a drug is lethality or death. In animals, we characterize this as the LD_{50}, the *median lethal dose*, the dose of the drug that kills 50% of the animals tested during a set period after an acute exposure. Ideally, the LD_{50} of a drug should be much larger than its ED_{50} because this would make the drug safer to use. The LD_{50} values may vary for the same drug given by different routes of administration because of differences in absorption and bioavailability from different administration sites.

The pharmacological therapeutic index (TI), also called the *therapeutic ratio*, of a drug is defined as:

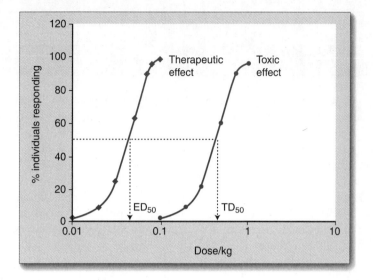

Figure 17.10. Quantal dose–response curves for the therapeutic effect and toxic effect of drug X. The ratio TD_{50}/ED_{50} gives the therapeutic index (TI) of the drug. Drug X has a TI = 10. Note that very little toxicity will be seen at a dose that gives therapeutic effect in greater than 90% of individuals.

$$\text{therapeutic index} = TI = \frac{LD_{50}}{ED_{50}} \quad \text{(Eq. 17.3)}$$

A large therapeutic index implies that a drug is safe. For example, a drug with a TI of 25 is safer than a drug with a TI of 8.

Because the LD_{50} cannot be determined in human subjects, clinicians instead define the TD_{50}, the median toxic dose, as the dose that produces a defined toxic effect in 50% of individuals. In this case the clinical therapeutic index is given by:

$$TI = \frac{TD_{50}}{ED_{50}} \quad \text{(Eq. 17.4)}$$

Here again the TI is a measure of the safety of the drug. A clinical TI of 5 means that the dose that produces a particular toxic effect (such as liver damage) in 50% of individuals is five times higher than the effective dose in 50% of individuals. We will use TI to mean the clinical TI for the remainder of the chapter.

Figure 17.10 illustrates the effective (therapeutic) and toxic dose–response relationships of drug X with a TI of 10. Drug X has considerable separation between these two dose–response curves, indicating that it has good safety. A general rule of thumb is that drugs with a TI less than 2 will show significant toxicity in some patients when used clinically at therapeutic doses. Thus, such drugs should be used only if the risk–benefit analysis for a particular patient is favorable. The selectivity of a drug is very important in determining its safety profile.

A drug can have many toxic effects of different degrees of severity. Relatively mild side effects like nausea, gastrointestinal upset, or headaches may occur at low doses whereas more serious toxic effects like liver or kidney damage may occur at higher doses. Therefore, a drug has different TD_{50} and TI values for each of its toxic effects.

Certain Safety Factor

The therapeutic index is not always a good measure of the safety of a drug because it compares only the midpoints of efficacy and toxicity dose–response curves.

Digoxin

Digoxin is among the top 50 most widely prescribed drugs in the United States, and has been used therapeutically for more than 300 years. It belongs to a class of drugs known as cardiac glycosides and is widely used in management of congestive heart failure, weakened heart, and irregular heart beat (arrhythmia). The common garden plant, the foxglove or *Digitalis purpurea,* is the source of digoxin.

Few drugs in clinical medicine have a therapeutic index as low as that of digoxin, or are a more frequent cause of adverse drug reactions. Digoxin toxicity is observed in a significant number of patients. Anorexia, frequently accompanied by muscular weakness, lethargy, vomiting, diarrhea, and abdominal pain, are common. The most serious and life-threatening ADRs are cardiac arrhythmias and disturbances of cardiac conduction, which may develop without warning.

One antidote for digoxin toxicity is digoxin immune Fab (Digibind, Digi-Fab), an antibody produced in sheep by immunization with a digoxin derivative. When given to patients with digoxin toxicity, the antibody binds to digoxin molecules, making them unavailable for binding at their receptors in the body. The affinity of digoxin for the antibody is higher than its affinity for its receptor. The net effect is to shift the binding equilibrium away from binding of digoxin to its receptors, thereby reversing its effects. The Fab–digoxin complex is then excreted by the kidneys.

These curves could have significant overlap, so that some patients might experience toxicity without significant therapeutic benefit even though the average patient is effectively treated.

This problem is apparent in the dose–response curves shown in Figure 17.11 for drug Y. Although the TI of drug Y is the same as that of drug X in Figure 17.8, drug Y is obviously not as safe as drug X. The reason for this is that we would need potentially toxic doses of drug Y to obtain desired effectiveness in some patients. Thus, TI alone is not useful for true determination of drug safety because it does not give any information about the slopes of the DRCs for therapeutic and toxic effects. If the therapeutic DRC is relatively flat, there may be significant overlap between the two curves even if TD_{50} and ED_{50} of a drug are quite different.

Ideally, we would like a drug that is effective in all individuals at a dose that does not produce toxic effects in any individual. This concept is characterized by a parameter called the certain safety factor (CSF) as follows:

$$TI = \frac{TD_{50}}{ED_{50}\ 95}$$

Here, TD_1 represents the *minimally toxic dose,* the dose that is toxic to only 1% of individuals, whereas ED_{99} represents the *maximally effective dose,* the dose that is effective in 99% of individuals. The percentages used here—1% and 99%—are just illustrations. In practice, one can establish the desired population percentage acceptable for both toxicity and effectiveness.

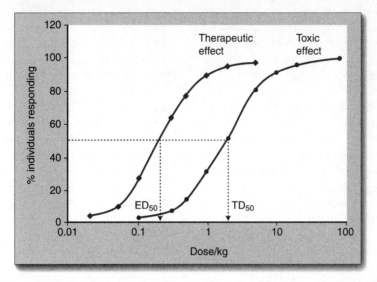

Figure 17.11. Quantal dose–response curves for the therapeutic effect and toxic effect of drug Y. The ratio TD_{50}/ED_{50} gives the therapeutic index (TI) of the drug. Drug Y has a TI = 10. Note that significant toxicity will be seen at a dose that gives therapeutic effect in greater than 90% of individuals.

The CSF is a measure of the overlap of the high end of the therapeutic DRC with the low end of the toxic DRC. A drug with a CSF of 1 can be dosed effectively to 99% of individuals while being toxic in only 1% of individuals. A higher CSF means that there is virtually no overlap between the two DRCs, and a maximally effective dose can be used with little chance of toxicity.

Risk Versus Benefit

A drug is usually considered safe if serious side effects or toxicity are unlikely when the drug is used at its *recommended* dosage in the *average* patient. This does not mean that there are no ADRs; it only means that the risk–benefit ratio of the drug is acceptable in most patients.

The TI and CSF are often used to predict the probability of toxicity in patients. When side effects or toxicity are likely, patients are given low doses to begin with and the dose is slowly boosted while monitoring the patient for ADRs. A drug that is safe in most patients may be toxic in a patient with a specific disease, impaired physiological function, or genetic predisposition.

KEY CONCEPTS

- Drug action at receptors or enzymes can be depicted as graphical dose–response relationships.
- Response plateaus at high concentrations or doses because receptors are saturated.
- Graded dose–response curves compare efficacy, potency, and toxicity of different drugs. They also reveal whether a drug is a full or partial agonist, or a competitive or noncompetitive antagonist.

- Quantal dose–response relationships are useful in illustrating the variability of drug response in a population.
- The safety of a drug can be illustrated by dose–toxic response relationships.
- The clinical therapeutic index of a drug is a ratio of the median toxic dose to the median effective dose.
- Dose–response and dose–toxic response curves are used together to define the risk–benefit of a drug and to select an appropriate dose.

ADDITIONAL READING

1. Katzung BG (ed). Basic and Clinical Pharmacology, 8th ed. McGraw-Hill/Appleton & Lange, 2000.

2. Mutschler E, Derendorf H. Drug Actions: Basic Principles and Therapeutic Aspects; CRC Press, 1995.

3. Brunton L, Lazo J, Parker K (eds). Goodman & Gilman's The Pharmacological Basis of Therapeutics, 11th ed. McGraw-Hill Professional, 2005.

4. Mycek MJ, Harvey RA, Champe PC. Lippincott's Illustrated Reviews: Pharmacology, 2nd ed. Lippincott Williams & Wilkins, 2000.

REVIEW QUESTIONS

1. Explain the important features of a concentration–response curve for a full and partial agonist. What are the similarities of this curve and a curve of enzyme activity? How do these curves change when the concentration is plotted on a logarithmic scale?

2. How does the concentration–response curve for an agonist change in the presence of competitive and noncompetitive antagonists?

3. How does the concentration–response curve for a substrate change in the presence of competitive and noncompetitive inhibitors?

4. What are the differences between a concentration–response relationship and a dose–response relationship? Why is the latter more useful in therapeutic application?

5. Explain the difference between potency and efficacy of a drug. How is this revealed in a dose–response curve?

6. What is meant by a selective drug? How can one determine selectivity from a dose–response curve?

7. Clarify the difference between the pharmacological therapeutic index and the clinical therapeutic index. Why is the latter more relevant to drug therapy?

8. Discuss why the certain safety factor is more appropriate in the choice of a drug dose than the clinical therapeutic index.

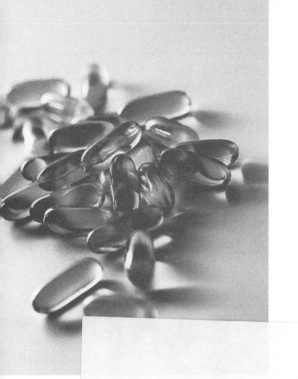

Section VI • **Drug Therapy**

QPS14.R4
2009

Therapeutic Variability

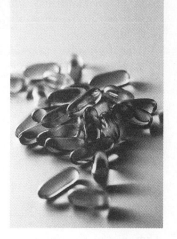

Earlier chapters have discussed what the body does to the drug (absorption, distribution, metabolism, and excretion [ADME] and pharmacokinetics) and what the drug does to the body (drug action and pharmacodynamics). Moreover, previous chapters have focused on the disposition and action of drugs in normal, relatively healthy individuals, suggesting that most patients process the drug in the same manner and that the drug works similarly in all individuals. In fact, the standard dose and dosing frequency of most drugs are based on the drug's behavior in an average patient population: approximately 18 to 65 years of age, weighing about 70 kg (150 lbs), with normal body functions.

However, patient attributes can affect the nature and degree of pharmacological response significantly. Not everyone responds to the same dose of a given drug in exactly the same manner at all times; variability in response to drug therapy is the rule rather than the exception for most medications. Even at the recommended standard doses of a drug, the *intensity* of the response is often different among patients because of individual differences in pharmacokinetics or pharmacodynamics. Even the *nature* of the response may vary in some patients, resulting in effects (such as drug allergy) not seen in the average patient. Alteration of physiological and pathological conditions in patients further complicates this picture.

Even the most successful drugs provide optimal benefits to only a fraction of patients. Variability in patient response to drug therapy must be taken into account to adapt drug treatment to individual patient needs.

Types of Therapeutic Variability

Therapeutic variability may be *interpatient,* i.e., between different people, or *intrapatient,* in which the drug response changes for a given person at different times. Many interwoven and overlapping factors contribute to variability. Scientists are reaching the conclusion that genetic variability among individuals is the primary underlying cause of altered response to drugs; we shall discuss genetic factors in detail in Chapter 20, Pharmacogenomics. Drug interaction, in which one drug influences the behavior of another, also contributes to therapeutic variability; this too, is the subject of a separate chapter (Chapter 19, Drug Interactions).

This chapter will deal with common and generally predictable factors contributing to therapeutic variability, such as:

- Pharmacokinetic factors that produce differing concentrations of the drug at the target receptor
- Pharmacodynamic factors that cause different pharmacological responses to the same drug concentration
- Immunological factors that result in allergic response

Other non–drug-related factors such as the personality, beliefs, and attitudes of both patient and clinician have been occasionally linked to therapeutic variability. We will not explore these in this book.

Many different factors contribute to therapeutic variability, and the same factor may cause pharmacokinetic as well as pharmacodynamic variability. Some common causes of variability can be anticipated by proper evaluation of a patient. In other cases, variability is unexpected and can result in therapeutic failure or toxicity.

Pharmacokinetic Variability

Pharmacokinetic variability refers to variability in delivery of drug to or removal of drug from sites of action involved in efficacy and/or toxicity. The obvious result of this is a change in the intensity of drug effect because either too much or too little drug reaches the site of action, and side effects because of higher than normal drug concentrations. Pharmacokinetic variability is particularly problematic for drugs with a narrow therapeutic range or *therapeutic window* (or low therapeutic index) because small differences may result in therapeutic failure or toxicity, as illustrated in Figure 18.1.

A patient who does not fit the "average" patient mold can show differences in absorption, distribution, metabolism, and excretion of drugs. Much of this can be anticipated, and appropriate changes in the dose or dosing schedule made before the initiation of drug therapy.

Pharmacokinetic variability may also be attributable to genetic effects, arising from alterations in certain biomolecules such as drug-metabolizing enzymes, and drug transporters that mediate drug uptake into and efflux from intracellular sites. Such genetic effects are often unpredictable, although new research is allowing clinicians to identify patients with an abnormal ADME profile for a certain drug. The relationship between genetic characteristics, drug effects, and toxicity is called *pharmacogenetics*; we shall discuss this in greater detail in Chapter 20, Pharmacogenomics.

Let us discuss common sources of pharmacokinetic variability.

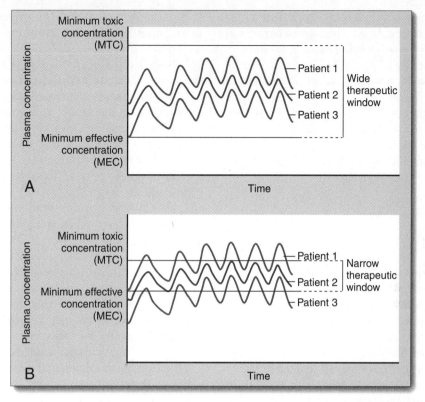

Figure 18.1. Effect of interindividual pharmacokinetic variability on the efficacy and toxicity of a drug with a wide (**A**) and narrow (**B**) therapeutic window, after multiple dosing in three patients.

Body Weight and Composition

Pharmacological effect depends on the concentration of drug reaching the site of action, which in turn depends on the drug dose and pharmacokinetics. The recommended standard dose of most drugs is typically based on a 70-kg adult male. If we assume ADME processes are functioning normally in an individual, then drug concentration at the site of action depends on dose and volume of distribution V. For a given dose, the greater the V, the lower the concentration in all tissues, including the site of action. This means that a given dose of drug gives lower tissue concentrations in large individuals compared with small ones. Thus, overweight individuals may need a higher than standard dose to achieve adequate tissue concentrations, whereas small individuals may need a lower than standard dose. Many drug products are available in multiple strengths (e.g., 10-, 20-, and 30-mg tablets) to allow dose adjustments in individual cases.

Although larger individuals generally require a higher dose to achieve therapeutic plasma or tissue concentrations, the difficulty lies in defining what large and small mean when referring to patients. A simple approach is to adjust doses based on body weight as follows:

$$\text{dose required} = \frac{\text{average dose}}{70 \text{ kg}} \times \text{weight of individual (kg)}$$

(Eq. 18.1)

Dose adjustments based on Equation 18.1 do not work for people who are extremely lean or obese because it does not account for dramatically altered body composition such as body fat and body water. Recall that V of drugs depends on drug lipophilicity. Thus, in an obese individual, a lipophilic drug may have an unusually large V, whereas the V of a hydrophilic drug may not be changed as dramatically. Consequently, doses for lipophilic and hydrophilic drugs may have to be adjusted by different factors in obese patients. In such cases, body surface area rather than body weight is often used to adjust dosage.

Age

Many drugs behave differently in children and the elderly compared with the average adult. Some of this difference is caused by variation in body size and composition, as discussed earlier. However, even when body size is taken into account, additional factors are responsible for increased sensitivity of the very young and the very old to drugs.

Special populations—the very young (infants and pediatrics) and the very old (geriatrics)—are usually excluded in clinical testing of drugs, and their response to drugs is generally unknown when a drug is first marketed. This is changing, however, and more and more drugs are now being tested in geriatric and pediatric populations to identify appropriate doses and dosing schedules.

Infants and Children. Infants constitute a very special subgroup of patients in which drugs must be used with extreme care. In addition to a much smaller body weight, there are significant physiological differences between infants and the average adult. The most important of these are:

- Increased permeability of all tissues, including the skin and blood–brain barrier
- Proportionately greater volume of body water, and a consequently higher V for certain drugs
- Lower rate of blood flow to most organs
- Decreased biotransformation as a result of underdeveloped metabolic enzymes

- Decreased renal clearance attributable to reduced glomerular filtration rate

Consequently, use of any drug in an infant must be carefully considered and the dose adjusted appropriately. At an age of about 1 year, metabolic and excretion functions are better developed, and the risk of using drugs in young children is less than in infants. At about 12 years of age, adult doses are often used. However, compensation for a lower body weight and altered body composition must always be considered when using all drugs in children.

Elderly. Many organ systems show a normal decline in function with age in the elderly population. Muscle mass decreases, whereas percentage of body fat rises. Absorption efficiency is usually only slightly reduced, but there are significant decreases in efficiency of metabolism and excretion of drugs. Hepatic effects include:

- Decreased hepatic mass
- Decreased hepatic blood flow
- Decreased enzyme activity

  Renal effects consist of:

- Reduced number of nephrons
- Reduced number of functioning glomeruli
- Decreased renal blood flow

The result is that plasma and tissue concentrations in geriatrics are often higher than expected, and sensitivity to the drug is increased.

Sex-Related Differences

Until the 1990s, health researchers used male subjects to determine safety and efficacy of new drugs and treatments. Reasons for this were concern about the potentially confounding effects of a woman's hormonal changes on treatment, the desire to protect a potential fetus, and fear of liability if a fetus was harmfully exposed. As a result, women of child-bearing age were systematically excluded from clinical trials. Treatment interventions, toxicity, and safety data were studied in men and then applied or assumed to be the same in women.

Sex. The discovery of differences between male and female response to disease and treatments has changed the landscape of new drug development. Women are now included in clinical trials unless the risk is unacceptable.

Sex-related differences in body weight and composition account for some pharmacokinetic variability. Women generally have a lower body weight and a higher proportion of body fat, and may therefore require a different drug dose. There is evidence that metabolic rates may also be different (usually lower) in women compared with men, requiring dosage adjustment. The issue of sex in drug safety becomes particularly important in women of childbearing age, and in pregnant and lactating women.

Pregnancy and Lactation. Many drugs administered to a mother during pregnancy and lactation may adversely influence the embryo, fetus, and infant. The placenta allows transport of many drugs from mother to embryo or fetus by passive diffusion, and drug concentrations in the embryo and in fetal circulation are often the same as those in the mother's circulation. Embryonic and fetal cells are highly sensitive to drugs, and severe toxic effects are seen when these are exposed to drugs. The type and extent of toxicity depend on the stage of embryonic or fetal development when exposure occurred.

The embryonic stage is the time between fertilization and the eighth week of pregnancy. Because major organ structures are being formed during this period, a major toxicity is teratogenicity, the ability of a drug to cause damage to a developing fetus, resulting in congenital malformation of various structures. Serious malformations result in a miscarriage. The fetal stage of development occurs after differentiation of major organ structures; here, toxic effects of drugs can be seen on already formed organ systems.

Many drugs, particularly lipophilic drugs, distribute readily into the breast milk of the mother during lactation. Infants in their first 3 months of life do not have fully developed enzyme systems for biotransformation and renal excretion of drugs. Thus, toxic levels may accumulate in nursing infants, resulting in a variety of effects depending on the drug.

Health and Disease

The overall health of the patient is critical in determining how a drug behaves and works in the body. Drugs are often used in patients whose organ systems are not functioning normally; particularly important are organs involved in drug elimination—the liver and kidney. Patients with impaired hepatic or renal function do not eliminate drugs readily, resulting in higher plasma levels and resultant potential toxicity. A change in dose or dosing frequency is often necessary in such patients.

Impaired circulation (resulting in lower blood flow rates to organs) seen in cardiovascular disease can affect all aspects of drug pharmacokinetics. Other factors such as body temperature, hydration or dehydration, and acidosis or alkalosis may also change the pharmacokinetics of some drugs. The dosage regimen for patients with disease often needs to be individualized on the basis of assessment of hepatic, renal, and cardiovascular function.

The nutritional status of a patient can influence drug pharmacokinetics. Malnutrition, vitamin deficiencies, or decreased protein synthesis may result in altered plasma protein and metabolic enzyme levels.

Pharmacodynamic Variability

Pharmacodynamic variability refers to variable drug effects despite equivalent drug delivery to the sites of action. It may reflect differences in the structure and function of target receptors or in the broad pathophysiological context in which a drug interacts with its target. The existence of pharmacodynamic variability means lack of a relationship between drug response and plasma concentration, and pharmacokinetic–pharmacodynamic correlations are not useful in these situations.

Sex-Related Differences

Physiological differences between men and women may result in altered pharmacodynamics of some drugs in women compared with men. For example, differences have been shown between men and women in both perception of and response to pain. Emerging scientific evidence points to sex-related pharmacological differences in opioid-receptor binding and in responses to certain opioid pain medications. These differences suggest the importance of developing sex-specific strategies for pain relief and highlight the need for further investigation of sex-related pain treatment.

Idiosyncrasy

A few individuals respond to drugs in a highly unusual and unpredictable manner, giving a response quantitatively much different than in the average patient. For example, some patients may have an intense response to a very small dose of the drug, whereas others may not respond to very high doses. The response may also be qualitatively different in some situations, with new pharmacological effects being observed. Such responses, referred to as drug idiosyncrasy or *idiosyncratic response,* are infrequent and believed to result from a genetically determined metabolic or enzyme deficiency that is not expressed under normal situations (e.g., hemolytic anemia occurring in patients with glucose-6-phosphate dehydrogenase deficiency after receiving an oxidant drug). These responses show a dose–response relationship, but not the same one shown by the average patient.

Circadian Rhythms

A circadian rhythm is the regular recurrence of a biological process or activity in cycles of about 24 hours. These cycles are set by a biological clock that seems to respond to recurring daylight and darkness. This clock, which lies in the brain, regulates organs like the liver, kidneys, and blood vessels by controlling circadian clocks within them; consequently, a daily reproducible pattern of peaks and troughs is seen in many physiological variables. The acknowledgment of circadian rhythms is philosophically different from the concept of homeostasis, which assumes that most physiological processes are in a state of equilibrium and do not change significantly with time.

It is now generally understood that there are circadian rhythms in many receptors, in signaling pathways, and in activity of enzymes. If these are targets of a drug, then pharmacodynamics of the drug can also be different at different times. There are a number of hormones that are primarily secreted in the morning, such as cortisol, catecholamines, plasma renin, aldosterone, and angiotensin. In contrast, other substances peak at the end of the day or at night, for example, gastric acid, growth hormone, prolactin, melatonin, follicle-stimulating hormone, luteinizing hormone, and adrenocorticotropic hormone.

There are consequences to the circadian changes in these hormones, and many common diseases show significant circadian variation in onset or exacerbation of symptoms. Asthma symptoms generally worsen during the night; in fact, estimates are that symptoms of asthma occur 50 to 100 times more often at night than during the day. Many circadian-dependent factors may contribute to the worsening of nocturnal asthma. For example, researchers have reported that cortisol (an anti-inflammatory ligand) levels were lowest in the middle of the night, and histamine (a mediator of bronchoconstriction) peaked at a level that coincided with the greatest degree of bronchoconstriction at 4 AM.

Because of its effect on physiological processes, circadian rhythm can affect all aspects of drug disposition and action and is one of the factors responsible for intraindividual variability of medications depending on time of administration. Many drugs display normal, reproducible daily variations in pharmacokinetics and pharmacodynamics. Circadian effects on drug pharmacokinetics have been related to time-dependent changes in the following processes and parameters:

- Gastrointestinal motility and intestinal absorption rates
- Intestinal enzyme activity
- Gastric acid secretion
- Hepatic drug metabolism activity and enzyme concentration
- Glomerular filtration rate
- Blood flow rate
- Urine pH

The narrower the therapeutic window for a specific drug, the more important the implication of circadian variation in plasma levels. Although most drug doses and dosing schedules have not yet taken into account such diurnal variation in drug action and disposition, mounting evidence suggests these factors must be considered in drug therapy.

For example, rhythmic changes in cell division may explain circadian variation in sensitivity of rapidly proliferating tumor tissues to chemotherapy. Many anticancer agents are most cytotoxic to normal tissues that are actively dividing during specific phases of the cell division cycle. Studies indicate the timing of cancer chemotherapy may be of practical importance in improving the therapeutic index of common cancer treatments. Corticosteroids and interferons are less toxic and no less effective when given, respectively, on awakening and just before sleep.

Drug Tolerance

Tolerance is the body's ability to adapt to the presence of a drug. The magnitude of the body's response to a particular drug depends on the concentration of drug at its site of action and the sensitivity of the target receptor to the drug. Tolerance may be defined as a state of progressively decreased responsiveness to a drug, as a result of which a larger dose of drug is needed to achieve the effect originally obtained by a smaller dose. Tolerance appears counterintuitive because addition of more of an activating ligand lessens the elicited response.

Tolerance may be pharmacokinetic in origin, but is most often related to drug pharmacodynamics. Pharmacokinetic tolerance develops when a drug induces its own metabolism and thus decreases concentration of drug at the site of action. Pharmacodynamic tolerance arises as a result of adaptive changes in receptor sensitivity in response to repeated exposure to a particular drug. The result is usually a decrease or loss of sensitivity to the drug, resulting in a decreased response. Adaptive changes may be related to receptor down-regulation, cellular adaptation, or *tachyphylaxis* (a rapidly decreasing response to a drug after administration of a few doses).

Drug Resistance

Drug resistance is defined as insensitivity or decreased sensitivity of cells to drugs that ordinarily cause growth inhibition (such as anti-tumor drugs) or cell death (such as anti-microbial drugs). It occurs despite administration of doses equal to or higher than those usually recommended but within limits of safety, and despite adequate absorption from the administration site.

Drug resistance may be classified as *intrinsic resistance,* in which the cell or organism is inherently insensitive to the drug and predisposed to respond poorly to it, or *acquired resistance,* in which

Chronopathology and Chronotherapeutics of Cardiovascular Disease

Chronopathology is the study of biological rhythms in disease processes and morbid and mortal events; a good example is seen in cardiovascular disease. Myocardial infarction, stroke, and sudden cardiac death occur with greater frequency between 6 AM and noon. These events can be explained by changes in multiple factors. With activation of the sympathetic nervous system before awakening, blood pressure and heart rate begin to increase. Blood pressure peaks between 6 AM and noon. These changes in blood pressure parallel the morning activation in catecholamines, renin, and angiotensin. Activity and sleep influence the level of blood pressure throughout the day, and blood pressure is generally lowest between midnight and 6 AM. At the same time, increase in catecholamines in the morning promotes platelet aggregation. This is especially important because fibrinogen also increases, whereas endogenous tissue plasminogen activator decreases, promoting a procoagulant state with increased blood viscosity.

The higher blood pressure and heart rate in the early morning increase shear forces in blood vessels and myocardial oxygen consumption, creating an environment for plaque rupture. Once plaque rupture occurs, thrombosis results, exacerbated by the procoagulant state in the early morning; the resulting consequence is a clinical event.

Chronotherapeutics is the purposeful control of plasma drug concentrations to match intrinsic disease rhythms to optimize therapeutic outcomes and minimize side effects. Optimum therapy is more likely when the right amount of drug is delivered to the correct target organ at the most appropriate time. In contrast, many side effects can be minimized if a drug is not present when it is *not* needed.

To achieve such customized dosing, scientists have developed *chronotherapeutic formulations* of drugs. Unlike conventional controlled-release formulations, which provide relatively constant plasma drug levels for 24 hours, chronotherapeutic formulations use various release mechanisms to provide varying plasma drug levels throughout the day. Currently, there are four chronotherapeutic antihypertensive products, two using verapamil and one each containing diltiazem and propranolol.

organisms or cells initially respond to the drug, but eventually some or all fail to respond because of an acquired resistant property.

Intrinsic Resistance. Intrinsic or primary resistance may occur as a result of systemic or cellular factors:

- *Systemic factors*: factors causing low drug concentration in the organism or tumor such as decreased absorption, increased elimination, or decreased distribution to the site of action because of functional membrane barriers (e.g., blood–brain barrier limits effective therapy of bacterial infections in the brain).

- *Cellular factors*: factors that affect ability of the drug to reach and interact with the drug target receptor or enzyme. Such factors include low intracellular levels of drug (owing to efflux proteins), low affinity of receptor for drug, absence of a particular receptor, or lack of activation of a prodrug to an active metabolite in the cell.

Acquired Resistance. Acquired resistance is usually related to genetic changes that alter the sensitivity of the target to a single drug (or to a chemically similar group of drugs) through a variety of mechanisms. Acquired resistance is an inheritable trait. It may be the result of induction by the drug of DNA mutations in some cells in the population. Alternatively, it may arise as a result of a drug selectively affecting the genetically susceptible cells within a population while not affecting a small number of resistant cells in the population. In both cases, the drug will be initially effective, but will become progressively less effective as acquired resistance develops.

Once a cell has developed acquired resistance, i.e., is altered such that it is partially or completely resistant to a drug, there is a selective advantage for its survival in a drug-containing environment. Selection is the process by which drug-resistant organisms or cells are enriched in a cell population. Consequently, with continued presence of drug, eventually only drug-resistant organisms or cells will survive, resulting in a resistant population.

Different drugs may share the same biochemical mechanism leading to development of resistance. *Cross-resistance* arises when cells become resistant to drugs that are chemically related or have the same mechanism of action. More problematic is *multiple drug resistance,* or multidrug resistance, in which cells become resistant to drugs with different chemical structures and mechanisms of action.

Several clinical approaches have been implemented to avoid or minimize resistance.

- Use of high doses to achieve adequate intracellular concentrations to inhibit or kill the intended organism or cell.

Because subtherapeutic concentrations encourage development of resistance, this approach reduces the probability that drug-resistant populations will develop.

- Combination therapy with two or more drugs with different mechanisms of action. The probability that DNA changes will emerge in the same cell resulting in resistance to both drugs is small. Thus, this approach reduces the probability of selection of a population of resistant cells.

- Cells resistant to one drug often exhibit increased sensitivity to another drug that acts by a different mechanism. Thus, knowledge of the mechanism of resistance to a drug can provide an approach to specifically target drug-resistant organisms or cells.

Immunological Variability

Drug allergy is a variability in drug response among individuals that is related to an immunological reaction and is seen only after a second or subsequent exposure of the patient to the drug. The effects are qualitatively different from the normal pharmacological effects of the drug. Allergic reactions to drugs do not show the usual dose–response relationships; even a small, subtherapeutic dose may be sufficient to cause allergy.

Drug Allergy

An allergic reaction is an adverse response to a drug as a result of a previous exposure to the same drug. Drug allergy is different from drug toxicity or idiosyncrasy in that it is not dose-dependent and not drug-specific. Thus, even therapeutic doses can cause an allergic reaction in some patients. Symptoms of drug allergy are similar for all drugs that cause an allergic response, and are not related to usual pharmacological effects of the drug.

Many macromolecules (such as foreign proteins) are viewed as antigens by the body, and their presence triggers formation

Multidrug Resistance

Multidrug resistance (MDR) occurs when cells become resistant to a broad range of structurally and functionally unrelated drugs after exposure to a single cytotoxic agent. This type of resistance is a serious problem in chemotherapy and in antiviral and antimicrobial therapy.

A number of different mechanisms can cause development of MDR, including increased drug efflux from the cell by ATP-dependent transporters, decreased drug uptake into the cell, or activation of biotransformation enzymes. However, MDR has most often been linked to the overexpression of P-glycoprotein (P-gp), a 170-kilodalton ATP-dependent membrane transporter that acts as a drug efflux pump.

Clinical observation has shown that MDR may develop after a course of chemotherapy (acquired resistance) or may be present on diagnosis (intrinsic resistance). MDR in chemotherapy has been associated with overexpression of P-gp transporters that act as efflux pumps to remove cytotoxic compounds from tumor cells, thereby preventing drugs from reaching therapeutic concentrations in the cell. The cytotoxic drugs most frequently associated with MDR are hydrophobic, amphipathic natural products, such as the taxanes (paclitaxel, docetaxel), vinca alkaloids (vinorelbine, vincristine, vinblastine), anthracyclines (doxorubicin, daunorubicin, epirubicin), epipodophyllotoxins (etoposide, teniposide), topotecan, dactinomycin, and mitomycin C.

Expression of P-gp is usually highest in tumors that are derived from tissues that normally express P-gp, such as epithelial cells of the colon, kidney, adrenal, pancreas, and liver. Such tumors may show resistance to some antitumor drugs even before chemotherapy is initiated. In other tumors, the expression of P-gp may be low at the beginning of treatment but increase after exposure to the drugs, resulting in the development of MDR.

Inhibiting P-gp as a way of reversing MDR has been extensively studied. Many P-gp inhibitors, both competitive and noncompetitive, have been identified, with the objective of administering the inhibitor along with the antitumor drug. However, clinical results have been disappointing. The inhibitors are either too toxic themselves, have a relatively low affinity for the transporter, or have other undesirable drug interactions.

---

of antibodies. Thus, many biopharmaceutical protein drugs have the potential of initiating antibody formation. However, small molecule drugs can also indirectly cause sensitization. This indirect effect occurs if the drug (or its metabolite) binds covalently to an endogenous protein (*hapten*), creating an antigen complex with specificity for the drug part of the complex. A subsequent exposure to the same drug then triggers an antigen–antibody response in the body, a chain reaction that is always the same regardless of drug.

The most important drug causes of immediate hypersensitivity reactions are antibiotics. Other common drugs that cause such reactions are insulin, enzymes (streptokinase and chymopapain), heterologous

Penicillin Allergy

Penicillin antibiotics are one of the most common causes of medication allergies. Penicillins are a family of antibiotics called β-lactams and include benzylpenicillin, penicillin V and penicillin G, amoxicillin, ampicillin, dicloxacillin, and naficillin. These drugs are generally used to eradicate many common bacterial infections such as skin, ear, sinus, and upper respiratory infections.

benzylpenicillin

Common allergic reactions to penicillin include rashes, hives, itchy eyes, and swollen lips, tongue, or face. Serious and occasionally fatal hypersensitivity (anaphylaxis) has been reported in patients on penicillin therapy. The anaphylactic reaction can develop within an hour of taking penicillin. Symptoms include difficulty breathing, hives, wheezing, dizziness, loss of consciousness, rapid or weak pulse, skin turning blue, diarrhea, nausea, and vomiting. Although anaphylaxis is more frequent after parenteral therapy, it also occurs in patients receiving oral penicillin.

Allergic reactions are more likely to occur in individuals with a history of penicillin hypersensitivity or a history of sensitivity to multiple allergens. Some people who are allergic to penicillin show cross-sensitivity to other closely related antibiotics, particularly other β-lactams. Drugs in this category include cephalosporins (e.g., cephalexin, cefprozil, and cefuroxime), carbapenems (e.g., imipenem), monobactams (e.g., aztreonam), and carbacephems.

The prevalence of penicillin hypersensitivity in the general population is not known. Before any penicillin therapy is initiated in a patient, it is important to make a careful inquiry concerning previous hypersensitivity reactions to penicillin, cephalosporins, or other antibiotics. Approximately 10% of hospitalized patients report a history of allergy to penicillin, and for this reason, many of these patients receive alternative antimicrobial drugs. The most reliable method for evaluating penicillin allergy is by skin testing to both major and minor determinants of penicillin.

If an allergic reaction occurs, the penicillin product should be discontinued immediately. Emergency treatment of penicillin allergy includes injections of epinephrine or intravenous administration of antihistamines and corticosteroids. Oxygen, intravenous steroids, and airway management, including intubation, are also administered as indicated.

antisera (equine antitoxins and antilymphocyte globulin), murine monoclonal antibodies, protamine, and heparin.

The first contact of the drug with a potentially allergic patient is called sensitization. On subsequent contacts, the body produces large amounts of histamine, an autacoid that causes potentially serious effects such as a skin rash, breathing difficulty, decrease in blood pressure and, ultimately, shock. This exaggerated immune response to a foreign agent such as an antigen or drug is called hypersensitivity. Symptoms may occur within seconds or minutes after the second drug exposure (*immediate hypersensitivity*) or may begin gradually with maximum effect in days or weeks after the second exposure (*delayed hypersensitivity*). The most serious manifestation of such an allergic reaction is called *anaphylaxis* or *anaphylactic shock*— a severe and life-threatening allergic reaction. Structurally similar drugs with the same determinant group (group recognized by the antibody) can show *cross-sensitivity,* in that an allergic response to the second drug is shown even without previous contact with it.

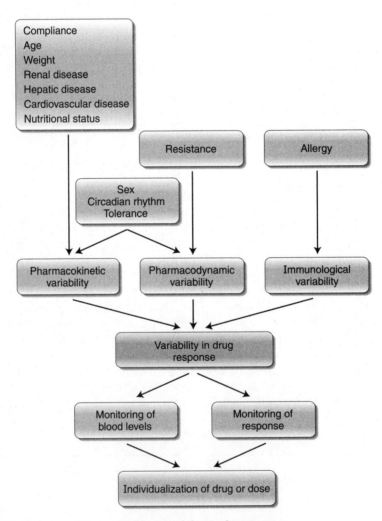

Figure 18.2. Summary of factors causing variability in drug response.

The predisposition of a patient to be allergic to a particular drug is partly genetic, but may be related to other factors such as duration of treatment or route of administration. Allergic reactions often occur without warning and cannot be predicted.

Drug Compliance

Compliance is the willingness and ability to follow a prescribed course of drug treatment. Medication noncompliance or nonadherence, i.e., the failure to take drugs on time in the doses and manner prescribed, is as dangerous and costly as many illnesses.

Noncompliance can be classified as either complete nonadherence (missing dosages) or partial adherence (prescribed dose is not completely administered) to a therapeutic regimen. Whether compliance is absent or partial, the outcome is a reduction of pharmacological effect or emergence of drug resistance. Some causes for noncompliance are:

- The patient is taking many medications (polypharmacy) on a complex dosing schedule and is unable to keep track of them.
- The cost of medications may cause the patient to miss doses or take reduced doses.

- Side effects may discourage the patient from taking the drug.
- The patient may lack understanding of a drug's benefits.

Although an obvious cause of therapeutic variability, noncompliance must be taken into account and strategies developed to encourage adherence to a dosing regimen.

Individualization of Therapy

The standard drug therapy, i.e., drug, dose, and dosing frequency, for a particular disease or condition is merely the starting point of treatment. Before the standard drug or dose is used, the patient needs to be assessed for factors discussed in this chapter to see whether this approach is suitable. Even if a patient is started on standard therapy, monitoring of response (efficacy, adverse effects) is necessary as therapy continues. For drugs with a narrow therapeutic window and in certain sensitive patients, blood levels may need to be monitored to ensure they are within the therapeutic range. The dose or the drug may have to be changed to individualize therapy to each patient. Figure 18.2 summarizes factors causing therapeutic variability and actions to be taken in these situations.

KEY CONCEPTS

- The standard dose of a drug is based on response of a majority of average patients.

- The effect of a particular dose of a particular drug is never the same in all persons, or even in the same person at different times. The standard drug or dose may need to be modified for the needs of a particular individual.

- Pharmacokinetic variability arises because of differences in ADME of the drug in patients.

- Pharmacodynamic variability is caused by differences in target re-

ceptors or in pathophysiology of the patient.

- Circadian rhythms are an important source of pharmacokinetic and pharmacodynamic variability.

- Drug tolerance and drug resistance can limit the therapeutic utility of a drug in some patients.

- Immunological variability, e.g., drug allergy, can cause serious adverse reactions in certain patients.

- Poor drug compliance is an important component of interindividual therapeutic variability.

ADDITIONAL READING

1. Rowland M, Tozer TN. Clinical Pharmacokinetics: Concepts and Applications, 3rd ed. Lippincott Williams & Wilkins, 1995.

2. Levine RR, Walsh CT, Schwartz-Bloom RD. Pharmacology: Drug Actions and Reactions, 6th ed. CRC Press-Parthenon Publishers, 2000.

3. Pacifici GM, Pelkonen O. Interindividual Variability in Human Drug Metabolism, 1st ed. Taylor and Francis, 2001.

4. Brunton L, Lazo J, Parker K (eds.). Goodman & Gilman's The Pharmacological Basis of Therapeutics, 11th ed. McGraw-Hill Professional, 2005.

REVIEW QUESTIONS

1. Why do patients respond differently to the same dose of a drug?

2. Why is pharmacokinetic variability particularly problematic for drugs with a narrow therapeutic range?

3. What factors can cause pharmacodynamic variability among patients?

4. What factors can cause variability in the same patient at different times?

5. Differentiate among drug toxicity, drug idiosyncrasy, and drug allergy.

6. Differentiate between drug tolerance and drug resistance. List the clinical approaches to minimizing drug resistance.

7. Differentiate between cross-resistance and multiple-drug resistance.

8. What is an allergic reaction to a drug? How does an allergic response differ from other responses seen after administering a drug?

9. What are the clinical approaches to ensuring that each patient is given the right dose of the right drug?

Drug Interactions

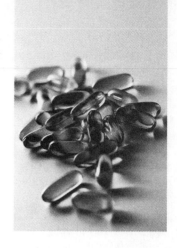

During development of a new drug, each compound is tested vigorously for pharmacokinetic, pharmacodynamic, and pharmaceutical properties to evaluate its safety and efficacy. An acceptable drug product is one that produces the desirable therapeutic effect in the recommended dosing range without serious adverse events. However, although each approved drug may be safe and effective on its own, this cannot be said definitively when drugs are used together.

In clinical practice, several drugs are often given to a patient concurrently (*polypharmacy*), either to treat multiple medical conditions or to use multiple approaches in treating a single disease. Whenever two or more drugs are coadministered there is a possibility of some type of interaction between them, i.e., a situation in which the action of one drug is altered by concurrent use of another drug. Unexpected drug interactions can cause severe adverse drug reactions (ADRs) in patients and may result in death. Drug interactions also contribute to therapeutic variability among patients given the same dose of the same drug and are particularly common in the elderly owing to age-associated changes in pharmacokinetics, pharmacodynamics, and high use of prescription and nonprescription medications. The health-care community is becoming increasingly aware of the role of drug interactions in loss of therapeutic effectiveness and increase in side effects. Many drug interactions can be predicted and prevented by making appropriate changes in dose or by choosing an alternative drug.

On the other hand, drug interactions can sometimes be exploited to enhance a drug's therapeutic effectiveness. A second drug is sometimes prescribed intentionally to modify effects of the first. Such an approach might be used to increase efficacy or reduce side effects of the primary drug. Thus, drug interactions are not necessarily to be always avoided; they just need to be anticipated and dealt with.

Interactions between foods and drugs are also possible because many physiological and biochemical pathways in the body (such as those for absorption, biotransformation, excretion, and transport) are shared by nutrients and drugs. The action of a drug may be altered by a food or nutrient, or vice versa. It is important to know whether safety or efficacy of a drug will be affected by coadministration with certain kinds of foods.

Drug–Drug Interactions

Interactions between drugs may be conveniently classified as:

- pharmaceutical drug interactions
- pharmacokinetic drug interactions
- pharmacodynamic drug interactions

Pharmaceutical interactions occur when two drugs react chemically or physically during administration or absorption so that the amount of drug available for absorption (of one or both drugs) is altered. *Pharmacokinetic interactions* arise when one drug changes the absorption, distribution, metabolism, or excretion (ADME) behavior of another drug. Finally, *pharmacodynamic interactions* develop when one drug increases or decreases the pharmacological effect of another.

Pharmaceutical Drug Interactions

Interactions that interfere with drug absorption as a result of chemical or physical reactions between drugs are called pharmaceutical drug interactions. Most of these occur during release or absorption after drug administration, such as in the stomach when two oral drugs are given concurrently. The main result of a pharmaceutical interaction is to reduce the concentration of drug available for absorption. This decreases the concentration gradient for absorption, thereby reducing the amount of drug absorbed and, therefore, its bioavailability. The more common causes of pharmaceutical interactions are discussed here.

Chelation

Chelating agents are compounds that can bind to a metal ion to form a salt or complex that is poorly absorbed; several drugs have chelating properties. Metal ions such as Ca^{2+}, Mg^{2+}, Al^{3+}, and Fe^{3+} are present in antacids, many nutritional supplements (vitamins and minerals), and foods (calcium in milk products and calcium-fortified products). When coadministered with metal ion-containing products, chelating drugs can combine with metal ions in the gastrointestinal (GI) tract to form complexes that are poorly absorbed.

A classic example of a chelation interaction occurs with orally administered tetracycline and fluoroquinolone (e.g., ciprofloxacin) antibiotics (Fig. 19.1). The acidic functional groups have the ability to chelate metal ions forming insoluble complexes, resulting in reduced bioavailability. Figure 19.2 shows a typical plasma concentration–time curve for tetracycline showing the effect of coadministration with a metal ion-containing product.

Separating administration of the interacting drugs by at least 2 hours can minimize this type of drug interaction. Chelating agents are often used as antidotes to treat heavy metal poisoning; ex-

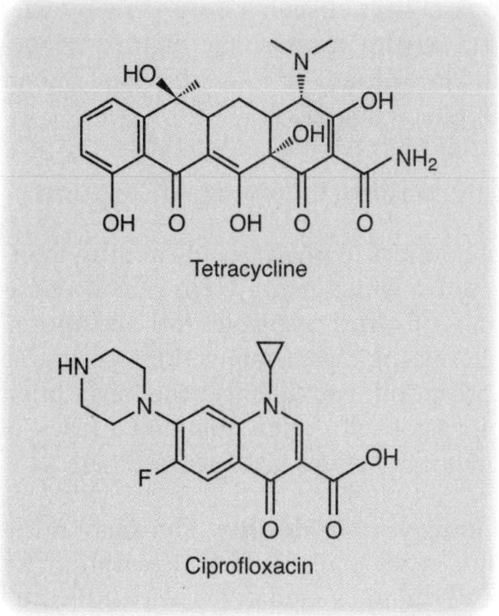

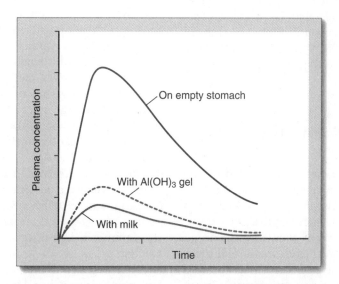

Figure 19.1. Structures of tetracycline and ciprofloxacin, two antibiotics that are capable of chelating metal ions.

amples are calcium disodium EDTA and dimercaprol.

Adsorption

Adsorption interactions are nonspecific and arise when molecules of a drug physically bind to the surface of another solid that acts as an adsorbent, reducing the concentration of drug available for absorption. Examples of adsorbents are antacids, antidiarrheal products (kaolin, bismuth subsalicylate), and ion exchange resins (colestipol and cholestyramine). These adsorbent medications disintegrate into many small solid particles in the GI tract after administration, providing a large surface area for adsorption. Cholestyramine adsorbs many drugs such as dicumarol, methotrexate, and digitoxin and decreases their absorption and bioavailability. Antacids adsorb and decrease absorption of digoxin and iron.

A solution to a drug interaction with an adsorbent is, once again, to separate administration of drugs and potential adsorbents by at least 2 hours. The adsorption mechanism can also be exploited for a beneficial use; adsorbents such as activated charcoal are used orally as antidotes to treat various types of poisoning.

Alteration of Gastric pH

Antacids, anticholinergic drugs, histamine (H_2) blockers, and proton pump inhibitors are used to decrease stomach

Figure 19.2. Plasma concentration–time curves for tetracycline showing the effect of coadministration with an antacid product ($Al(OH)_3$ gel) or with calcium-containing food (milk), compared with administration on an empty stomach. Plasma levels are significantly lower when tetracycline is administered with a product containing metal ions.

acidity and increase stomach pH. This alteration of gastric pH can influence the ionization of other coadministered weak acid and weak base drugs and change the ratio of their ionized to un-ionized forms in the GI tract. This change could, in turn, influence dissolution, absorption rate, and bioavailability of the drug after oral administration.

For example, absorption of iron salts, ketoconazole, or ampicillin administered in ester form requires a low gastric pH for adequate dissolution. If omeprazole, a proton-pump inhibitor that increases stomach pH, is coadministered with these drugs, it can interfere with their absorption.

Incompatibilities

Some drug products such as intravenous (IV) solutions are mixed together before administration for convenience, but may be incompatible with each other when combined. These incompatibilities can be considered a type of pharmaceutical interaction. For example, phenytoin precipitates in the IV bag as an insoluble salt when added to dextrose solutions, and is consequently unavailable to control seizures. Amphotericin precipitates if it is administered in saline and can cause serious complications. Gentamicin is incompatible with most β-lactams in IV fluids, resulting in loss of antibiotic effect.

Pharmacokinetic Drug Interactions

Most drug interactions are pharmacokinetic in nature, involving an alteration of absorption, distribution, biotransformation, or excretion of one drug by another. They can occur anytime while the drug is in the body. Although many pharmacokinetic interactions have been studied, documented, and can be anticipated, unexpected interactions arise frequently. From a pharmacokinetic standpoint, the major effect of such a drug–drug interaction results in unusually high or unusually low plasma or tissue levels of one or all interacting drugs.

Interactions Involving Absorption

In contrast to pharmaceutical drug interactions, which mainly change concentration of drug available for absorption, pharmacokinetic interactions affecting absorption can change the absorption process itself. Some common causes of such interactions are discussed here.

Change in GI Motility. The small intestine is the major site of absorption for orally administered drugs; very little drug is absorbed from the stomach. Therefore, the longer a drug remains in the stomach, i.e., the longer its *gastric emptying time,* the slower it is absorbed. Conversely, the shorter the gastric emptying time, the faster a drug can be absorbed. Drugs such as phenytoin and morphine inhibit gastric emptying and increase gastric emptying time. Other agents such as metoclopramide, erythromycin, and reserpine speed up gastric emptying and decrease gastric emptying time. Therefore, drugs that alter gastric emptying can affect the absorption rate of other concurrently administered drugs. Some drugs, particularly anticholinergics and laxatives, affect the small intestines by changing its *motility,* i.e., they change peristaltic activity that moves intestinal contents down the tract. This will also affect residence time in the GI tract and potentially influence bioavailability and absorption rate.

Alterations in GI residence time by one drug can influence absorption of another oral drug administered to the patient. In general, drugs that decrease GI motility (e.g., anticholinergics) reduce the rate but not the extent of absorption of concurrently administered drugs; reduction in rate may cause delay in achieving desired blood levels. The extent of absorption also may be reduced in some cases. An example is reduction in GI motility caused by the antihistamine chlorpheniramine. When the drug levodopa (used in Parkinson's disease) is coadministered with chlorpheniramine, there is a decrease in levodopa absorption. The reduction in GI motility allows greater degradation of levodopa in the GI tract, decreasing the amount available for absorption.

Medications that increase GI motility considerably (such as laxatives) may reduce both extent and rate of absorption of other drugs, resulting in lower blood levels and poor bioavailability. This occurs because the drug spends an insufficient time in the small intestines to be completely absorbed.

Alteration of Intestinal Flora. Some oral antibiotics reduce the bacterial flora in the large intestines. These bacteria are responsible for metabolism of certain drugs (e.g., digoxin) and deconjugation of other drugs (e.g., oral contraceptives) that enter the large intestines during enterohepatic recycling. In the case of digoxin, concomitant administration with antibiotics (such as erythromycin or tetracycline) may result in higher blood levels than expected. When oral contraceptives and antibiotics are given together, a lack of deconjugation decreases reabsorption back into the circulation, lowering blood levels below the therapeutic range.

Saturation of Carrier-Mediated Absorption. A few drugs rely on active transporters in the intestinal wall for their absorption. If another substrate for this transporter is also present in the intestinal contents, competition may arise, reducing absorption of one or both substrates.

Interactions Involving Distribution

The main interaction affecting distribution is displacement of one drug from plasma protein binding by another. Binding of drugs to plasma proteins is the norm rather than an exception. Such interactions are therefore quite common, and occur when drugs compete with each other for the same binding sites on plasma proteins. The result is that the drugs displace one another from the protein, increasing free drug concentrations in plasma.

How much displacement is seen depends on relative affinities of the drugs for the protein. Increase in free drug concentrations in plasma means more drug is available to distribute into tissues, increasing the volume of distribution (V). A higher free drug concentration in plasma also means elimination (metabolism and excretion) rates of the displaced drug will increase, resulting in an increase in renal and hepatic clearances. This will serve to rapidly decrease plasma concentration of free drug, counteracting the increase caused by the displacement of drug from plasma proteins. Therefore, if the patient has normal liver and kidney functions, and if the drugs have wide therapeutic ranges, the transitory increase in plasma concentrations of free drug is not usually clinically important.

The risk of interactions as a result of plasma protein displacement is significant primarily for drugs that are highly protein-bound (>90%) and have a small volume of distribution. Such interactions may also be a problem for patients with impaired liver and kidney functions, or for drugs with narrow therapeutic ranges. For example, valproic acid reportedly displaces phenytoin from plasma proteins, causing increased adverse reactions attributable to phenytoin.

Sometimes, such interactions occur when a metabolite of one drug displaces a second drug from its plasma protein-binding site. Thus, in dealing with drug interactions, one needs to consider all drug-related species in the circulation.

Interactions Involving Excretion

Renal excretion of a drug can be affected by a coadministered drug for many different reasons. The second drug can alter any of the contributing processes of renal clearance, such as reabsorption, tubular secretion, glomerular filtration rate, or renal blood flow.

Modification of Urine pH. The effects of urine pH on tubular reabsorption of weak acids and bases have been discussed in Chapter 12, Drug Excretion. Compounds that lower urinary pH (such as ammonium chloride) can increase excretion rate of basic drugs and decrease excretion rate of acidic drugs. Compounds that elevate urinary pH (such as sodium bicarbonate) have the opposite effect. For example, excretion of antihistamines and amphetamines (weak bases) is decreased by sodium bicarbonate and increased by ammonium chloride. Conversely, excretion of weak acids such as aspirin and phenobarbital is decreased by ammonium chloride and increased by sodium bicarbonate. Such modifications in urinary pH are often intentionally used to increase excretion rates of drugs after an overdose.

Regular administration of antacids has also been shown to increase urine pH and decrease excretion rates of basic drugs, which are less ionized at high pH. The result is higher blood levels of these drugs, with potential toxic effects.

Alteration of Tubular Secretion. Tubular secretion from plasma into urine is an active transport process involving specific transporters for weak acids and weak bases. Thus, one weak acid (or base) can compete with another for these transporters, thereby reducing tubular secretion rate, decreasing renal clearance, and consequently increasing plasma concentrations. For example, weak bases such as acetylcholine, histamine, morphine, and atropine compete with each other for tubular transporters and can reduce each other's excretion.

A classic example for such an interaction is with the drug probenecid, a weak acid that blocks tubular secretion of other weak acids. Therefore, probenecid

can reduce renal clearance of many drugs such as penicillins, cephalosporins, and sulfonamides. In fact, probenecid is administered concurrently with some antibiotics when high antibiotic levels in plasma and tissue are required.

Interactions Involving Biotransformation

The majority of serious drug–drug interactions are caused by interference of metabolism of one drug by another because of inhibition or induction of metabolic enzymes. In general, drugs with a low extraction ratio are more affected by these interactions than drugs with a high extraction ratio. Moreover, interactions involving biotransformation have more serious consequences for drugs with a narrow therapeutic range.

We have learned that oxidation by CYP450 is the most common pathway for phase I metabolism of many drugs. Thus, it is no surprise that most biotransformation interactions involve inhibition or induction of CYP450 isozymes, particularly the six subfamilies responsible for metabolism of a majority of drugs; the CYP3A family is the most important of these.

Enzyme Induction. Most enzyme induction situations arise when a substance increases the cellular biosynthesis of enzymes that metabolize another drug. When the level of metabolic enzymes is increased by induction, possible effects are:

- decreased duration of action of the drug owing to increase in its rate of biotransformation
- loss of therapeutic effect of the drug because plasma concentrations are lower than the minimum effective concentration
- increased concentration of metabolites of the drug, which is important if a metabolite has therapeutic or toxic effects

Barbiturates and other drugs such as carbamazepine, rifampin, and phenytoin are known to induce hepatic enzymes and increase drug biotransformation. For example, phenobarbital increases metabolism of warfarin and decreases its anticoagulant activity. The dose of warfarin is usually increased to compensate for this. However, if phenobarbital is subsequently discontinued, the warfarin dose has to be reduced to avoid toxic effects.

Many drugs induce their own metabolism after repeated administration (*auto-induction* or *self-induction*); this may result in development of tolerance. Some inducing agents can also produce physiological changes that affect drug metabolism. For example, some barbiturates increase hepatic blood flow and bile flow, consequently increasing metabolic rates.

Enzyme Inhibition. Enzyme inhibition is, by far, the mechanism most often responsible for life-threatening drug interactions. If biotransformation of a drug is impeded as a result of inhibition of an enzyme predominantly responsible for its metabolism, possible effects are:

- High plasma levels, resulting in increased pharmacological activity. This may or may not be a problem depending on the therapeutic window for the drug. If plasma levels rise above maximum safe concentration (MSC), increased toxicity may also be seen.
- In cases when biotransformation of a prodrug is impeded, less of the active drug will be formed, presumably resulting in lower therapeutic effectiveness.
- If the major metabolic pathway of a drug is impeded, secondary pathways may become more favorable, resulting in higher concentrations of usually uncommon metabolites. If these metabolites are toxic, a new pattern of side effects may be observed.

For example, cimetidine inhibits oxidative biotransformation reactions, thus elevating blood levels of drugs (such as theophylline, benzodiazepines, phenytoin, and warfarin) metabolized by this pathway.

Consider two drugs metabolized by the same isoform of CYP450. If these two drugs are dosed simultaneously, it is apparent they will competitively inhibit each other's metabolism, and plasma levels of both drugs may be higher than if each drug were dosed alone. Which drug will be affected more will depend on their relative plasma concentrations and enzyme affinities. Many drugs, such as erythromycin, clarithromycin, ketoconazole, and certain antidepressants, inhibit hepatic CYP450 enzyme systems. Table 19.1 shows some important inducers and

TABLE 19.1. Some Important Inhibitors and Inducers of CYP3A	
CYP3A Inhibitors	*CYP3A Inducers*
Ketoconazole	Carbamazepine
Itraconazole	Rifampin
Fluconazole	Rifabutin
Cimetidine	Ritonavir
Clarithromycin	St. John's wort
Erythromycin	
Troleandomycin	
Grapefruit juice	

Terfenadine and Fexofenadine

CYP3A4 has been the basis for most of the fatal drug interactions that have gained so much publicity in recent years. Terfenadine (Seldane), one of the first nonsedating antihistamines marketed, is metabolized by CYP3A4 to its metabolite fexofenadine, which has the same pharmacological activity as terfenadine. Many commonly used drugs such as ketoconazole are also metabolized by CYP3A4 and can inhibit it. When CYP3A-mediated metabolism of terfenadine is inhibited by concurrent administration of ketoconazole, terfenadine accumulates to high levels. At these levels, terfenadine blocks potassium channels in the heart, which play an important role in repolarization of the heart. Once these channels are blocked, the QT interval on the electrocardiogram can be prolonged, and a potentially lethal arrhythmia, called *torsades de pointes*, can develop.

For terfenadine as well as for other drugs such as astemizole and cisapride, recognition of torsades de pointes in association with the drug and its interactions ultimately led to withdrawal of these drugs from the market. Fexofenadine (Allegra), the active metabolite of terfenadine, has equal potency at the histamine receptor but is more than 50 times less active in blocking potassium channels in the heart. Therefore, unlike terfenadine, it does not cause torsades de pointes. Allegra is now on the market and used clinically for allergic rhinitis.

inhibitors of CYP3A4, the enzyme involved in metabolism of most drugs.

Pharmacodynamic Drug Interactions

Pharmacodynamic drug interactions arise when one drug alters tissue sensitivity or responsiveness to another drug, resulting in additive or opposing effects. We have considered the principles behind these types of interactions in Chapter 16, Mechanisms of Drug Action. Pharmacodynamic interactions may result in additivity, potentiation, or antagonism.

Additivity

Additivity, or summation, is the most common type of pharmacodynamic drug interaction and occurs when two drugs acting on the same receptor or effector system show an additive effect. Examples of drug regimens with potential additive interactions are insulin plus a sulfonylurea (both agents lower blood glucose levels), or concurrent use of two central nervous system (CNS) depressants (such as antianxiety drugs, antipsychotics, certain antihistamines, or alcohol), producing excessive sedation.

Potentiation

Potentiation or synergism is seen when the combined effect of two drugs is greater than the sum of their individual effects, and requires that the two drugs act at different receptors or effector systems. True synergism is relatively rare; most of the time, summation is mistaken for synergism.

Antagonism

Antagonism, or inhibition, occurs when one drug (the antagonist or inhibitor) diminishes or prevents the action of another (usually the agonist or substrate).

Antagonism can be further classified as competitive, noncompetitive, functional, or chemical; these were discussed in detail in Chapter 16, Mechanisms of Drug Action. An antagonistic drug interaction may occur, for example, when an antihypertensive agent and fludrocortisone are given (the antihypertensive agent decreases blood pressure, whereas fludrocortisone may elevate it).

Clinically Serious Interactions

Because most drugs use similar ADME pathways and often work at similar receptors, the possibility of two drugs interacting in some way is high. Hundreds of drug interactions have been reported in the pharmaceutical and medical literature. However, the clinical significance of the interaction is not always apparent, and it may be possible to coadminister interacting drugs if the interaction is not clinically relevant.

Clinicians have identified the main drug interactions that are particularly problematic in long-term care settings. Each of these drug interactions involves medications that are commonly used in long-term care in the elderly, and each has the potential to cause significant harm if not managed appropriately. They are listed in Table 19.2. Drugs on the list are those that are used frequently in older adults in the long-term care setting, and have a potential for adverse consequences if used together. Because of individual variability, not every patient who takes these medications together will experience an adverse reaction. However, these combinations have the potential to produce serious side effects.

Food–Drug Interactions

Many foods and beverages contain substances capable of interacting with drugs because they often share the same ADME pathways. The most common of these interactions are summarized here.

Administration with Meals

Dosing drugs during a meal is often recommended to reduce gastric irritation and for convenience of remembering a dosing schedule. However, food may change absorption of many drugs by slowing gastric emptying, binding with drugs, decreasing access to absorptive sites on the intestinal mucosa, altering pH of gastric contents, or changing dissolution rate. Food reduces rate or extent of absorption of many antibiotics and of drugs such as alendronate, astemizole, captopril, and didanosine. These drugs should be taken on an empty stomach. Absorption of some lipophilic drugs (e.g., theophylline) is improved when they are taken with a high-fat meal; the fat presumably accelerates dissolution rate of the drug by providing a lipid medium and increasing GI residence time.

Alcohol

Alcohol has so many pharmacokinetic and pharmacodynamic interactions with drugs that simultaneous intake of alcohol and any drug is strongly discouraged.

Alcohol is a CNS depressant and can have an additive pharmacological interaction when taken with other CNS depressant drugs. Alcohol also causes vasodilation and can result in hypotension when taken with vasodilator drugs.

Alcohol is oxidized by mixed-function oxidase (MFO) enzymes and competes with drugs for metabolism with this enzyme system. Chronic alcohol consumption can also induce certain MFO enzymes, resulting in production of higher concentrations of toxic metabolites of certain drugs. An example is

TABLE 19.2. Most Serious Drug Interactions in the Elderly

Drug 1	Drug 2	Adverse Effect	Mechanism
Warfarin (anticoagulant)	NSAIDs (e.g., naproxen, ibuprofen)	Serious GI bleeding	NSAIDs destroy protective lining of stomach and decrease platelet aggregation
Warfarin (anticoagulant)	Macrolide antibiotics (e.g., erythromycin, azithromycin)	Increased effects of warfarin, with potential for bleeding	Macrolides inhibit the metabolism of warfarin. Warfarin action may also be prolonged owing to reduction in intestinal flora by macrolides, causing a decrease in production of vitamin K for clotting factor production
Warfarin (anticoagulant)	Quinolone antibiotics (e.g., ciprofloxacin, ofloxacin, and norfloxacin)	Increased effects of warfarin, with potential for bleeding	Exact mechanism is unknown. Probable causes are reduction in intestinal flora and decreased warfarin clearance
Warfarin (anticoagulant)	Phenytoin	Increased effects of warfarin and phenytoin	Currently unknown, but probably a genetic basis involving liver metabolism of warfarin and phenytoin
ACE inhibitors (e.g., captopril, enalapril)	Potassium supplements	Elevated serum potassium levels	ACE inhibition results in lower aldosterone production and decreased potassium excretion
ACE inhibitors (e.g., captopril, enalapril)	Spironolactone	Elevated serum potassium levels	Unknown, possibly an additive effect
Digoxin	Amiodarone	Digoxin toxicity	Exact mechanism unknown. Amiodarone may decrease digoxin clearance, resulting in prolonged digoxin activity. May also be an additive effect on sinus node of heart
Digoxin	Verapamil	Digoxin toxicity	Synergistic effect of slowing impulse conduction and muscle contractility, leading to bradycardia and possible heart block
Theophyllines (e.g., theophylline, aminophylline, and oxtriphylline)	Quinolones (e.g., ciprofloxacin, ofloxacin, and norfloxacin)	Theophylline toxicity	Inhibition of hepatic metabolism of theophylline by quinolones

GI, gastrointestinal; NSAIDs, nonsteroidal anti-inflammatory drugs; ACE, angiotensin-converting enzyme.

metabolism of acetaminophen, which produces higher levels of a toxic metabolite when alcohol is consumed by the patient. Alcohol also depletes glutathione supply in the liver, decreasing glutathione conjugation of drugs and their metabolites.

Grapefruit Juice

Drugs that undergo oxidative metabolism by CYP450 enzymes in the intestinal wall or liver (particularly by CYP3A4) have the potential for an interaction with grapefruit juice. Grapefruit juice contains various bioflavonoids and furanocoumarins, which may bind to the CYP3A4, impairing first-pass metabolism either by inactivation or inhibition of the enzyme. The net effect of this inhibition seems to be a selective down-regulation of CYP3A4. Grapefruit juice thus improves oral absorption of several important medications by inhibiting CYP3A4 in the enterocytes of the intestinal wall, which are responsible for presystemic metabolism of many drugs. Extensive consumption of grapefruit juice may inhibit hepatic CYP450 as well, further increasing bioavailability. Drugs affected by this interaction include calcium-channel blockers (i.e., felodipine) and HIV-protease inhibitors (i.e., saquinavir). One glass of grapefruit juice or half a grapefruit can significantly increase blood levels of these drugs, resulting in increased therapeutic effect or increased toxicity.

However, grapefruit juice can also inhibit absorption of other drugs, including vinblastine, cyclosporine, digoxin, and fexofenadine. A study performed in cellular models shows that grapefruit juice activates P-glycoprotein (P-gp) -mediated efflux pumps in intestinal epithelial cells. This effect partially counteracts the CYP3A4 inhibitory effects of grapefruit juice, reducing the absorption and bioavailability of susceptible drugs from the small intestines. The consequences are lower blood levels and reduced therapeutic efficacy. The combination of effects of grapefruit juice on CYP3A4 and P-gp may explain why the effect of grapefruit juice on drug absorption is unpredictable and highly variable.

Other Food Ingredients

Tyramine is a natural component of foods and beverages such as cheese, alcoholic drinks, yeast extracts, and pickled herring. It is normally metabolized by the enzyme monoamine oxidase (MAO) in the liver. Drugs that inhibit MAO (such as the antidepressants phenelzine and tranylcypromine) will reduce metabolism of tyramine, resulting in tyramine accumulation, which causes a subsequent release of norepinephrine from adrenergic neurons. This can cause a hypertensive crisis in patients as a result of a sudden elevation in blood pressure.

Dietary sources of vitamin K, such as spinach or broccoli, may increase the dosage requirement for warfarin by pharmacodynamic antagonism of its effect. Patients should be counseled to maintain a consistent diet during warfarin therapy.

Sometimes, eating certain foods may minimize a drug's side effects. For example, many antibiotics destroy not only infectious organisms, but also the natural intestinal bacteria that maintain critical balances. These imbalances can result in diarrhea and vaginal yeast infections. Research has shown that eating foods that contain active *Lactobacillus acidophilus* bacteria (found in most yogurts) can help eliminate these side effects.

Some other common drug–food interactions are listed in Table 19.3.

Drug–Herbal Interactions

Changes in dietary habits favoring diets rich in fruits and vegetables, and a significant rise in the consumption of dietary supplements and herbal products, have substantially increased human exposure to *phytochemicals,* chemical substances found in plants or plant-derived products. It is, therefore, not surprising that herbal remedies and other nutritional supplements can interact with each other and with prescription drugs. Phytochemicals have the potential to both elevate and suppress CYP450 activity. Such effects are more likely to occur in the intestine, in which high concentrations of phytochemicals are achieved. Alteration in CYP450 activity will influence, in particular, the fate of drugs that are subject to extensive presystemic and first-pass metabolism. Moreover, it is increasingly apparent

TABLE 19.3. Some Common Drug–Food Interactions	
Drugs	*Effect(s) of Food*
Acetaminophen, aspirin, digoxin	Delayed absorption
	Reduced absorption
ACE inhibitors (captopril and moexipril)	Significant decrease in plasma concentration
Fluoroquinolones (ciprofloxacin, levofloxacin, ofloxacin, trovafloxacin), tetracycline	Decreased absorption with antacids (especially magnesium and aluminum) and iron supplements
Didanosine (ddI)	Food, especially acidic foods or juices, significantly decreases absorption
Saquinavir, griseofulvin, itraconazole, lovastatin, spironolactone	Food, especially high-fat meals, improves absorption
Famotidine	Delayed absorption
	Reduced absorption
Ketoconazole	Acidic foods and drinks significantly increase absorption
Iron, levodopa, penicillins (most), tetracycline, erythromycin	High-carbohydrate meals decrease absorption

ACE, angiotensin-converting enzyme.

that phytochemicals can also influence the pharmacological activity of drugs by modifying their cellular uptake through interaction with drug transporters. Thus, phytochemicals have the potential to alter the effectiveness of prescription and nonprescription drugs, either impairing or exaggerating their pharmacological activity.

For example, ingestion of St. John's wort has resulted in several clinically significant interactions with drugs metabolized by CYP1A2 or CYP3A, including indinavir (Crixivan) and cyclosporine (Sandimmune and Neoral). An interaction with digoxin (Lanoxin) has also been reported, which may be mediated by interference with a P-gp efflux pump. These interactions are believed to be related to induction of the CYP isozyme or the drug efflux transporter, and have caused decreased plasma levels of drugs. In the case of cyclosporine, subtherapeutic levels resulted in transplant organ rejection. Warnings about St. John's wort drug interactions have been extended to oral contraceptives, because there is a possibility of breakthrough bleeding and potential for loss of contraceptive effect.

Table 19.4 lists some interactions between drugs and herbal products that have been reported in the literature and that pose a potential risk. Many more drug–herbal interactions probably exist but have not yet been reported.

Drug–Disease Interactions

Certain drugs show altered behavior and properties when administered to patients with specific disease states. The effect of renal disease on elimination of drugs primarily cleared renally (as unchanged drug) is generally predictable, and there are clinical guidelines for dosage adjustment of many drugs in renal disease.

Severe liver disease is associated with reduced hepatic clearance and higher plasma levels of drugs extensively metabolized by the liver. Although a decrease in liver function reduces clearance of most drugs, the change is relatively small and usually not clinically relevant except in patients with near terminal liver disease.

TABLE 19.4. Some Interactions Between Drugs and Herbal Products That Have Been Reported in the Literature and That Pose a Potential Risk

Drug	Herbal Product	Potential Adverse Drug Interactions
Alprazolam	Kava	Synergistic CNS activity of alprazolam
Digoxin	Licorice	Significantly elevated plasma digoxin concentration
	Hawthorn	Increased cardiac toxicity
	Ginseng	Significantly elevated plasma digoxin concentration
	St. John's wort	Reduced plasma digoxin concentration
Lithium	Broom, buchu, dandelion, juniper	Increased plasma concentration of lithium
Estrogen	Herbal tea	Increased estrogen plasma levels
Paroxetine and other SSRIs	St. John's wort	Confusion, nausea, weakness, and fatigue
Phenelzine	Ginseng (Siberian)	Insomnia, headaches, irritability, and visual hallucinations
Spironolactone	Licorice	Hypokalemia and muscle weakness
Theophylline	St. John's wort	Increased plasma theophylline concentration
Warfarin	Ginkgo biloba, garlic, feverfew, and cayenne	Increased risk of bleeding or bruising
	Ginseng (Siberian)	Decreased anticoagulant activity
	Licorice	Increased risk of bleeding
	Alfalfa	Decreased anticoagulant activity
	Vitamin E (doses of 200 IU/day)	Increased anticoagulant activity and increased platelet aggregation inhibition, increased risk of bleeding
	Ginger	Increased anticoagulant activity, prolonged bleeding

CNS, central nervous system; SSRIs, selective serotonin reuptake inhibitors.

Heart failure reduces hepatic blood flow and causes a reduction in clearance for drugs such as lidocaine or propranolol that are usually extensively cleared by the liver. Acute myocardial infarction reduces clearance of some drugs such as lidocaine.

Dealing with Interactions

The first consideration in prescribing a new drug to a patient is to determine what medications (prescription, over-the-counter, and herbal) the patient is already taking. If interaction is a potential problem, a drug that does not interact with currently used therapy can be chosen from several reference guides available to the clinician. If use of an alternative agent is not possible, existing therapy may need to be modified (either with a different drug or different dose) to allow for use of the newly prescribed agent. When these two choices are not possible, the patient should be warned of potential increased or decreased drug response or adverse effects, and monitored as necessary.

KEY CONCEPTS

- Polypharmacy can result in drug interactions that cause serious side effects in patients.

- Coadministered drugs can alter each other's pharmaceutical, pharmacokinetic, or pharmacodynamic properties.

- Common pharmaceutical interactions involve reduction in the amount of drug available for absorption, usually from the GI tract.

- Pharmacokinetic interactions involve one of the ADME processes; alterations of elimination (metabolism or excretion) of one drug by another are the most common interactions.

- Pharmacodynamic interactions are a result of additivity, potentiation, or antagonism of one drug by another.

- Food and nutritional supplements can interact with drugs and either enhance or reduce their effectiveness, or cause adverse reactions.

- Herbal and nonprescription medications can interact with many prescription drugs, and should be considered in evaluation of drug interactions.

ADDITIONAL READING

1. Tatro DS. Drug Interaction Facts 2004. Facts and Comparisons, 2003.
2. McCabe BJ, Wolfe JJ, Frankel EH. Handbook of Food–Drug Interactions. CRC Press, 2003.
3. Levy RH, Thummel KE, Trager WF. Metabolic Drug Interactions, 1st ed. Lippincott Williams & Wilkins, 2000.
4. Rodrigues AD. Drug–Drug Interactions, 1st ed. Marcel Dekker, 2001.

REVIEW QUESTIONS

1. Why are drug interactions most often encountered in the elderly?
2. Explain which pharmaceutical drug interactions can increase, and which can decrease, the absorption rate or bioavailability of drugs.
3. How do interactions involving distribution occur? Why are these clinically significant for only a few types of drugs?
4. What types of drugs modify urine pH, and why can this alter excretion of other drugs?
5. Discuss the consequences of enzyme induction and inhibition on plasma levels of interacting drugs.
6. Explain how administration with meals can increase or decrease the bioavailability of certain drugs.
7. How does coadministration of grapefruit juice alter plasma levels of certain drugs?
8. Which types of drug interactions can be minimized by separating administration of interacting drugs by 1 to 2 hours? What types of interactions will not be avoided by this approach?
9. What are some common clinical approaches to minimizing drug interactions in patients?

Pharmacogenomics

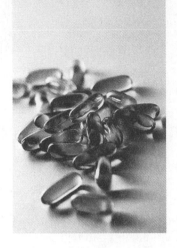

Patients often respond quite differently when given the same dose of a drug; variability in response to drug therapy is the rule, not the exception. Chapter 18, Therapeutic Variability, discussed common physiological and environmental factors that cause differing drug effects among patients. However, even when these factors are taken into account, there remains a large variability in individual drug response.

Interindividual variability in response to drugs complicates new drug discovery and approval. How does one weigh the benefit-to-risk ratio of a drug, taking into account the entire population that might use it? Such questions often result in potentially beneficial drugs never coming to market because of toxicity in a subgroup of subjects, or in the withdrawal of useful drugs from the market when serious adverse events are seen in a small percentage of patients. If the origin of variability in drug response could be identified and compensated for, all drugs could be safe and effective in the correctly chosen patient.

Environment, diet, age, lifestyle, and state of health can influence how an individual reacts to a drug, but the response also has a genetic component that can make a drug therapeutic in one patient, ineffective in a second, and toxic in a third.

Extent of Interindividual Variability

Even the most successful drugs provide optimal benefits to only a fraction of patients; some patients show no benefit, whereas others experience unacceptable toxicity. For example, studies have shown up to 30% of patients do not respond to 3-hydroxy-3-methylglutaryl coenzyme A (HMG-CoA) reductase inhibitors (statins like atorvastatin), up to 35% do not respond to β-blockers (e.g., propranolol), and as many as 50% do not respond to tricyclic antidepressants (e.g., desipramine). Variability is particularly evident in cancer chemotherapy, in which response rates and cure rates are low and serious adverse effects are common. Popular antihypertensive drugs correctly lower the blood pressure in some individuals, have no effect in some, and cause deadly side effects in others.

Even for patients who are helped by a particular drug, optimal doses can vary widely among individuals. For example, the daily therapeutic dose varies 20-fold for warfarin, and 40-fold for propranolol. The variability in dose and response is very apparent for the common cholesterol-lowering drug simvastatin. It lowers LDL (low-density lipoprotein) levels in patients by an average of 41% at the recommended 40-mg dose, 47% at an 80-mg dose, and 53% at a 160-mg dose. However, even at the highest dose of 160 mg, about 5% of patients show only a 10 to 20% reduction and 6% of patients show no LDL lowering at all. Even at the low dose of 40 mg, about 2% of patients have significant side effects. These numbers illustrate the interindividual variability in drug response, even for very successful and relatively safe drugs. As with many drugs, the reasons for such variability are still unknown, making drug dosing a proposition requiring vigilant monitoring and professional judgment. It is hoped that pharmacogenomics will offer answers to clinicians looking for the right drug for the right patient.

The existence of large population differences with smaller intrapatient variability is consistent with inheritance as a determinant of drug response. Understanding an individual's genetic makeup is believed to be the key to designing and using drugs with greater efficacy and safety.

Genetic factors are also very important in determining health and illness. Many diseases, whether infectious diseases, cardiovascular disease, or cancer, have a genetic component. Genetic research will enable us to identify the genes that cause disease and the individuals who are at risk, and will suggest therapeutic approaches. Analyzing genetic variations will also allow selection of patients who might be helped by a treatment, and those who may show resistance or adverse reactions.

To understand the influence of genetic factors on disease and drug therapy, let us first briefly review how genes control the expression of proteins.

Review of Genetics

Chromosomes

Our genetic material is located primarily in structures called chromosomes contained in the nucleus. Humans have 23 pairs of chromosomes for a total of 46. One pair (chromosome pair 23) is made up of the sex chromosomes—females have two X chromosomes whereas males have an X and a Y chromosome. The other 22 pairs of chromosomes (1 through 22) are called *autosomes*.

Each chromosome contains a single DNA molecule, composed of two polynucleotide strands that wind about each other into a double helix, often compared with a spiral ladder. The sides of the ladder are composed of two sugar-phosphate backbones, and each rung of the ladder consists of two paired bases, one from each strand. The helix is stabilized by van der Waals forces, hydrogen bonds between the base pairs, and hydrophobic interactions between the bases and surrounding water. The hydrogen bonding between base pairs is such that the most energetically stable DNA configuration is achieved when adenine (A) pairs with thymine (T) and guanine (G) pairs with cytosine(C); A–T and G–C are called *complementary base pairs*. Each human chromosome can contain as many as 300 million base pairs.

Genes

A gene is a precise sequence of DNA on a chromosome that encodes information for a particular characteristic or function. Different sequences of base pairs contain different coded messages. The coded information is contained in triplets or *codons,* such as ATG. Almost all genes have one primary function: they code for proteins. The process of *transcription* converts DNA to mRNA, and *translation* converts the mRNA to a functional protein. The *genetic code* is the correspondence between the codons in DNA with the amino acids that are ultimately assembled into protein. It is the precise sequence of these codons that results in the synthesis of different proteins.

Less than 10% of human DNA is believed to contain functional genes. Between genes are other DNA sections called *regulatory regions* that control gene activity. There are also long stretches of random DNA, or noncoding DNA, that has no apparent function.

Each gene is found at a specific location or *locus* on a chromosome. A gene can have two alternative forms, or **alleles**, one copy from each parent on each chromosome pair. If both chromosomes have the same allele occupying the same locus on the two chromosomes, the individual or cell is referred to as **homozygous** for this allele; if the alleles at the two loci are different, the condition is referred to as **heterozygous** for both alleles. Alleles are often responsible for alternative traits, and some alleles are dominant over the other in the pair.

The majority of genes are the same for all humans. In fact, even chimpanzees are more than 98% genetically similar to humans. Individual gene sequences in people may differ to the extent of about 1 in 1,000 base pairs, which at first seems to be too small to account for all the differences we see in humans. However, these small differences can result in significant differences in the protein they code for, and an infinite number of DNA sequence variations. In the broadest sense, human genetic variation refers to the differences in DNA sequence among individuals.

The Human Genome

The *genome* is all the genetic information of an organism. The human genome consists of about 30,000 known genes, a small number considering the complexity of humans. This means that other factors such as the environment play an important role in human biology. The *genotype* refers to the genetic makeup or genome of an individual; it can pertain to all genes or to a specific gene. By contrast, the *phenotype* results from interaction between the genotype and the environment. It is a composite of the characteristics shown by a cell, an individual, or an organism under a particular set of environmental conditions.

Gene Expression

The genetic code or genotype does not control all biological functions. Some of the differences among species and among individuals are also a result of differences in *gene expression* rather than dissimilar genes because not all genes are expressed all the time. In its simplest terms, gene expression is the manifestation of the genotype of an organism into the phenotype, involving execution of the instructions held in the genes into a final, functioning protein.

One can think of the genome as a book of recipes and gene expression as the selection of recipes for a meal. Very different meals can result depending on which recipes from the same book are used at a particular time. A small difference in timing and level of gene expression could account for many interindividual differences. Variability in *mRNA* expression patterns rather than in the DNA itself may help find the cause of some diseases and of variable response to drugs. Thus, an understanding of gene expression may be as useful in understanding disease and in approaches to drug therapy as knowledge of DNA sequence.

Changes in protein structure can occur as a result of differences in DNA transcription into mRNA or translation of the mRNA into protein. The gene transcript (mRNA) can be spliced in different ways before translation into protein. After translation, many proteins are chemically changed through posttranslational modification, mainly through the addition of carbohydrate and phosphate groups. Such modification plays a vital role in modulating the function of many proteins but is not directly coded by genes. As a consequence, the information from a single gene can encode as many as 50 different protein species.

Genetic Variation and Disease

Genomic research has provided a vast amount of information linking gene activity with disease.

Types of Genetic Variation

Mutation

One type of genetic variation is a **mutation**, a permanent change or structural alteration in the DNA. Mutations are a result of random chance events or can be caused by external factors, including environmental insults such as radiation and mutagenic chemicals.

Mutation refers to a genome variation that is present in less than 1% of the population and is usually harmful. However, some mutations may have no physiological or biochemical effect if they occur in the noncoding part of DNA. Occasionally, a mutation can be beneficial and improve the organism's chance of survival, contributing to adaptation and evolution of a population over time. Such beneficial mutations usually become polymorphisms if they persist in the gene pool, as discussed a little later.

A *germline mutation* or *hereditary* mutation is an inheritable change in the DNA that occurred in a germ cell (a cell that will become an egg or a sperm) or the zygote at the single-cell stage. Such a mutation is incorporated into every cell of the body of the resulting offspring. Germline mutations play an important role in many genetic diseases. They are also involved in certain types of cancer (e.g., eye tumor retinoblastoma and Wilms tumor, a childhood malignancy of the kidney).

By contrast, an *acquired mutation* is a change in a gene or chromosome that occurs in a single cell after conception. This change is then transmitted to all cells descended from the altered cell, giving rise to a clone of cells marked by the mutation. Acquired mutations occur in general body cells as opposed to germ cells, and are not passed on to descendants. Many diseases arise as a result of acquired mutations; for instance, the great majority of people who get breast cancer or colon cancer have not inherited such altered genes. Inherited forms of cancer represent only perhaps 5 or

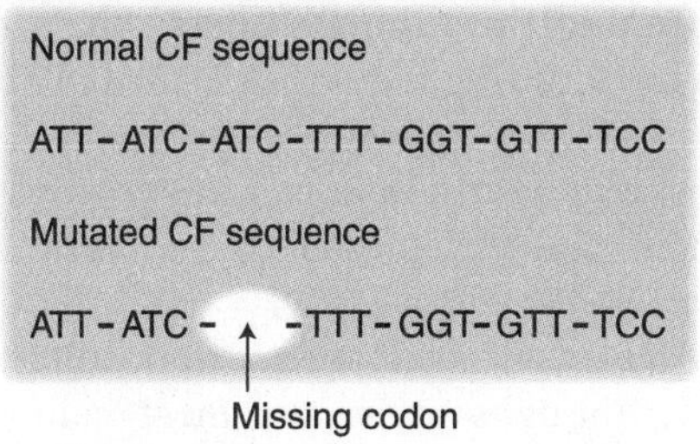

Figure 20.1. Example of a mutation causing cystic fibrosis (CF). A codon (ATC) that codes for the amino acid phenylalanine has been deleted in the mutated CF gene, resulting in an abnormal CF protein that does not have phenylalanine in this position. Individuals with the abnormal protein develop CF.

10% of all cancers. This is true even for families that have several members with cancer; certain cancers are so common that some clusters are bound to happen purely by chance. Cases that are diagnosed at older ages, in particular, are more likely to be caused by acquired mutations.

Many mutated genes make physiologically important proteins that do not function correctly and are, therefore, directly responsible for disease. For example, a change in a single amino acid in the normal hemoglobin protein causes sickle cell anemia. Figure 20.1 illustrates a mutation that causes cystic fibrosis (CF). By searching for mutations, scientists can identify and understand the molecular genetic basis for disease. A flaw in virtually any gene may potentially result in a disease, or in an altered response to a drug.

Genetic Polymorphism

Another kind of genetic variation is a polymorphism, a variation in the DNA that occurs with an appreciable frequency in the population and is too common to be caused merely by a new mutation. In general, polymorphisms have a frequency of at least 1% in the general population. Polymorphisms that occur at a lower frequency are called mutations or genetic variants.

Polymorphisms probably begin as germline mutations but become common in a certain patient population because of inheritance. Polymorphisms are generally more benign than mutations, and many polymorphisms persist in the gene pool because they confer a survival advantage to the individuals in certain environments. However, the same polymorphism may result in another detrimental trait.

An example is the gene for sickle cell disease, in which a mutation occurred thousands of years ago. The altered gene was passed on to offspring and became common in malarious areas because it gave individuals a selective advantage against malaria. However, the altered gene is also responsible for making abnormal hemoglobin, so children who inherit an altered gene from both parents have sickle cell anemia. Children who inherit only one altered gene have no symptoms of the disease, but can pass on the genetic predisposition trait to their offspring.

Polymorphisms are particularly important in certain ethnic groups and races. Glucose-6-phosphate dehydrogenase (G6PD) is an enzyme normally present in red blood cells that protects these cells from oxidative stress. G6PD deficiency is a sex-linked polymorphism that affects 400 million people worldwide; about 10% of black men and fewer black women have G6PD deficiency. Inheriting the G6PD deficiency gene is believed to also protect against malaria. However, the polymorphism causes life-threatening hemolytic anemia, in which red blood cells burst. This anemia develops only under specific conditions—eating fava beans, inhaling certain types of pollen, contracting certain infections, or taking certain drugs. Some drugs that potentiate hemolytic anemia in people with G6PD deficiency are chloroquine, pamaquine and primaquine, aspirin, probenecid, and vitamin K.

Single-Nucleotide Polymorphism. The most common form of genetic polymorphism is a single-nucleotide polymorphism

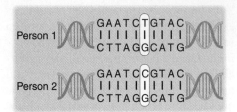

Figure 20.2. Illustration of a single-nucleotide polymorphism in a DNA sequence. In this case, a T in the general population (person 1) has been replaced with a C in a small subgroup of the population (person 2).

(*SNP*), a change of one base pair at a specific point in the DNA molecule. This occurs when a single nucleotide, such as an A, replaces one of the other three nucleotides—C, G, or T. An example of an SNP is the alteration of the DNA segment AAGGTTA to ATGGTTA, where the second "A" in the first segment is replaced with a "T." Figure 20.2 illustrates the concept of an SNP. Other less common sources of genetic variation are duplications or deletions in a single base pair or in multiple base pairs in the DNA.

SNPs account for the vast majority of genetic differences among individuals, and there are large databases that have collected such SNP information. Although SNPs can occur anywhere in the genome, their locus is important in determining the ultimate effect. SNPs can occur in coding regions of DNA (cSNPs), in regulatory regions of DNA (rSNPs), or most commonly, in noncoding regions, in which case they are referred to as *anonymous* SNPs.

SNPs that occur in the noncoding region, thought to be the most common type of SNPs, have no known effect on gene function. Even among cSNPs, *synonymous* SNPs do not change the amino acid sequence of the encoded protein and are not expected to have any functional consequences. Only *nonsynonymous* SNPs, those that result in a code for a different amino acid, have the potential of influencing propensity to disease or drug response. The magnitude of their effect will depend on how much the two amino acids differ and how this difference changes protein structure, folding, and active site configuration. There are an estimated 200,000 cSNPs present in the human genome.

Figure 20.3 shows one approach for locating disease-susceptibility genes in individuals using SNP association studies.

Monogenic Diseases

Human genetics first focused on the identification of genes that cause monogenic diseases or *single-gene disorders*,

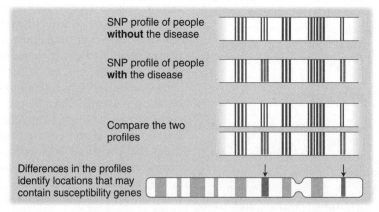

Figure 20.3. Association studies for locating disease susceptibility genes in individuals using single-nucleotide polymorphisms (SNPs). The process involves looking at particular genes or variations in two groups (e.g., affected patients and control subjects) to establish an association with a phenotype by finding significant genetic variations in the two groups.

Linkage

Scientists have found that long blocks of DNA have traveled from one generation to the next with little genetic shuffling. Along any given stretch of chromosome, the genetic variation within these blocks comes in only four or five patterns in different people. These DNA segments often contain one or more genes that make important proteins, many gene regulatory segments, and many fragments with no known function.

Linkage refers to the tendency for DNA segments that are located close to each other on the same chromosome to be inherited together. One of the segments may be the gene of interest whereas the other is a *marker*—a segment of DNA with an identifiable physical location on a chromosome whose inheritance can be followed. A marker can be a gene or a section of DNA with no known function. The closer together two segments are on a chromosome, the lower the probability that they will be separated during DNA repair or replication processes, and hence the greater the probability that they will be inherited together.

Thus, the marker is typically unrelated to the phenotype of interest, but is nonetheless useful for predicting the phenotype owing to the marker's proximity to the gene that is functionally producing the phenotype. Markers are often used as indirect ways of tracking the inheritance patterns of genes that have not yet been identified, but whose approximate locations are known. Because SNPs occur frequently throughout the genome and tend to be relatively stable genetically, they serve as excellent biological markers to track disease-linked genes.

those caused by a defect in just one gene. Scientists currently believe single-gene mutations cause approximately 6,000 inherited diseases. These conditions include a number of lung and blood disorders, such as cystic fibrosis, Huntington's disease, sickle cell anemia, and hemophilia. Although rare, as a group these monogenic disorders still affect millions of people worldwide. The precise molecular defects that result in more than 100 of these disorders have now been characterized. The study of monogenic disorders has led to important advances in early diagnosis, understanding the disease process, and finding potential cures.

Most monogenic diseases, with very few exceptions, occur regardless of the environment; if an individual inherits a mutation that causes the disease, it will manifest itself regardless of the person's lifestyle and living conditions.

Monogenic diseases can be classified as X-linked, autosomal recessive, or autosomal dominant. The defective version of the gene responsible for the disease is known as a mutant allele or a disease allele. X-linked diseases are monogenic disorders that are linked to defective genes on the X chromosome (the sex chromosome). X-linked alleles can be dominant or recessive. Only a few disorders (e.g., X-linked hypophosphatemia) have a dominant inheritance pattern. Examples of X-linked recessive disorders are hemophilia A and Duchenne muscular dystrophy. Autosomal disorders are those caused by defects in chromosomes 1 through 22. Autosomal recessive diseases (e.g., cystic fibrosis and sickle cell

TABLE 20.1. Some Common Monogenic Disorders, the Chromosome Where the Mutation is Located, and the Type of Mutation

Disorder	Mutation	Chromosome
Color blindness	P	X
Cystic fibrosis	P	7
Down syndrome	C	21 (extra chromosome)
Hemophilia	P	X
Klinefelter syndrome	C	X (extra chromosome)
Spina bifida	P	1

P, point mutation, or any insertion or deletion entirely inside one gene; C, whole chromosome extra, missing, or both.

anemia) require an individual to have two disease alleles. Autosomal dominant diseases (e.g., Huntington's disease) can be manifest when there is only one disease allele.

Table 20.1 lists some common monogenic disorders.

Polygenic Diseases

Attention is now turning to more common **polygenic diseases** or complex diseases, those that arise as a result of defects in several genes. Such diseases or disorders are often a result of a combination of genetic flaws in alleles of multiple genes. Polygenic disorders include common conditions that affect many millions of people, such as asthma, heart disease, adult-onset diabetes, migraine, and Alzheimer's disease. Depression and other mental illnesses are also believed to be the result of alterations in several genes at once. These diseases do not show the clear patterns of inheritance seen in monogenic diseases because genotype does not necessarily translate into phenotype. However, complex diseases still tend to cluster in families, but not in the predictable manner shown by monogenic diseases.

Many common polygenic diseases are a result of a complex interaction between a combination of flawed **susceptibility genes** and external environmental factors (such as a person's diet, air pollutants, tobacco smoke, and exposure to allergens). Susceptibility genes contribute to an individual's risk of developing a specific disease, but usually are not enough to cause the disease. Different alleles of a gene may be associated with different degrees of susceptibility or risk. The *APOE* gene on chromosome 19 is one example of a disease susceptibility gene. An individual who has two copies of one variant allele of *APOE* is more likely to develop Alzheimer's disease at an earlier age than an individual with a different *APOE* genotype. Infectious diseases reveal even more complexity, because manifestation of the disease involves the genome of the individual, the genome of the infectious invader, and environmental influences on both.

The relative importance of genetics versus environment as determinants of disease varies across a broad spectrum. In some diseases, external factors appear to be more important, whereas in others intrinsic predispositions prevail. Susceptibility genes may influence the age of onset of a disease, contribute to its rate of progression, or help to protect against it. Understanding the rules of their inheritance and their roles in disease is a complicated challenge. Researchers believe genetic factors account for much of the susceptibility of an individual to a disease; environmental factors may determine whether the disease actually manifests itself. For example, if two individuals with the same genetic susceptibility to a

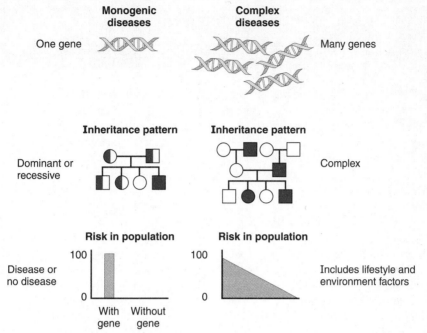

Figure 20.4. Difference between simple monogenic diseases and complex polygenic diseases. Monogenic diseases arise owing to a defect in one gene and have a fairly predictable inheritance pattern. Polygenic diseases develop as a result of defects in several genes, any combination of which can be inherited, giving rise to a complex inheritance pattern. Monogenic diseases show a clear relationship between genotype and phenotype; a person either has the disease or does not. The correlation between genotype and phenotype is complex in polygenic diseases, and is further complicated by the influence of one or more lifestyle and environmental factors. Persons may have different degrees of susceptibility or risk for the disease, and the exact degree of risk cannot be determined with any certainty.

particular disease grow up in two entirely different environments, one that contributes to disease and one that does not, only the individual in the disease-contributing environment will manifest the disease. Thus, early knowledge about disease susceptibility may make it possible to control environmental and lifestyle factors to prevent disease, or to initiate prophylactic or early treatment.

Figure 20.4 illustrates the difference between monogenic and polygenic diseases.

Genetic Variation and Response to Drugs

Some genetic variations are responsible for the disease itself, as we have just dis-

cussed. Other types of genetic variations, although not involved in the disease process, can influence the pharmacokinetic behavior or pharmacodynamic response to a drug in an individual. Genetic variation refers not only to gene alterations leading to protein structure modifications but also to gene regulation that results in the synthesis of different amounts of protein. A drug's behavior in the body is a result of complex interactions with a variety of endogenous cellular proteins such as receptors, metabolizing enzymes, transporters, and binding and carrier proteins. Small but important genetic polymorphisms among individuals can result in differences in structure or amount of these proteins among individuals, leading to dramatic differences in the way each person responds to a drug.

Genetic Testing

Genetic tests can be performed to confirm a suspected diagnosis, to predict the possibility of future disease, to detect the presence of a carrier state in unaffected individuals (whose children may be at risk), and to predict response to drug therapy. Many different types of body fluids and tissues can be used in genetic testing. For DNA screening, only a very small sample of cellular material such as blood, skin, bone, or other tissue is needed. Even the small amount of tissue at the bottom end of a human hair is usually enough. Most tests look for DNA variants; other types of genetic tests look for the actual protein encoded by the gene. Such functional gene tests, which detect protein rather than DNA, show not only that a mutated gene is present but also that it is actively making an abnormal protein or no protein at all.

The most widespread type of genetic testing is prenatal and newborn screening. Biochemical, chromosomal, and DNA-based genetic tests are widely used for the prenatal diagnosis of conditions such as Down syndrome. Newborns are tested for phenylketonuria (PKU), an inherited autosomal recessive metabolic disorder caused by a genetic variation of the enzyme that metabolizes phenylalanine. High levels of phenylalanine in blood can lead to mental retardation if not treated early in life with a special, restricted diet. The test uses a blood sample from the baby to look for the presence of excessive phenylalanine, rather than looking for the mutated gene itself.

Most of the currently available gene-specific tests for disease are for identifying monogenic disorders; the test for cystic fibrosis, for instance, looks for 32 different mutations in the *CFTR* gene.

There are fewer tests available for polygenic disorders, but the number is growing. Most of these disease susceptibility tests are currently recommended only in families in which there is a strong history of the disorder. For instance, *BRCA1* and *BRCA2* testing is only offered to individuals with a strong family history of breast and ovarian cancer. Women with the *BRCA1* breast cancer susceptibility gene have an 80% chance of developing breast cancer by the age of 65. The risk is high but not certain. Moreover, family members who test negative for the *BRCA1* susceptibility gene are not exempt from breast cancer risk; over time, they can acquire breast cancer-associated genetic changes at the same rate as the general population.

A few genetic tests to predict drug response are available, such as the test for estrogen receptors in breast tumors to determine whether the drug Herceptin will be effective. Tests to predict drug responsiveness for cancer, heart disease, asthma, and other disorders are under development.

Pharmacogenetics and Pharmacogenomics

The field of pharmacogenetics, which is about 40 years old, is the study of genetically determined variability in the response of individuals to drugs. Much of the research in this area has focused on genetic variations affecting hepatic metabolizing enzymes, particularly the CYP450 family. Pharmacogenetics attempts to identify those individuals within the population who are susceptible to possible alterations in drug metabolism so that this may be taken into account during development of a therapeutic regimen. The ability to identify hereditary differences in metabolism allows drugs to be prescribed in a more efficacious and safe manner to begin with, without having to adjust dosage after observing an undesired patient response. Many pharmacogenetic studies have explained drug idiosyncrasy, which is the abnormal response to a drug in a few patients, resulting in serious toxicity. Most idiosyncratic reactions are now known to arise because of genetic variation in metabolizing enzymes.

Although the field of pharmacogenetics began with a focus on drug metabolism, it now encompasses the entire spectrum of drug disposition, including a growing list of transporters that influence drug absorption, distribution, and excretion.

Pharmacogenomics is the study of the effect of an individual's genetic inheritance on the body's response to drugs. It is a broader study of multiple genes and their alleles, of the entirety of expressed and nonexpressed genes in any given physiological state and how they affect all aspects of pharmacokinetics and pharmacodynamics. Although the terms pharmacogenetics and pharmacogenomics are often used interchangeably and are synonymous for all practical purposes, pharmacogenomics uses a genome-wide approach while pharmacogenetics generally focuses on specific interindividual differences.

Consequences of Genetic Variation

The pharmacokinetic behavior of a drug and the pharmacodynamic response of an individual are directly related to drug–protein interactions and, to a lesser extent, to interactions of the drug with other biomolecules. Thus, a more complete understanding of genetic variability in drug therapy may be gained by looking directly at polymorphisms in cellular proteins. Interindividual differences in

drug response may be caused by sequence variants in genes encoding drug-metabolizing enzymes, drug transporters, or drug targets.

Drug-Metabolizing Enzymes

Genetic polymorphisms in drug-metabolizing enzymes give rise to distinct population subgroups that differ in their ability to carry out certain biotransformation reactions. These differences can lead to changes in enzyme levels or enzyme activity in particular groups of people. Structurally altered enzymes can exhibit either an increased or decreased Michaelis constant K_m or maximum velocity V_{max}, or both. There are more than 30 families of drug-metabolizing enzymes in humans, almost all with polymorphic variants. Many of these polymorphisms translate into functional changes in the enzymes encoded, although all variations in enzyme structure may not lead to clinically significant differences in metabolizing ability.

Gene amplification gives rise to "super-enzymes" that are extremely efficient in metabolizing a drug; this can result in a patient population resistant to the drug because it is eliminated very rapidly. *Gene deletion* leads to a deficiency in the enzyme, giving rise to a patient population that is a *slow metabolizer* of a particular drug. Figure 20.5 shows a typical frequency distribution of normal metabolizers and slow metabolizers of a drug. Genetic alteration can also cause absence of a metabolizing enzyme or a complete lack of activity of the encoded enzyme. In this situation, plasma drug concentrations can quickly reach toxic levels even at standard therapeutic doses.

CYP Enzymes. Much work has been done with the CYP450 family of enzymes, which is responsible for the biotransformation of most drugs. There appears to be a relatively high incidence of polymorphism in the six most common CYP drug-metabolizing enzymes

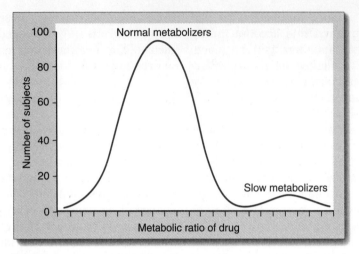

Figure 20.5. A typical bimodal graph showing the frequency distribution of normal metabolizers and slow metabolizers of a drug. The *x* axis is the metabolic ratio, defined as the ratio between parent drug concentration and metabolite concentration in plasma. The higher the ratio (slow metabolizers) the greater the probability of adverse drug reactions. A small percentage of the population are slow metabolizers of the drug in this example. Trimodal graphs, showing three different metabolic subgroups, are also seen for some drugs.

(CYP1A2, CYP3A4, CYP2A6, CYP2C9, CYP2C19, and CYP2D6). For example, almost 20 SNP variants of CYP2D6 have been found; this enzyme is responsible for biotransformation of more than 50 different drugs, from cough medications to antihypertensives, including amitriptyline, fluoxetine, haloperidol, and propafenone. The CYP2D6 metabolism of the antihypertensive drug debrisoquine is used as an index of CYP2D6 activity. This drug has been used in population studies to classify individuals as "poor metabolizers," "intermediate metabolizers," "extensive metabolizers," or "ultrarapid metabolizers" of CYP2D6 substrates. Approximately 1 to 10% of people in various ethnic groups are poor metabolizers of drugs that are substrates for CYP2D6.

Other Enzymes. Other enzyme systems are affected by SNPs as well. For example, SNPs are responsible for a number of variants of the enzyme *N*-acetyl-transferase-2, which plays a role in the phase II acetylation of several drugs, including isoniazid. In particular, a rapid-metabo-

lizing and a slow-metabolizing variant can be distinguished, the corresponding individuals being known as "rapid acetylators" and "slow acetylators," respectively. Rapid acetylators require high doses of the drugs concerned whereas slow acetylators need smaller doses. This is because the drug persists longer and in higher concentrations in the cells of patients with the slow-metabolizing variant of the enzyme. It was observed that therapeutic failure rates for pulmonary tuberculosis treated with isoniazid were higher in rapid acetylators than in slow acetylators, presumably because the duration of action of isoniazid was shorter.

Clinical Implications. One way to identify slow metabolizers of a particular drug is to monitor blood levels after dosing. Unusually high drug levels may be a sign of slow metabolism as a result of an enzyme defect. However, drug level monitoring is expensive and inconvenient, and high drug levels may be caused by other physiological problems as well.

Genotyping of individuals to identify genetic polymorphisms of drug-metabolizing enzymes is a more direct approach and may be widely available some day. Using such genotype information may not be self-evident, however. Many drugs are metabolized by more than one type of reaction, and more than one enzyme is involved. Additionally, each enzyme may have several possible polymorphisms, not all of which may be clinically important. Thus, identification of an individual with a polymorphism in a particular enzyme may shed little light on how to plan drug therapy.

In general, clinically significant genetic polymorphisms of drug metabolism occur when the metabolic pathway subject to polymorphism is a major route of elimination for the drug, if the drug has a narrow therapeutic range, or if the drug is a prodrug that must be activated to produce pharmacologically active metabolites.

Many pharmaceutical companies are trying to get around the issue of slow metabolizers in a different way. For example, because of the high incidence of CYP2D6 polymorphism, pharmaceutical companies are designing drugs with structures that do not involve CYP2D6 for biotransformation.

Drug Targets

Pharmacodynamic effects can lead to interindividual differences in drug effect despite the presence of appropriate concentrations of drug at the intended site of action. Here, effects of the drug are modulated by variations in how the target molecule, or another downstream member of the target molecule's signal transduction pathway, responds to the drug. In contrast to the wealth of information available on the genetic polymorphism of metabolizing enzymes, the importance of polymorphism in influencing receptor structure and the pharmacodynamics of a drug is yet to be well understood.

Mutations in receptor genes can make receptors *hyporesponsive* or *hyperresponsive*. A hyporesponsive receptor is one

less susceptible than normal to up- or down-regulation, whereas the opposite is true for a hyperresponsive receptor. However, not all mutations in receptor genes are problematic in drug therapy. In fact, some mutations can be beneficial by making the receptor more responsive to the drug, whereas others may not significantly influence drug–receptor interactions at all.

For example, asthmatic patients with a certain genotype of the β_2-adrenergic receptor do not respond to the most commonly prescribed inhaled drug, albuterol. The gene in this case carries the information for the β_2-adrenergic receptor at which the drug acts. If the base present at position 16 of this gene is adenine, albuterol is able to exert its effect. If, on the other hand, guanine is present at this position, the receptor fails to perform its function and the drug is inactive.

Tumors often express unusual combinations of genes compared with normal cells. For example, individuals with breast cancer exhibit *BRCA1* or *BRCA2* mutations. The classification of cancer tumors on the basis of their mRNA expression profiles may be very valuable as a diagnostic tool and may help to select the best therapy.

Genotyping of infectious agents such as bacteria and viruses is also expected to be useful in selecting the best therapy. Many infectious agents mutate and become resistant to certain antimicrobial or antiviral drugs. For example, the HIV-AIDS virus in a patient can be genotyped to determine whether it is resistant to certain drugs. Selection of the appropriate drugs for the patient can make therapy more successful and less expensive.

There are also several cases of genetic variability in signal transduction or other downstream proteins influencing drug response. An example is angiotensin-converting enzyme (ACE) inhibitors, which block conversion of angiotensin I to angiotensin II and prevent breakdown of bradykinin. Polymorphism in the G protein–coupled receptor of bradykinin results in cough, one of the side effects of ACE inhibitors. Thus, although the polymorphism is not directly in the protein that is the target of ACE inhibitors, it influences the overall response of these drugs.

Transporters

Many transport proteins are involved in the absorption, distribution, and excretion of drugs so that their genetic variation will contribute to variability in drug disposition among individuals. Transport proteins may also be implicated in pharmacodynamics if they are themselves drug targets. Because many drug transporters are still unknown and the functions of many transporters have not been fully defined, much work needs to be done before we can understand the impact of transporter polymorphisms on drug disposition and response.

Among the most extensively studied transporters involved in drug disposition is P-glycoprotein encoded by the human *ABCB1* gene (also called *MDR1*) on chromosome 7. It is believed a polymorphism of the multidrug-resistant efflux protein MDR1 can explain the differences in oral absorption and target organ accumulation of several drugs. For example, a variation in the *MDR1* gene results in low expression of the transporter and, consequently, high plasma levels of digoxin after oral dosing.

The serotonin transporter, which is the target of serotonin reuptake inhibitor drugs, is another transporter known to show genetic variation that is related to drug response. Studies have documented an association between genotype and antidepressant response.

Clinical Applications of Pharmacogenomics

Many aspects of interindividual variability in drug efficacy and toxicity can be traced back to genetic variability. One of the goals of pharmacogenomics is to identify the precise subgroup of patients that will benefit from a particular drug. The reverse situation—trying to identify those at risk for toxicity from a certain drug—is also important. Screening tests to identify the presence or absence of critical genes are being developed, and will help to identify the optimal drug for a given patient. Figure 20.6 shows one way that pharmacogenomics will influence future drug therapy.

For example, it is estimated in various studies that only 20 to 40% of Alzheimer's patients benefit from the drug tacrine. Researchers have discovered that patients with the gene subtype *ApoE4* are less likely to benefit from the drug. Such knowledge helps to target the use of tacrine, facilitates valid data analysis of clinical trials of Alzheimer's therapies, and will promote investigation of new therapies specifically for *ApoE4* carriers.

The anticipated benefits of pharmacogenomics on future drug therapy are numerous:

- *Advanced screening for disease:* Knowing one's disease susceptibility will allow a person to make lifestyle and environmental changes at an early age to avoid or lessen the severity of a genetic disease. Prior knowledge of a patient's disease susceptibility will allow physicians to monitor and initiate therapy at the appropriate stage of the disease.
- *Targeted drugs:* Pharmaceutical companies will be able to design drugs based on the proteins, enzymes, and RNA associated with diseases, facilitating therapies better targeted to specific diseases with maximum therapeutic effects and minimal damage to healthy cells.
- *Choice of drug:* Instead of the standard trial-and-error method of matching patients with the right drugs, physicians will be able to analyze a patient's genetic profile and prescribe the best available drug therapy from the beginning. This will speed recovery time, decrease likelihood of adverse effects, and increase safety.

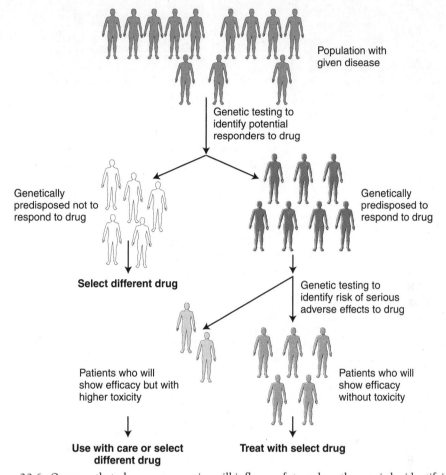

Figure 20.6. One way that pharmacogenomics will influence future drug therapy is by identifying the right drug therapy for the right patient.

- *Choice of dose:* The current practice of basing doses on patient weight and age will be replaced with doses based on a person's genetics—how an individual's pharmacokinetics handles a drug. This will maximize efficacy and safety.
- *Designing "universal" drugs:* Some scientists believe that pharmacogenomics could be used to design drugs that are intentionally not affected by, or bypass, common polymorphisms among individuals. Such drugs could be given safely to all patients and ensure both efficacy and safety.

Figure 20.7 illustrates the approach to discovering targeted drugs using pharmacogenomic and genetic information.

Proteomics

The elucidation of the human genome and numerous pathogen genomes will have a profound impact on our understanding of human disease and its treatment. The Human Genome Project has given scientists the structure and sequences of thousands of genes that encode for hitherto unknown proteins. About 30,000 genes could well translate into one million proteins. In most cases, gene sequence reveals little about the protein structure or its role in disease. Although many of these proteins will belong to well-characterized families with predictable biological functions, many others will be entirely novel with unknown structure and function.

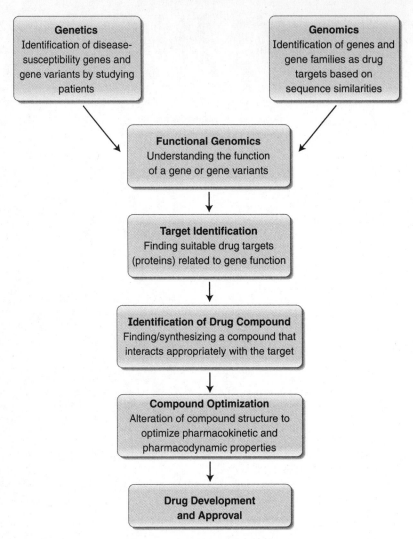

Figure 20.7. Use of genetic and genomic strategies in new drug discovery. It will be useful to combine genetic and genomic strategies and to focus on identification of targets that will lead to new and effective drugs. Genomics and genetics complement each other by providing focus and speed to target identification.

The term proteome refers to all the proteins expressed by a genome, and proteomics is the systematic identification of proteins in the body and the determination of their role in biological functions. Although an individual's genome remains unchanged to a large extent, the proteins in any particular cell change dramatically as genes are turned on and off in response to the environment. The dynamic nature of the proteome has led to the term *functional proteome* to describe all the proteins produced by a specific cell at a particular time. Although there may be more than 100,000 proteins in humans, only a fraction of these are expressed in any given cell type. Only certain genes in a cell are active at any given moment, and as cells mature, many of their genes become permanently inactive. It is the pattern of active and inactive genes in a cell and its resulting protein composition that determines what kind of cell it is and what it can and cannot do.

To discover the relevance of a protein to a disease process, scientists must catalog where, when, and to what extent a protein is expressed, and how these parameters are altered in the disease state. If all the proteins present in a cell at any one time were known, it would indicate which genes were currently expressed and producing these proteins. If this cataloging process were repeated at various stages in a cell's life cycle, it would yield a biochemical time line of the particular physiological process of interest.

Many human diseases occur because of irregularities in protein interactions that can be related directly to alterations in protein structure. However, not all proteins are going to be involved in producing disease. The true value of genome sequence information will only be realized after a function has been assigned for each of the encoded proteins; this is the task of proteomics.

Ultimately, it is believed proteomics will help to identify new disease markers and drug targets, which will then help to design compounds that prevent, diagnose, and treat disease. The future of biotechnology and medicine will be impacted greatly by proteomics, but there is still much to do before patients can realize the potential benefits. Genome sequencing was a large but finite problem; there are a fixed number of genes in the human genome. But the human proteome involves or impacts hundreds of tissues, thousands of diseases, hundreds of cell types all in combination, and it all changes by the second. This makes sequencing the proteome a problem of much greater complexity.

Most drugs work by interacting with proteins in some way, but all the known drugs affect only about 300 to 500 human proteins. That leaves more than 100,000 human proteins with unknown functions, waiting for drugs that might interact with them. These novel proteins offer a tremendous opportunity to investigate new pathways for disease and to identify new molecular targets to address unmet therapeutic needs. If one could make chemical compounds that interfere with the synthesis of the protein, the resulting changes in the organism would help to understand the protein's role. The chemical compound structure could then be appropriately fine-tuned to yield a drug.

Promise of Pharmacogenomics

The statement "no single drug fits all patients" is the new maxim in drug therapy. The emerging challenge for the pharmaceutical sciences is to understand why individuals respond differently to drug therapy, and then to design drugs taking this variability into account. Many pharmaceutical companies have begun to direct their research activities toward achieving individualized medicine; the approach is now toward finding the "right" patient population for a given drug.

In the near future, genetic analysis may help us to get to individualized medicine: the right drug for the right patient at the right time. By understanding the molecular basis of individual variation in drug response, we will be able to focus on the patient as an individual and identify the drug and dose most suited for the patient at that time. We also know environmental factors will play an important role in the success of the therapy. The complete understanding of the environmental and molecular basis of drug response will be a long, complicated but exciting process.

KEY CONCEPTS

- Genetic variation arises as a result of mutations or polymorphisms. Mutations are relatively rare, whereas a polymorphism is a genetic variation present in at least 1% of the population.
- Single-nucleotide polymorphisms (SNPs) are the most common type of polymorphism and arise from an alteration of one base pair in a gene.
- Monogenic disorders occur because of a genetic defect in one gene. Most monogenic diseases manifest themselves regardless of the individual's lifestyle or environment.
- Polygenic or complex disorders are the most prevalent illnesses and arise because of a complex interaction of defects in several susceptibility genes and the individual's environment and lifestyle.
- Genetic variation can influence an individual's response to drugs by affecting drug pharmacokinetics or pharmacodynamics.

- Polymorphisms of drug-metabolizing enzymes can give rise to distinct subgroups (slow, intermediate, and fast metabolizers) in the population.
- Variations in drug targets (receptors, enzymes) or their signal-transduction pathways can affect drug pharmacodynamics.
- Genetic variability of transporters can influence absorption, distribution, metabolism, or elimination, or pharmacodynamics, of a drug.
- Pharmacogenomics will have a large impact in improving drug therapy outcomes for patients, and in developing new drugs with better safety and efficacy profiles.
- Proteomics, the characterization of the structure and function of all the proteins in the body, promises to be the next major advance in this area.

ADDITIONAL READING

1. Licinio J, Wong M-L (eds). Pharmacogenomics: The Search for Individualized Therapies. Wiley-VCH, 2002.

2. Pharmacogenomics: Applications to Patient Care: Modules 1–3. American College of Clinical Pharmacy, 2004.

3. Weber W. Pharmacogenetics, 1st ed. Oxford University Press, 1997.

REVIEW QUESTIONS

1. Describe three causes of mutations in DNA. How is a germline mutation different from a somatic mutation?

2. Describe the major types of genetic variation, including mutations and single-nucleotide polymorphisms.

3. How are mutations different from genetic polymorphisms? What is meant by a single-nucleotide polymorphism (SNP)?

4. Do all mutations and genetic polymorphisms lead to disease? Why not?

5. Elaborate on the effect of genetic variability on drug-metabolizing enzymes, drug transporters, and drug targets.

6. Why are polygenic disorders more complex than monogenic disorders?

7. How does the environment influence the probability of getting a disease? What is meant by susceptibility genes?
8. How can SNPs influence the metabolism, transport, and action of a drug?
9. Why are SNPs in *CYP* genes particularly relevant in variability of drug response among individuals?
10. What are the benefits of a pharmacogenomic approach to drug research and therapy?
11. Why is the proteome as important as or more important than the genome for understanding disease and for the discovery and development of new drugs?

Section VII • **Special Topics**

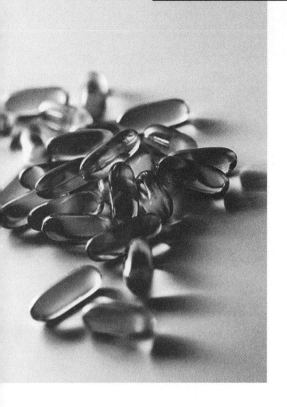

Biopharmaceuticals

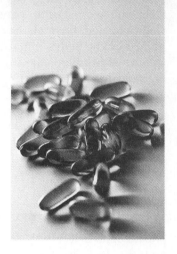

Most drugs on the market are small molecules with molecular weights less than 1,000. However, an increasing number of new drugs are macromolecules such as polypeptides and proteins and the trend is expected to continue. Most of these macromolecular agents cannot be manufactured by conventional chemical methods and have to be made using biological procedures. A **biopharmaceutical** is defined as a therapeutic agent manufactured by a biological process rather than by chemical synthesis.

Currently marketed biopharmaceuticals include proteins that occur naturally in our bodies (therapeutic proteins) as well as nonnatural proteins (therapeutic antibodies). **Therapeutic proteins** are naturally occurring or slightly modified natural proteins that are administered to patients as drugs. Some therapeutic protein drugs, such as insulin for the treatment of diabetes, are quite old. Newer therapeutic proteins include tissue plasminogen activator (TPA) to break down blood clots and interferon-β for relapsing multiple sclerosis.

A variation on the theme of protein drugs is the class of therapeutic antibodies. An **antibody** is a protein produced by the body's immune system in response to foreign invaders such as bacteria and viruses. In contrast to most cellular proteins whose characteristics are predetermined by the genes that encode them, the body generates antibodies dynamically, and their characteristics are refined by the body's immune system to match the profile of the invader with a high degree of specificity. Antibodies made by biotechnology are often used as drugs or as drug-targeting systems.

In its broadest definition, the term biopharmaceutical also includes vaccines and gene therapy.

Biotechnology

Most biopharmaceuticals are made using biotechnology, any process that uses living organisms or parts of living organisms to make or modify useful products. *Pharmaceutical biotechnology* is the integration of natural sciences and engineering sciences to use organisms, cells, or their parts to make therapeutic products. Therapeutic agents made by biotechnology fall into several broad areas depending on the type of technology used. The major biotechnology techniques and the resulting therapeutic agents are:

* Recombinant DNA techniques to make therapeutic proteins in cell tissue culture
* Transgenic animals to make therapeutic proteins
* Hybridoma techniques to make monoclonal antibodies

Genetic Engineering

Genetic engineering is the process of moving genetic information from one chromosome to another or from one organism to another. It includes a group of techniques for locating the desired gene, isolating it, and then moving it into the genome of another cell or organism to produce a desired protein. Genetic engineering is an umbrella term that covers a wide range of methods to change genetic material in a living organism.

Before the advent of genetic engineering, biopharmaceutical drug supplies were extremely limited because the proteins had to be obtained from natural sources. For instance, insulin was collected from slaughtered pigs and human growth hormone was obtained from human cadavers. A number of therapeutic proteins and protein-based drugs are now readily available commercially as a result of progress in biotechnology and genetic engineering.

There are several reasons for manipulating the DNA of a cell or organism, such as:

* repairing a genetic defect, as with gene therapy
* enhancing an effect already natural to that organism (e.g., increasing growth rate)
* increasing resistance to disease or external damage (e.g., in food crops)
* causing an organism to perform an unnatural function (e.g., enabling bacteria to produce human insulin, or sheep to produce human blood-clotting protein)

Therapeutic Proteins

Therapeutic proteins represent a class of drugs that allow management of diseases not treated adequately with conventional small molecule drugs. Proteins can be used in therapy in two ways. In one application, large amounts of a particular protein drug may be given to suppress a process that contributes to the disease or trauma. For example, fibrinolytics (clot-destroying drugs such as Activase and Retavase) are used in facilitative therapy for the treatment of heart attacks. When administered in large doses, their natural biological function can be used to dissolve blood clots. Another application is in replacement therapy; the therapeutic protein replaces or supplements a protein that is deficient or defective in a patient. For example, insulin is used as replacement therapy to compensate

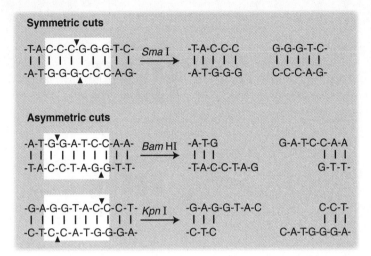

Figure 21.1. Examples of restriction enzymes with the recognition sequence (white box) and the sites of cuts (arrows). Restriction enzymes such as *Sma*I cut the DNA strand symmetrically, yielding *blunt ends*, whereas *Bam*HI and *Kpn*I cut the DNA strand asymmetrically, leaving *sticky ends*.

for the lower levels of insulin made by the pancreas of diabetic patients.

Recombinant DNA Technology

Recombinant DNA (rDNA) is DNA that has been created artificially (outside a cell) by joining DNA from two or more sources into a single molecule. It is made using recombinant DNA technology, a body of techniques for cutting apart and splicing together different pieces of DNA.

Biotechnology got a tremendous boost with the discovery of restriction enzymes (also called restriction endonucleases) that cleave DNA strands into shorter nucleotide segments. A majority of these enzymes have been isolated from bacteria in which they serve to protect bacteria by destroying invading DNA molecules. Several thousand restriction enzymes have been identified, each with the ability to cut DNA at specific recognition sequences that are generally four, five, or six base pairs in length. Restriction enzymes hydrolyze the backbone of DNA between deoxyribose and phosphate groups, leaving a phosphate group on the 5′ ends and a hydroxyl on the 3′ ends of

both strands. Examples of the recognition sequence and cut sites of restriction enzymes are shown in Figure 21.1.

The creation of recombinant DNA next requires recombining these cut fragments of DNA from different sources into a new and, hopefully, useful DNA molecule. Joining linear DNA fragments together with covalent bonds is called *ligation*—creating a phosphodiester bond between the 3′ hydroxyl of one nucleotide and the 5′ phosphate of another. The enzyme used to join DNA fragments is DNA ligase, which can join DNA fragments with blunt or complementary "sticky" ends. Any pair of complementary sequences will bond even if one fragment comes from human DNA and the other from a bacterial DNA. It is this ability of stickiness that allows production of recombinant DNA molecules composed of DNA from different sources. Figure 21.2 illustrates the process of creating a recombinant DNA molecule.

To be useful, the recombinant DNA needs to be cloned, or replicated many times. A clone is DNA, a cell, group of cells, or organism descended from and genetically identical to a single common ancestor. Cloning can be done *in vitro*,

The restriction enzyme cuts
both DNA strands at the same site

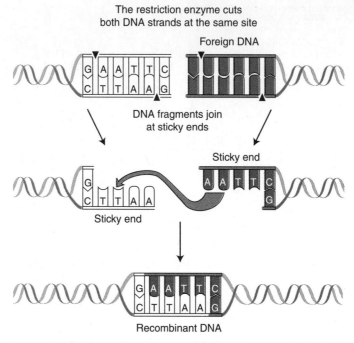

Figure 21.2. An overview of the creation of a recombinant DNA molecule. In this example, complementary sticky ends are generated by the action of the restriction enzyme *Eco*RI (obtained from *E. coli*) on two DNA molecules from different organisms. These sticky ends are then joined together by DNA ligase to create the new recombinant DNA molecule.

via the polymerase chain reaction (PCR), or *in vivo* (inside the cell) using unicellular prokaryotes (e.g., *Escherichia coli*), unicellular eukaryotes (e.g., yeast), or mammalian tissue culture cells.

When the rDNA is inserted into hosts such as bacterial, yeast, or mammalian cells, the host is *transformed*, i.e., its genotype is modified by introduction of DNA from another source. The transformed host can now make the protein of interest encoded by the rDNA. To make sufficient quantities of a biopharmaceutical, many cells of the transformed host are needed; these are produced by cloning the cells (allowing them to reproduce asexually). Thus, using genetic engineering techniques, the gene for a protein drug of interest can be transferred into another organism that will produce large amounts of the drug. The steps involved the production of a biopharmaceutical by recombinant DNA technology are as follows:

1. The gene for the therapeutic protein of interest is isolated on a strand of human DNA.

2. The DNA is cut at specific points by restriction enzymes.

3. The cut DNA segment, containing the gene of interest, is inserted into a *vector.* A vector is a piece of DNA capable of independent growth; commonly used vectors are bacterial plasmids (circular pieces of extrachromosomal bacterial DNA) and viruses. Restriction enzymes are used to cut open the vector DNA, the gene of interest (foreign DNA) is inserted, and DNA ligase splices the human DNA segment into the vector DNA, creating a recombinant DNA.

4. The rDNA is inserted into host cells (bacteria, yeast, or mammalian cells). Once inside the cell, a plasmid rDNA including the gene of interest can become integrated into the genome of the host cell and its function can be expressed. Viral vectors use the

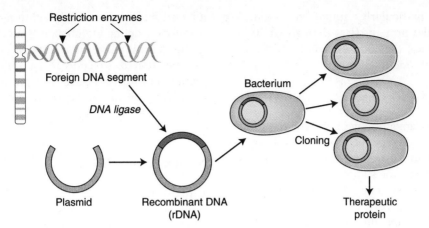

Figure 21.3. The overall process of making a recombinant DNA therapeutic protein.

mechanism of viral infection of a host to get the viral rDNA with the gene of interest into the host cell. Once the DNA has entered the cell, the viral DNA becomes incorporated into the host genome just like the plasmid DNA.

5. The host cells process the encoded instructions in the rDNA and make the desired therapeutic protein. If the rDNA fails to integrate into the host genome, it is not expressed and does not affect the host cell.

6. As the host cells are allowed to multiply, the rDNA is passed on to the daughter cells by cloning. Thus, these cells become "factories" for the production of the protein coded for by the inserted DNA.

7. The therapeutic protein is then isolated and purified.

Figure 21.3 shows an overview of this process. Using procedures like this, many human genes have been cloned, making it possible to produce large amounts of human therapeutic proteins.

Bacterial Hosts

Many bacteria can readily acquire new genes by taking up DNA molecules like plasmids from their surroundings. The ability to deliberately transform the common bacterium E. coli has made possible the cloning of select human genes to produce biopharmaceuticals. Large amounts of bacterial cells can be grown easily in commercial-sized fermenters to give useful quantities of therapeutic proteins.

The first successful therapeutic products of recombinant technology were proteins like insulin and growth hormone. An inexpensive, easy-to-grow culture of genetically engineered bacteria like E. coli can manufacture these protein drugs. This has made it possible to produce virtually unlimited amounts of such human proteins in vitro.

However, bacterial hosts, being prokaryotic, present some disadvantages. There is a possibility of the presence of pyrogenic (fever causing) and endotoxin (immunogenic) contaminants from bacterial cell membranes in the final product. Additionally, the exact human protein may not be produced because bacteria do not perform posttranslational modifications such as phosphorylation and glycosylation (the addition of complex branched saccharides). Most proteins of biological and therapeutic significance are glycoconjugates; examples include tumor necrosis factor (TNF), blood factors (VII, VIII, IX), erythropoietin, and tissue plasminogen activator.

Proteins such as insulin are not glycosylated in their native state and can be expressed by hosts with different glycosylation machinery. Thus, bacterial hosts are particularly suited to producing smaller proteins (less than about 30 kilodaltons) that do not require posttranslational modification.

Yeast Cell Hosts

Yeasts are attractive hosts for the production of therapeutic proteins and have been used to express recombinant proteins to overcome the shortcoming of bacterial expression systems. The most obvious advantage in yeast over prokaryotic systems is the capability of processing diverse posttranslational modifications required to produce "authentic" and bioactive mammalian proteins. In addition, yeast expression systems have the following advantages: high level of protein secretion, rapid growth rate, ease of large-scale production, ease of genetic manipulation, lower cost compared with animal expression systems, lack of endotoxins, lytic viruses, and no known pathogenic relationship with man. Yeasts are also capable of expressing larger molecular weight proteins (greater than 50 kilodaltons).

Saccharomyces cerevisiae, a common and safe yeast used in baking and brewing, was the first to be used for the production of recombinant proteins such as interferon and hepatitis surface antigen. But *S. cerevisiae* often causes super-high glycosylation in expressing glycosylated proteins, so several different yeast hosts have been identified that offer the characteristics well suited to the expression of a particular protein. *Pichia pastoris* is a yeast that has been extensively used for this purpose.

Even when posttranslational modification patterns generated by yeasts are different than those desired, they can sometimes be changed by altering experimental conditions such as culture pH, culture medium, fermentation method, oxygen and metal ion concentration, and additive agent.

Another very useful protein engineering technique to control glycosylation and phosphorylation of proteins is *site-directed mutagenesis.* This technique introduces a deliberate change (mutation) in the rDNA molecule so that a codon can be altered to code for a different amino acid, to introduce new glycosylation sites, or to modify restriction enzyme sites for manipulation of DNA.

Mammalian Cell Hosts

Difficult-to-express proteins and proteins requiring "complete authenticity" (matching glycosylation and amino acid sequence) can only be produced using host cells of higher organisms like mammals. Mammalian cells also contain chaperonins to help fold proteins properly. Prediction and consistency of glycosylation, however, continues to be an issue with mammalian hosts as well.

Genetically engineered Chinese hamster ovary (CHO) cells have been used extensively for this purpose. These cells can perform the posttranslational processing necessary for the secretion of a biologically active recombinant protein. In addition, CHO cells have a very low susceptibility to contamination by human viruses, usually a potentially serious problem in the manufacture of recombinant products. However, because CHO cells are not of human origin, even glycoproteins produced in CHO are often glycosylated differently compared with their native human counterparts, and further genetic engineering is needed to produce the correct protein.

Biopharmaceuticals made successfully by mammalian host cells include factor IX, factor VIII, interferon-γ, interleukin 2, human growth hormone, and TPA. Unfortunately, mammalian hosts are difficult and expensive to grow and transfect, and the cultures are often of lower cell densities and have slower growth rates. Mammalian cells also carry the risk of containing oncogenes or viral DNA, so recombinant protein products from them must be tested more extensively.

Transgenic Animal Hosts

Cloned genes can also be expressed *in vivo* if introduced into the germline of an animal. Mice and fruit flies are the most commonly used animal hosts. An animal that is genetically engineered by insertion of a foreign gene into its genome is called a transgenic organism, and the introduced engineered gene is a *transgene*. The protein encoded by the transgene is secreted into the animal's milk, eggs, or blood, and then collected and purified. Livestock such as cattle, sheep, goats, chickens, rabbits, and pigs have already been modified in this way to produce several useful proteins and drugs.

The first transgenic animals were developed to advance basic biomedical research by genetically modifying lab rats, mice, rabbits, and monkeys to give them characteristics that mimic human diseases. This research rapidly advanced the understanding of oncogenes—genes responsible for causing cancers. Moreover, researchers now seek ways to genetically modify the organs of animals, such as pigs, for possible transplantation into humans.

Before the advent of cloning, microinjection of fertilized eggs was the only method for producing transgenic animals. Using this approach to produce a group of transgenic animals was a long and expensive process because only a small number of animals acquired the transgene in their genome and not all of these passed it on to their offspring. Cloning dramatically improved the *pharming* technology; when one suitable transgenic animal has been raised, an unlimited number of genetically identical animals can be produced rapidly.

Transgenic animals are now being used for the production of therapeutic proteins that require complex posttranslational modifications or are needed in large quantities. Milk production by mammals has been the target for production of these proteins. The DNA for the therapeutic protein drug is coupled with a DNA signal directing milk production

in the mammary gland. This rDNA is injected into a fertilized animal embryo (cow, sheep, goat, or mouse). The embryos are then implanted into recipient females where, hopefully, they survive and are born normally.

The new gene, present in every cell of the offspring transgenic animal, functions only in the mammary gland so the protein drug is made only in the milk. The farm animal becomes a production facility for the therapeutic protein, which is secreted into the milk. The overall process is illustrated in Figure 21.4. Because of the long time periods involved in the development of a mature animal and the low success rates, obtaining biopharmaceuticals from transgenic animals is currently very expensive.

Therapeutic products being produced from the milk of transgenic animals or waiting for final U.S. Food and Drug Administration (FDA) approval include factor IX, a blood-clotting factor deficient in hemophiliacs; an α-antitrypsin, the shortage of which makes people more likely to get emphysema; and TPA, which dissolves blood clots.

Types of Therapeutic Protein Products

Several recombinant therapeutic proteins are on the market today. They include proteins with a variety of biological functions, such as hormones, cytokines and growth factors, enzymes, and clotting factors.

Many hormones are proteins or peptides and can be made using recombinant techniques. We have already discussed the role of hormones as important chemical messengers in our bodies in Chapter 15, Ligands and Receptors. Insulin was the first hormone target of biopharmaceutical development; several types of recombinant human insulin and recombinant insulin analogs are now available. Some other important examples of recombinant hormones are shown in Table 21.1.

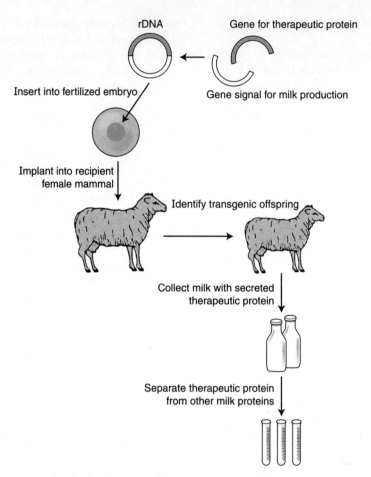

Figure 21.4. Process for the development of a transgenic animal that secretes a therapeutic protein into milk.

Recombinant cytokines and related growth factors form another group of therapeutic proteins. Cytokines are molecules that control reactions between cells and activate immune system cells such as lymphocytes and macrophages mediating proliferation or differentiation. We have mentioned cytokines as endogenous chemical messengers in Chapter 15, Ligands and Receptors. Cytokine is a general name; other names include lymphokines (cytokines made by lymphocytes), monokines (cytokines made by monocytes), chemokines (cytokines with chemotactic activities), and interleukins (cytokines made by one leukocyte and acting on other leukocytes). Cytokines may exhibit autocrine, paracrine, or in

some cases endocrine action. Some important recombinant cytokine biopharmaceuticals are listed in Table 21.2.

Enzymes are very important players in almost all biochemical processes and common targets during drug design. They can also be used as drugs, and some examples of recombinant therapeutic enzymes are listed in Table 21.3.

Clotting factors are a series of different proteins that act together to form a blood clot shortly after platelets have broken at the site of the wound. The factors have Roman numeral names, e.g., VII, VIII, IX, X, XI, and XIII. Defects in genes that code for any of these factors result in genetic diseases such as hemophilia, which results from a defect in the

Transgenic Plants

Plant biotechnology was developed to improve agricultural products but is now being used to manufacture biopharmaceuticals for human health. The number of proteins successfully expressed in plants is large and is expected to grow rapidly in the future. A new term, *pharming*, is now being used, a combination of the words *farming* and *pharmaceuticals*, to describe the combination of methods of agriculture with advanced biotechnology. Another term for this technology is *molecular farming*.

Plants are an attractive alternative to other expression systems (bacterial, yeast, or mammalian cultures, or transgenic animals) because large amounts of biopharmaceuticals can be produced easily and inexpensively. The most important advantage is the low cost of production, estimated to be 2 to 10% of the cost of microbial fermentation and 0.1% of the cost of mammalian cells. Other advantages of growing biopharmaceuticals in plants is that the drug can be delivered directly as food, and plant systems allow for proteins free from human pathogens.

Molecular farming requires that DNA for encoding the protein of choice be introduced into the plant of choice. A variety of crops are being used, such as corn, soybean, canola, alfalfa, tobacco, tomatoes, potatoes, and safflower. In the example of tobacco, the drug is actually manufactured in the tobacco leaves, which are then harvested, the juice is collected, and the proteins are purified and developed as an injectable drug. If the drug is made in a food plant, such as corn or soybeans, it is possible that the plant material could be fed directly as an orally delivered product after some additional processing. Several plant-derived biopharmaceuticals for treatment of human diseases are in advanced stages of testing, including recombinant gastric lipase for the treatment of cystic fibrosis and antibodies for the prevention of dental caries and treatment of non-Hodgkin's lymphoma.

There are a few obstacles with transgenic plant-based biopharmaceutical production. One is the low product yield, i.e., the low concentration of drug in plant tissues, such as a leaf or a seed. Much research is focusing on increasing these yields. Another is the slightly different glycosylation process in plants compared with mammals. New approaches for the modification of glycosylation activities in plants are being developed so that the glycoproteins better mimic those of humans. Finally, the impact of pharmaceutical plants on the environment and potential cross-contamination with food crops must be considered.

gene for factor VIII or IX. Examples of recombinant clotting factors are summarized in Table 21.4.

Therapeutic Antibodies

Antibody proteins are produced in our bodies as a defense against infection. Most antibodies are immunoglobulins (Ig), a type of glycoprotein synthesized and secreted by B cells (also called B lymphocytes) of the immune system after they bind to their specific antigen. T-helper cells are also often necessary for production of the antibody. The terms antibody and immunoglobulin are often used interchangeably. Unfortunately, the

TABLE 21.1. Examples of Some Recombinant Hormone Products

Biopharmaceutical	Action	Disease/Condition
Insulin	Assists in cellular uptake of glucose	Type 1 and type 2 diabetes
Glucagon	Controls glycogen metabolism in liver; opposes the action of insulin	Severe hypoglycemia in patients with diabetes Diagnostic procedures involving the gastrointestinal system
Growth hormone (rHGH, somatotropin)	Stimulates growth Mediates protein, lipid, and carbohydrate metabolism	Idiopathic short stature in children Adult growth hormone deficiency Women with Turner syndrome
Follicle-stimulating hormone (Follitropin alfa)	Induces ovarian follicular growth and maturation	Women with ovulatory dysfunction

TABLE 21.2. Examples of Some Recombinant Cytokine Biopharmaceuticals

Biopharmaceutical	Action	Disease/Condition
Interferons (rIFN-α, -β, -γ)	Act against viruses and uncontrolled cell proliferation	AIDS-related Kaposi's sarcoma Hairy cell leukemia Hepatitis B
Interleukins (rIL 1–7)	Stimulates T lymphocytes	Cancers; cancer immunotherapy
Granulocyte colony-stimulating factor (G-CSF; e.g., filgrastim)	Stimulates bone marrow to produce neutrophils	Control of infections during immunosuppressive therapies
Granulocyte-macrophage colony-stimulating factor (GM-CSF; e.g., sargramostim)	Stimulates bone marrow to produce neutrophils and macrophages	Control of infections during immunosuppressive therapies, e.g., cancer, AIDS, transplants
Hematopoietic growth factors (erythropoietin, rEPO)	Stimulates production of red blood cells by the bone marrow	Anemia

TABLE 21.3. Examples of Some Recombinant Enzyme Biopharmaceuticals

Biopharmaceutical	Action	Disease/Condition
Human DNAse I, rhDNAse	Reduces viscosity of cystic fibrosis sputum	Cystic fibrosis
Tissue-type plasminogen activator (TPA; e.g., altepase, reteplase)	Prevents blood clotting at inappropriate locations and times	To dissolve blood clots in heart attacks, strokes
β-glucocerebrosidase (imiglucerase or miglustat)	Metabolizes a lipid called glucocerebroside	Gaucher disease (genetic deficiency of β-glucocerebrosidase)

TABLE 21.4. Examples of Some Recombinant Clotting Factors		
Biopharmaceutical	*Action*	*Disease/Condition*
Recombinant factor VII (rfVIIa)	Replaces deficient or missing factor	Factor VII deficiency; excessive bleeding
Recombinant factor VIII (rFVIII)	Replaces deficient or missing factor	Hemophilia A (genetic deficiency of factor VIII)
Recombinant factor IX (rFIX)	Replaces deficient or missing factor	Hemophilia B (genetic deficiency of factor IX)

immune system is often unable to mount an antibody response large enough to remove the infected or injured cells, which leads to disease.

Almost all cells (human or otherwise) display a range of surface antigens. Some are found on a variety of cell types whereas others, called unique surface antigens (USAs), are specific to a given cell type. Antibodies produced against USAs bind selectively to the surface of these cells. In effect these antibodies are "magic bullets" capable of selectively targeting specific cell types such as cancer cells, virally infected cells, or microbial cells at an infection site.

Therapeutic antibodies are precisely targeted biopharmaceuticals that recognize and bind to a cell surface antigen and then trigger a biological response. Each therapeutic antibody recognizes a different protein and can be used alone, in combination with a chemotherapeutic agent, or as a carrier of toxins or radioisotopes (for radiation therapy). After binding to the targeted site, the therapeutic antibody may perform one of several functions. It may activate cell membrane receptors and change a cell's function, block the growth of a tumor, recruit the body's immune system to attack a target, or sensitize a cancer cell to chemotherapy.

Antibody Structure

Immunoglobulins are heavy plasma proteins usually with added sugar chains. The basic unit of each antibody is a monomer, a Y-shaped molecule with two identical heavy glycoprotein chains and two identical light glycoprotein chains connected to each other by disulfide bonds (Fig. 21.5). The amino acid sequence of both heavy and light chains at the tips of the Y varies greatly among different antibodies and is the antigen-binding region. This region, composed of 110 to 130 amino acids, provides the specificity for binding antigen. Each antibody molecule has two identical antigen-binding sites.

Heavy chains can exist as five different types (called γ, δ, α, μ, and ε); these types are used to define the different immunoglobulin classes (IgG, IgD, IgA, IgM, and IgE, respectively). Each heavy chain has a *constant region,* which is the same for all immunoglobulins of the same class, and a *variable region* that differs among immunoglobulins made by different B cells, but is the same for all immunoglobulins of the same B cell. Light chains exist in two types, γ and κ, and all antibodies have one or the other type. Each light chain has one *constant region* and one *variable region.*

Once the heavy and light chains are assembled, however, the areas or domains of the antibody become more important than the individual chains. Each half of the forked end of the Y-shaped molecule is called a Fab (fragment, antigen binding) region, containing the antigen-binding ends of one light chain and one heavy chain. If an antibody molecule is enzymatically cleaved it yields two Fab fragments and one Fc fragment (fragment

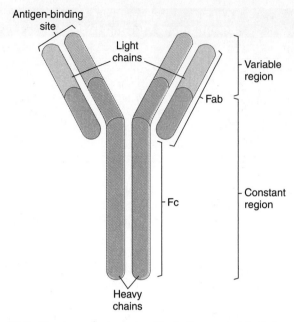

Figure 21.5. Structure of a typical antibody (immunoglobulin) molecule.

crystallizable), composed of the stem of the Y with constant regions of the heavy chains. The Fab region has great diversity so that antibodies can be made to recognize any and every antigen the body encounters, whereas the constant Fc region defines the class of antibody (IgG, for example). The Fc portion also provides for a long half-life of antibodies in the bloodstream, an important factor in the efficacy of therapeutic antibodies.

Polyclonal Antibodies

When an antigen is injected into a mouse or a human, some of the immune system's B cells start producing antibodies that bind to that antigen. Each B cell produces only one kind of antibody, but different B cells produce structurally different antibodies that bind to different parts of the antigen. This mixture of antibodies is known as polyclonal antibodies. Although the mixture contains immunoglobulins of different structures, each of the antibodies in the mixture is specific to the one antigen it was made in response to. This specificity of

antibodies makes them attractive as therapeutic agents.

Monoclonal Antibodies

The conventional method of making an antibody was to inject a laboratory animal with an antigen and then, after antibodies had been formed, to collect those antibodies from the blood serum (antibody-containing serum is called *antiserum*). There are two problems with this method: it yields antisera that contain undesired substances and it provides a very small amount of usable antibody. Another important disadvantage is that these antibodies are polyclonal, meaning that they are derived from a preparation containing many kinds of cells and therefore are a mixture of many different immunoglobulin structures.

A monoclonal antibody (MAb) is an antibody with uniform structure and specificity derived from a single clone of cells. MAbs are produced in the laboratory by cells created through the fusion of an antibody-producing cell (such as a

B lymphocyte) with an immortal tumor cell to produce a hybrid cell (hybridoma) that expresses properties of both cells. The hybridoma cells are all identical because they derive from a single cell and multiply rapidly, creating a clone that produces large quantities of the antibody. This application of recombinant DNA technology allows the production of large amounts of identical, pure antibodies. An overview of monoclonal antibody production is illustrated in Figure 21.6.

Chimeric, Humanized, and Human Antibodies

The main difficulty of using an animal such as a mouse to make antibodies is that mouse (or *murine*) antibodies are considered foreign by the human immune system, which mounts an immune response against them by producing human anti-mouse antibodies or HAMA. The anti-mouse antibodies cause the therapeutic antibody to be quickly eliminated from the patient and can also cause serious side effects.

This drawback has been somewhat addressed by a couple of approaches. The first is to fuse the DNA that encodes the antigen-binding region of the mouse antibody to the DNA that codes for the constant region of a human antibody using genetic engineering. Mammalian cell cultures are then used to express this new DNA and produce half-mouse and half-human antibodies. Depending on the proportion of human sequences in the final molecule, the

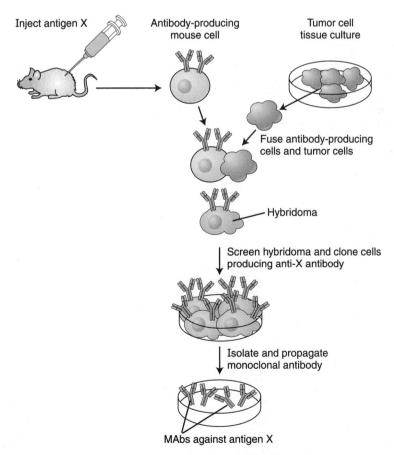

Figure 21.6. A schematic of murine monoclonal antibody (MAb) production using hybridomas.

resulting product is called either a chimeric antibody (approximately 70% human sequences) or a humanized antibody (greater than 90% human sequences). The presence of the human sequences helps reduce any immune response by the patient against the antibody itself.

Fully human antibodies are now being developed. One approach is to make use of transgenic mice in which mouse antibody gene expression is suppressed and replaced with human antibody gene expression. These mice have the ability to make fully human monoclonal antibodies, avoiding the need to humanize murine monoclonal antibodies. The human genes in these transgenic mice are stable and are passed on to offspring of the mice.

Figure 21.7 illustrates the differences among murine, chimeric, humanized, and human monoclonal antibodies.

Fusion Proteins

A fusion protein is one created through genetic engineering by removing the stop codon from the DNA sequence of the first protein, then appending the DNA sequence of the second protein to it. Cells will then express the new DNA sequence as a single protein. Although not antibodies themselves, recombinant DNA technology has facilitated the development of fusion proteins that contain antibody domains fused to therapeutic proteins. One example is etanercept for rheumatoid arthritis, a fusion protein of the human TNF receptor attached to the Fc portion of human IgG. It is produced in Chinese hamster ovary cells.

Antibody Fragments

Monoclonal antibodies are large molecules and have difficulty penetrating solid tumors. This has spurred the development of antibody fragments, especially Fab fragments. Such fragments, because of their smaller size, are capable of more readily penetrating solid tumors and should therefore show increased efficacy for treating cancers. Studies have shown that whereas intact IgG molecules take about 50 hours to travel 1 mm through a solid tumor, a Fab fragment can travel the same distance in about 16 hours. Antigen-binding Fab fragments can be made by direct proteolytic cleavage of intact antibodies, or by genetic engineering.

Applications of Monoclonal Antibody Products

Pharmaceutical companies have brought several genetically engineered monoclonal antibody drugs and related products to market in the United States and Europe, and many more are in development. Table 21.5 lists examples of important monoclonal antibodies and related products used in therapy and diagnostics.

However, the specificity of antibody therapy is a disadvantage from a commercial viewpoint. The market is potentially small, because every patient may

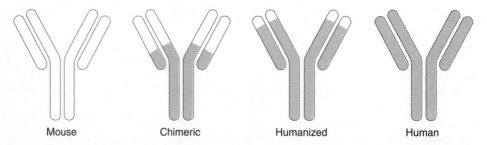

Figure 21.7. Differences among murine, chimeric, humanized, and human monoclonal antibodies.

TABLE 21.5. Examples of Some Important Monoclonal Antibodies and Related Products Used in Therapy and Diagnostics

Monoclonal Antibody	Type	Action	Disease/Condition
Therapeutic monoclonal antibodies			
Muromonab	Murine	Directed against T-lymphocyte surface antigen CD3	Reversal of acute kidney transplant rejection
Adalimumab	Human	Directed against tumor necrosis factor (TNF)	Rheumatoid arthritis
Infliximab	Chimeric (mouse–human)	Directed against tumor necrosis factor (TNF)	Rheumatoid arthritis
Etanercept	Humanized (fusion protein)	Directed against tumor necrosis factor (TNF)	Rheumatoid arthritis
Herceptin	Humanized	Directed against HER-2, a growth factor receptor found on some breast cancers	Metastatic breast cancer
Daclizumab	Humanized	Directed against interleukin 2 receptor	Prevention of acute kidney transplant rejection
Abciximab	Chimeric Fab fragment	Inhibits platelet aggregation	Prevention of reclogging of coronary arteries after angioplasty
Palivizumab	Humanized	Directed against respiratory syncytial virus	Lower respiratory tract infections
Diagnostic monoclonal antibodies			
Nofetumomab	Murine Fab fragment	Directed against carcinoma-associated antigen	Detection of small cell lung cancer
Arcitumomab	Murine Fab fragment	Directed against human carcinoembryonic antigen	Detection of recurrent or metastatic colorectal cancer
Imciromab pentetate	Murine MAb fragment	Directed against human cardiac myosin	Myocardial infarction imaging

require a different product. Even in one patient, a single antibody will probably not recognize all tumor cells; combinations of antibodies may be needed. As a result, MAbs are much more extensively used as diagnostic and research reagents, and their introduction into human therapy has been slower than initially expected.

On the horizon are *bispecific* antibodies and antibody fragments (BsAbs). As the name implies, these antibodies are engineered to bind to two different, specific antigens; they can be designed so that one antigen-binding site targets a unique surface antigen on a cancer cell while the other either binds a therapeutic agent or attracts immune effector cells to the target cell surface.

Challenges with Biopharmaceutical Development

Although biopharmaceuticals are attractive conceptually because they represent naturally derived products for treatment of disease, there are some major obstacles in their development. Even if biotechnology can now successfully produce large quantities of the pure protein, delivering the drug to the patient in a safe, accurate, convenient, and reproducible manner can be a challenge. The unique chemical and physical properties of macromolecules, as compared with small molecule drugs, present formidable difficulties in purification, separation, analysis, formulation, storage, and administration to the patient. Even if these problems are overcome, the body often treats proteins differently than it treats small molecules, limiting their plasma half-life.

Stability

Proteins are large and unstable molecules; the instability of proteins can be classified as chemical or physical. Both physical and chemical instability can cause a therapeutic protein to lose its activity or to develop a potential for toxicity. The primary structure of proteins, defined by peptide bonds between amino acids, is susceptible to degradation and cleavage by chemical reactions, causing *chemical instability*. Covalent bonds can be broken through hydrolysis reactions—either in the product or *in vivo*—and the protein can be cleaved into two or more chemically different molecules. This type of chemical stability problem is similar to that seen for small molecule drugs with amide or ester linkages.

Physical stability issues are unique to macromolecular and protein drugs and are usually not seen in small molecule drugs, so let us examine them more closely. Denaturation of a protein can be defined as any modification of secondary, tertiary, or quaternary structure of the protein molecule. Denaturation is therefore a process by which hydrogen bonds, hydrophobic interactions, and salt linkages are broken, and the protein goes from its native, folded state to an un-

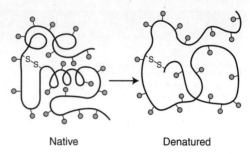

Native   Denatured

Figure 21.8. Denaturation of a protein in solution. The active, native protein (on the *left*) can be denatured by heat or agitation to yield a partially or completely unfolded structure (on the *right*). The denatured protein is not active and can adsorb to the container, aggregate with itself, and precipitate out.

folded chain with no specific three-dimensional structure (Fig. 21.8) Because denaturation reactions are not strong enough to break peptide bonds, the primary structure remains unchanged after a denaturation process.

The unfolding of a folded protein often results in hydrophobic amino acid residues, previously buried inside the folded structure, being exposed to water. This can have several other consequences. One is adsorption, in which the unfolded protein molecules stick to the sides of the product container, reducing their aqueous concentration. Changes in the residues exposed on the surface can also cause self-association of several protein molecules into a larger complex or aggregate. The aggregate may remain in solution, or may be insoluble enough to cause precipitation.

Denaturation is accelerated by heat (thermal denaturation) and agitation (mechanical denaturation). Susceptibility of a protein to thermal denaturation depends on several factors, such as temperature, presence of water, and additives in the aqueous solution. This type of stability problem can be minimized by storing protein solutions under refrigeration, and by using appropriate additives (salts, sugars, and glycerol). Many proteins denature and precipitate when solutions are agitated or shaken because of incorporation of air bubbles and adsorption of protein molecules to the air–liquid interface, where they can undergo conformational changes. Shaking protein solutions vigorously is to be avoided.

Chemical and physical instability decreases the concentration of the native, active protein in the product as a function of time. In addition, the degradation products may cause serious adverse reactions owing to their immunogenic potential. As a consequence of the greater instability of protein drugs as compared with small molecule drugs, protein drug products have a shorter shelf life and often need to be refrigerated. Freezing is generally to be avoided, however, because it can further compromise protein physical stability.

Formulation and Delivery

For biological activity, protein drugs need to retain not only their primary structure but also their secondary, tertiary, and quaternary structures during manufacture, formulation, and storage. The active, folded structure of most proteins depends strongly on the environment (solvent, pH, temperature, and so forth) around the molecule. This restricts the types of solvents and excipients that can be used in protein formulation; many protein formulations are simple aqueous solutions.

Even when refrigerated, many aqueous solutions of proteins do not have an adequate shelf life for practical use. Only a few biopharmaceuticals can be stored as aqueous solutions for 2 or more years at refrigerator temperatures.

To overcome these stability issues, a majority of the biopharmaceutical proteins currently on the market are stabilized by **lyophilization** (or *freeze-drying*), a technique that converts an aqueous solution of a protein into a solid. Water greatly facilitates thermal denaturation of proteins, so that removing it to make dry protein powders dramatically reduces protein denaturation.

A dry powder is also safe from mechanical denaturation.

The lyophilization process involves rapid freezing of a solution at low temperature followed by rapid dehydration by sublimation in a high vacuum. Freeze-drying is often used to preserve biological specimens or to concentrate macromolecules with little or no loss of activity. The process often requires inclusion of a *lyoprotectant,* an excipient added to prevent denaturation of the protein during lyophilization. When reconstituted with an appropriate solvent such as saline or a buffer, a successfully lyophilized protein will dissolve rapidly into its active, folded configuration. Lyophilized proteins can be stored for relatively long periods of time.

Most proteins cannot be administered orally because the peptide bond is unstable in the acidic stomach and in the presence of gastric and intestinal enzymes. Additionally, proteins are generally too large and too polar to be absorbed from the intestinal tract. The most common route of administration has been by injection, although recent advances suggest that inhalation, nasal delivery, or delivery through the oral cavity (buccal or sublingual) will be viable administration routes in the near future.

Immunogenicity

The therapeutic use of biopharmaceuticals derived from both human and non-human sources has been associated with **immunogenicity**, the potential for immune rejection of the administered drug and serious adverse reactions in patients. Such responses occur because the body views the protein as an antigen, and mounts an immune response by producing neutralizing antibodies. This not only reduces or eliminates the therapeutic activity of the drug but also can cause reactions such as allergic shock. In addition, contaminants (such as fetal bovine serum or cell media components) in biopharmaceuticals often enhance the production of neutralizing antibodies.

Scientists initially believed that immunogenicity was a result of using foreign proteins, such as insulin derived from pigs and cows. It was believed that the problem would disappear with the advent of recombinant technology that produces protein that is identical or nearly identical to human protein. However, although serious immune responses have been reduced, immunogenicity related to biopharmaceutical drugs still persists as a potentially serious problem. Some of the common factors responsible for causing immunogenicity with the use of biopharmaceuticals are summarized here.

Sequence Differences

Therapeutic proteins derived from non-human sources may have a somewhat different amino acid sequence than the human protein. This may result in an immune reaction, although, as discussed, this problem has been minimized by rDNA technology. However, even rDNA-derived proteins with a sequence identical to the human version do sometimes show immunogenicity. Conversely, some proteins with a slightly different sequence from the human sequence may not lead to enhanced immunogenicity.

Posttranslational Modifications

We have discussed the importance of posttranslational modifications in determining the biological activity of a protein. If a protein is not, say, glycosylated, in the same way as the human protein, it may not show biological activity but may be immunogenic. Thus, the host cell used for the recombinant protein preparation has a significant bearing on immunogenicity; for example, the fact that natural interleukin 2 is less immunogenic than the one made by *E. coli* is

related, in part, to the inability of bacteria to glycosylate proteins.

Formulation Issues

As discussed above, formulating and manufacturing a practical and stable protein product involves the use of several excipients. These excipients may induce an immunogenic reaction, either by themselves or in combination with the biopharmaceutical. Degradation products resulting from chemical and physical instability are particularly problematic in biopharmaceutical products because the body views them as foreign proteins. Since many biopharmaceuticals are used in immunologically compromised patients, even a small amount of a potentially immunogenic substance may pose a serious risk.

Disposition

Therapeutic proteins are typically administered by intravenous injection of a protein solution. Once administered, efficacy and duration of effect depend on the pharmacokinetics and pharmacodynamics of the protein. The same factors that limit the shelf life and stability of protein products also limit the length of time that the active protein circulates in the body. We have also seen that an immune response can occur that removes the protein from circulation and limits the efficacy of the protein. In addition, a multitude of enzymes that degrade proteins are present all over the body and rapidly attack the protein to break it down into smaller fragments. These processes contribute to the short duration of action of many therapeutic proteins.

Scientists have been examining ways to prolong the half-life of proteins in the body after administration. Therapeutic proteins have been modified chemically by the covalent addition of polymers, dextrans, or other sugars, or by cross-linking to other proteins. All of these

PEGylation

A solution to many problems in the disposition and toxicity of proteins is PEGylation, the attachment of a flexible strand or strands of polyethylene glycol (PEG) to a protein. PEGs are neutral, water-soluble, nontoxic polymers available in a wide range of molecular weights. They are extensively hydrated in water and have a large exclusion volume, meaning that other molecules and cells cannot approach the hydrated structure too closely. PEGs used for PEGylation are approximately in the same molecular weight range as the protein to be PEGylated.

PEGylation is generally achieved by forming covalent bonds between an amino or sulfhydryl group on the protein and a chemically reactive group (e.g., carbonate, ester, aldehyde) added to the PEG molecule. PEGylated proteins can be considered prodrugs because the protein–PEG linkage must be broken in the body to obtain the active protein drug. However, it appears that random attachment can alter the biological activity of the protein, so careful consideration must be given to the sites to which PEG is attached.

Currently available PEGylated products include peginterferon alfa-2a (an antiviral and antineoplastic agent), pegfilgrastim (for chemotherapy-induced neutropenia), and pegadenosine deaminase (for enzyme replacement).

The advantages of protein PEGylation include enhanced solubility and physicochemical stability, improved distribution, reduced renal clearance, slower rate of metabolism, and longer plasma half-life. For example, attachment of one or two 10- to 20-kilodalton PEG molecules can increase the circulating half-life of small proteins severalfold. By increasing the biological half-life and improving the efficacy of therapeutic proteins in the body, PEGylation can reduce the frequency of injections a patient requires. Modifying proteins with multiple PEGs can also mask immunogenic sites and prevent neutralizing-antibody formation to certain proteins and therapeutic enzymes.

modifications aim to extend circulation time or avoid immunogenicity or toxicity.

Vaccines

Disease-causing organisms, in addition to producing an illness, induce an immune response in the infected host as a result of the synthesis of appropriate antibodies. If these two effects of disease-causing organisms can be separated, a vaccine can be made to provide protection against the disease. A vaccine is any preparation of dead or weakened pathogens, or their products, that when introduced into the body stimulates the production of protective antibodies or T cells without causing the disease. Several different approaches have been used to generate vaccines.

Inactivated Vaccines

One approach is to kill the organism using chemicals or heat to produce *inactivated* or *killed* vaccines such as the Salk polio vaccine and vaccines against typhoid, cholera, plague, and hepatitis A. Such vaccines are stable and safe; they cannot revert to the virulent (disease-causing) form. However, most inactivated vaccines stimulate a relatively weak immune response and require several doses (boosters) over the years. The flu shot is an inactivated vaccine, as are the vaccines for cholera, plague, and hepatitis A.

Live, Attenuated Vaccines

Some vaccines contain live microorganisms that have been attenuated or weakened. These *live* or *attenuated* vaccines generate a strong immune response because the microorganisms continue to multiply in the body of the host. Examples are vaccines against measles, mumps, and rubella. Although live vaccines require special handling and storage to maintain their potency, they produce both antibody-mediated and cell-mediated immunity and generally require only one booster dose. However, such vaccines carry the greatest risk because they may mutate back to the virulent form at any time, resulting in induction of the disease rather than in protection against it. Most live vaccines are injected; some, however, such as the Sabin polio vaccine, are given orally. In addition some attenuated vaccines can be given nasally, such as one for influenza.

Toxoids

In some diseases the protein toxin liberated by the organism is dangerous rather than the organism itself. Vaccines called *toxoids* containing inactivated toxins from the disease-producing organism are useful in such cases; examples are the diphtheria and tetanus vaccines. Formalin, a solution of formaldehyde and sterile water, is most often used to inactivate toxins and produce toxoids.

Conjugate Vaccines

Another approach uses only the antigenic part of the disease-causing organism, such as the capsule, flagella, or part of the protein cell wall, to produce an *acellular* vaccine. For example, the bacteria that cause pneumococcal pneumonia and certain types of meningitis have special outer coats. These coats disguise antigens so that the immature immune systems of infants and younger children are unable to recognize these harmful bacteria. In a conjugate vaccine, proteins or toxins from a second type of organism, one that an immature immune system can recognize, are linked to the outer coats of the disease-causing bacteria. This enables a young immune system to respond and defend against the disease agent.

Subunit Vaccines

Subunit vaccines contain purified antigens or antigenic fragments rather than whole organisms, and are often able to evoke an immune response with fewer side effects than a vaccine made from the whole organism. Subunit vaccines can be made by taking apart the actual microbe, or they can be made in the laboratory using genetic engineering techniques. Today, subunit vaccines are used against pneumonia caused by *Streptococcus pneumoniae* and against a type of meningitis. Subunit vaccines are safe for immunocompromised patients because they cannot cause the disease.

Recombinant Vector Vaccines

Recombinant vaccines are those in which genes for desired antigens are inserted into a vector, such as a weakened virus or bacterium. The vector expressing the antigen may be used as the vaccine, or the antigen may be purified and injected as a subunit vaccine. Advantages of recombinant vaccines are that the vector can be chosen to be not only safe but also easy to grow and store, reducing production cost.

An example of a recombinant vaccine currently in use in humans is the hepatitis B virus (HBV) vaccine. Hepatitis B surface antigen is produced from a gene transfected into yeast cells and purified for injection as a subunit vaccine. The vaccinia virus, the virus that causes cowpox, is now used to make recombinant vector vaccines. The vaccinia virus containing several genes from the human immunodeficiency virus (HIV) is currently being tested as a vaccine for acquired immune deficiency syndrome (AIDS).

Gene Therapy

Gene therapy is the transfer of genetic material into the cells of an individual, resulting in a therapeutic benefit to the individual. It involves the intentional modification of genetic material with the aim of preventing, diagnosing, or curing a disease. These modifications include the correction of a genetic defect resulting from the absence or alteration of a protein, or the addition of genetic information to modify cellular characteristics.

Gene therapy usually involves fixing a defective gene in a cell by the insertion of a functional gene or group of genes. Because genes control synthesis of proteins, gene therapy aims to treat, cure, or prevent disease by changing the expression of a person's genes or providing a missing protein via delivery of the gene for that protein. It uses agents that either interact with the gene products (proteins) or are gene products themselves, and allows modification of specific genes without having to alter the disease phenotype. The result of gene therapy is the permanent treatment of disease, hopefully with few or no side effects.

Gene Delivery

Successful gene therapy requires two main components: a therapeutic gene and a suitable gene delivery system—a way to get the correct genes into the correct cells. Although several therapeutic genes have been identified, all gene therapy strategies share a common problem—the need for a selective delivery vehicle to target genes to desired cells. Even when the gene delivery system reaches target cells, it has to be internalized and reach the cell nucleus for transcription of the delivered DNA, a process called *transfection*. The gene needs an appropriate *transfection vector* to introduce the gene into the body, carry it to its target, and allow it to be internalized and expressed in the cell.

A good gene delivery system should be:

- Able to reach the desired target tissues
- Efficient at introducing genes into recipient cells
- Able to achieve long-term or short-term expression as needed
- Nontoxic to the patient (low potential for immune response, tissue damage)
- Able to deliver a variety of genes
- Able to deliver the right concentrations of the gene
- Convenient to administer by acceptable means

Transfection Vectors

A carrier called a transfection vector must be used to deliver the therapeutic gene to the patient's target cells; vectors used in gene therapy can be either viral or nonviral.

Viral Vectors. Viral vectors are viruses that carry a modified or foreign gene, and currently offer the most efficient method for gene transfer. They infect the target cell and transfer the therapeutic gene using their natural biological mechanisms. A primary requirement is that the virus must be unable to replicate and have no lytic (ability to rupture a cell) activity. Some common viruses used as vectors in gene therapy include:

- Retroviruses
- Adenoviruses
- Parvoviruses

- Herpesviruses
- Poxviruses

The most successful viral vector so far has been the adenovirus, a group of DNA-containing viruses that can infect most cell types.

Nonviral Vectors. Viruses, although the vector of choice in most gene therapy studies, present several potential problems for the patient: toxicity, immune and inflammatory responses, and gene control and targeting issues. In addition, there is always the fear that the viral vector may recover its ability to cause disease once inside the patient. This has reduced their initial popularity as gene delivery vectors.

The problems with viral vectors have encouraged research into nonviral or synthetic vectors for gene delivery. The simplest approach is direct introduction of therapeutic DNA into target cells. This approach is of limited application because it can be used only with certain tissues and requires large amounts of DNA.

Liposomes and polycationic carriers have been studied as vectors to deliver genes. The assumption is they will hone in on appropriate target cells (e.g., cancer cells) throughout the body, enter the cell by endocytosis, and successfully integrate the desired gene into the DNA of these cells. The major challenge is overcoming the many barriers the delivery system encounters before and after reaching the target cells.

Types of Gene Therapy

There are three main types of gene therapy:

- *Gene-replacement therapy* supplies cells with healthy copies of a missing or flawed gene that encodes for production of a specific protein missing or underexpressed in the cell.
- *Suicide gene therapy* provides "suicide" genes to target cancer cells for destruc-

tion; these genes make the cancer cells more susceptible to chemotherapeutic agents.
- *Antisense gene therapy* provides a single-stranded gene in an *antisense* (backward) orientation to block production of harmful proteins.

Modes of Gene Therapy

Gene therapy can be carried out *ex vivo* or directly *in vivo* (Fig. 21.9).

Ex Vivo Gene Therapy

Ex vivo therapy involves removing cells from the patient's blood or bone marrow and growing them in the laboratory under conditions that encourage them to multiply. The desired gene is then inserted into the cells using recombinant techniques as discussed previously. The successfully altered patient cells are selected out, encouraged to multiply, and returned to the patient's body via the bloodstream. The hope is that they will replicate and produce functional descendants for the life of the transplanted individual. The *ex vivo* approach is best suited for diseases in which the desired cells can be extracted from readily accessible locations such as the blood or liver. The advantages are that the therapy involves injecting the patient's own cells rather than a potentially immunogenic foreign substance.

In Vivo Gene Therapy

In vivo gene therapy generally involves injection of a product that contains a therapeutic gene together with a vector, usually a virus. This approach is useful in diseases for which the target cells cannot be easily removed and replaced as in *ex vivo* therapy. The great advantage of *in vivo* therapy is it does not need the special techniques for removing, manipulating, and returning a patient's

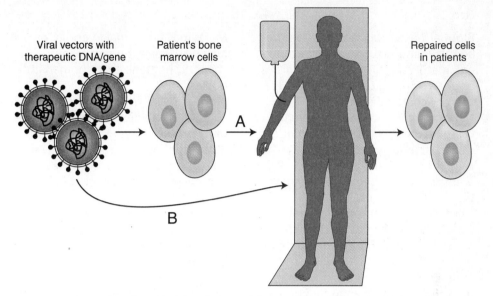

Figure 21.9. Examples of *ex vivo* (**A**) and *in vivo* (**B**) gene therapy. In *ex vivo* therapy, cells (such as bone marrow cells) are removed from the patient, and the desired gene or DNA is inserted into them using recombinant techniques. The modified cells are then injected into the patient. *In vivo* gene therapy involves injecting a vector containing the therapeutic DNA directly into the patient.

cells. However, the vector carriers have a difficult task: they must deliver the genes to enough cells for results to be achieved, and they have to remain undetected by the body's immune system.

Adenovirus is a good vector for this approach because it can infect cells *in vivo*, rather than requiring manipulation of cells *in vitro*. To become a vector, the virus is first genetically engineered by removing all viral DNA except for the minimum necessary for the virus to live and infect cells. Viral vectors like these are harmless and typically cannot live on their own. A copy of the desired gene (such as the cystic fibrosis gene) is then inserted into the virus *in vitro*, making a recombinant virus. The rDNA is then "packaged" by mixing it with all of the protein components of the virus along with some viral enzymes that assemble the virus. This creates a complete, intact virus with the new rDNA inside. The new virus carrying the desired gene is cloned to make many copies of itself and can be used for gene therapy.

Limitations to Gene Therapy

Monogenic disorders (arising from defects in a single gene) are the best candidates for gene therapy. Unfortunately, most commonly occurring disorders, such as heart disease, high blood pressure, Alzheimer's disease, arthritis, and diabetes, are polygenic (caused by variations in many genes) and will be especially difficult to treat effectively with gene therapy.

Stimulating the immune system in a way that reduces the effectiveness of gene therapy is a potential risk. Furthermore, the immune system's enhanced response to foreign invaders it has seen before makes it difficult for gene therapy to be repeated in patients.

The therapeutic DNA introduced into target cells must be integrated into the genome and remain functional. The altered cells must be long-lived and stable. These conditions prevent gene therapy from achieving guaranteed long-lasting benefits, and patients will have to undergo multiple rounds of gene therapy before such therapy can become a cure for any condition.

KEY CONCEPTS

- Biopharmaceuticals are therapeutic agents manufactured by biotechnology methods (using living organisms or parts of living organisms) rather than by chemical synthesis.
- Most biopharmaceuticals are made using recombinant DNA techniques using bacterial, yeast, or mammalian cells as hosts. Transgenic plants and animals are also being used to make biopharmaceuticals.
- Glycosylation differences among various hosts need to be taken into account when making a human biopharmaceutical.
- Therapeutic proteins are naturally occurring or slightly modified proteins that are administered to patients as biopharmaceutical drugs for replacement or facilitative therapy.
- Therapeutic antibodies are proteins made in response to an antigen, and are used as biopharmaceuticals or as drug-targeting systems.
- Monoclonal antibodies (MAbs) are made using hybridoma technology.

- MAbs may be animal in origin, or may be partially human as in chimeric, humanized, or human antibodies.
- Biopharmaceuticals are large molecules with chemical and physical stability problems.
- Most biopharmaceuticals are available as aqueous solutions or as lyophilized solids designed to be reconstituted before use.
- Vaccines are preparations of dead or weakened pathogens, or their toxins, that stimulate the production of protective antibodies without causing the disease.
- Gene therapy is the transfer of genetic material into the cells of an individual with the objective of fixing a defective gene.
- One of the primary challenges in gene delivery is finding safe and effective delivery vectors. Common vectors are viruses, although nonviral vectors are being studied.

ADDITIONAL READING

1. Crommelin D (ed). Pharmaceutical Biotechnology, 2nd ed. CRC Press, 2002.
2. Walsh G. Biopharmaceuticals: Biochemistry and Biotechnology. John Wiley & Sons, 2003.
3. Kayser O, Müller R (eds). Pharmaceutical Biotechnology: Drug Discovery and Clinical Applications. John Wiley & Sons, 2004.
4. Rho J, Louie S (eds). Handbook of Pharmaceutical Biotechnology. Pharmaceutical Products Press, 2003.

REVIEW QUESTIONS

1. How are proteins used as drugs in therapy?
2. Explain the terms biotechnology, biopharmaceuticals, and genetic engineering.
3. Briefly discuss the steps involved in making a therapeutic protein by recombinant DNA technology.
4. Compare different host cell types for the manufacture of recombinant proteins. What advantages do transgenic animals provide in the

manufacture of recombinant proteins?

5. Describe the structure of a monoclonal antibody. What is the difference between monoclonal and polyclonal antibodies?

6. Outline the manufacture of monoclonal antibodies using hybridoma technology. How can these MAbs be made more compatible with humans?

7. Explain the sources of protein instability and how formulation techniques can minimize instability.

8. Briefly describe the denaturation process and its consequences.

9. Why are most biopharmaceuticals administered by nonoral routes?

10. What factors are responsible for the short duration of action and immunogenicity of biopharmaceuticals?

11. What are the differences between *in vivo* and *ex vivo* gene therapy?

12. Why are vectors needed to transport DNA during gene therapy?

Drug Discovery, Development, and Approval

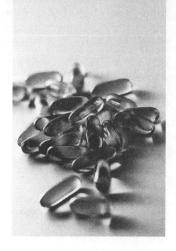

The drug research and development process is complex, lengthy, and expensive. It is also risky, in that there is no guarantee the end result will be a marketable drug product. Every pharmaceutical and biopharmaceutical product must undergo rigorous scientific testing and scrutiny to ensure it is safe and effective for its intended use before receiving approval for marketing in the United States. For every 10,000 compounds synthesized or isolated as potential drugs, only one on average will successfully complete all the requirements to make it to the market. Compounds drop out of the process for several reasons, the most common ones being:

- Lack of efficacy
- Unacceptable toxicity
- Poor pharmaceutical properties, such as chemical instability, low aqueous solubility, poor cell permeability, and unacceptably high clearance

Early identification of potentially problematic drug candidates is extremely important, and pharmaceutical companies use *in vitro* and *in vivo* screens to identify and eliminate such compounds from the development process as early as possible. Currently, the estimated average cost of bringing a new drug to market is $800 million, and the average length of time from discovery to patient is 10 to 15 years. As lengthy and complicated as the process is, however, it has been remarkably successful in bringing safe and effective drugs to market.

In the United States, the Food and Drug Administration (FDA) regulates the development of new drugs and their subsequent marketing.

The FDA

One of the FDA's primary functions is to promote and protect public health by helping safe and effective drug products reach the market in a timely manner, and to monitor these products for continued safety after they are in use. In addition to conventional drugs, the FDA regulates related products like biologicals (biopharmaceuticals, blood products, and tissues for transplantation), medical devices, and veterinary drugs, as well as most food products (except meat and poultry) and animal feed. In addition, the FDA monitors the safety of cosmetics, other medical and consumer products, and devices that emit radiation (such as cell phones, microwave ovens, and lasers).

The FDA has also taken on some new responsibilities in the war on terrorism. In the area of drugs, the FDA has been asked to improve the availability of drug products to prevent or treat injuries caused by biological, chemical, and nuclear weapons.

FDA Centers

The FDA is organized into several centers, each with its own areas of responsibility. Figure 22.1 shows an FDA organizational chart with the various FDA centers and offices. The Center for Drug Evaluation and Research (CDER) and the Center for Biologics Evaluation and Research (CBER) are the two most involved in the review, approval, and monitoring of human

pharmaceuticals. The CDER is responsible for regulating human drugs, including most biopharmaceuticals. It evaluates prescription, generic, and over-the-counter (OTC) drug products for safety and effectiveness before they can be marketed. The CDER also monitors all human drugs and biopharmaceuticals once they are on the market, and removes products from the market that may not be manufactured properly or may cause harm to patients.

The CBER regulates biologics not reviewed by the CDER, such as vaccines, blood and blood products, gene therapy products, and cellular and tissue transplants, including stem cell therapy, xenotransplantation, and transgenic plants and animals whose products will result in new vaccines and therapeutics. Many biopharmaceuticals fall under the responsibilities of both the CBER and the CDER.

Two related arms of the FDA should also be mentioned here. The Office of Regulatory Affairs (ORA) is responsible for monitoring sites and facilities in which human pharmaceuticals are manufactured. The Center for Veterinary Medicine (CVM) regulates drug products intended for veterinary use only.

Evolution of FDA Regulations

The drug regulatory system in the United States is continuously evolving. Drug product regulations introduced in the early years came about as a result of public demand that caused Congress to pass a series of bills. The current FDA authority to regulate pharmaceutical products comes from the 1938 *Federal Food, Drug, and Cosmetic Act,* a law that has undergone many changes over the years. The Code of Federal Regulations, or CFR, is the book in which all final regulations are codified.

Some of the major milestones that came before and after the 1938 Act are summarized here.

- *Food and Drugs Act (1906):* This first drug law mandated that marketed drug products meet standards of strength

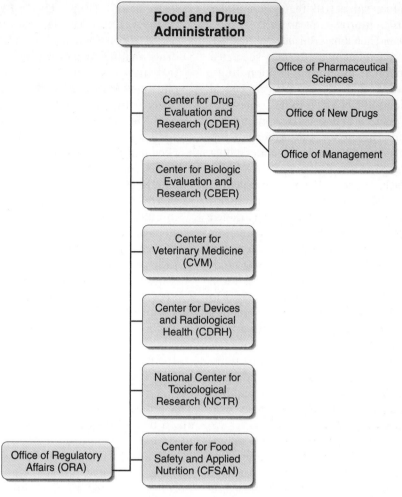

Figure 22.1. Organizational chart of the U.S. Food and Drug Administration. The CDER is responsible for human drugs, including most biopharmaceuticals, whether prescription, generic, or over-the-counter (OTC). The CBER regulates some biopharmaceuticals and other biologics such as vaccines, blood products, and gene therapy.

and purity, but evidence of safety or effectiveness of the drug product was not required. The FDA had to prove a product's labeling was false and fraudulent before it could be removed from the market.

- *Federal Food, Drug, and Cosmetic (FD&C) Act (1938)*: The 1906 Act was revised in 1938 by a bill enacted by Congress. This revision was prompted by the death of 107 people from a poisonous ingredient in the product "Elixir Sulfanilamide." Pharmaceutical manufacturers now had to prove that a

drug product was safe before it could be marketed.

- *Public Health Service (PHS) Act (1944)*: This act was the legal basis for licensing of biologic products and established the mechanism for marketing approval of a biologic drug product. The difference between a biologic and drug, which was once quite clear, has become blurred with the advent of biotechnology and resulting biopharmaceuticals. Thus, most biologic products also meet the definition of "drugs" under the FD&C Act, and are therefore subject to regulation under FD&C Act provisions as well.

- *Durham-Humphrey Amendment (1951):* This amendment to the Act separated prescription and nonprescription drugs, requiring that certain pharmaceutical products be labeled "for sale by prescription only." It defined prescription drugs as those unsafe for self-medication and which should be used only under a doctor's supervision.

- *Kefauver-Harris Drug Amendments (1962):* Congress passed these amendments to tighten control over marketed drugs. A pharmaceutical company now had to prove not only the safety but also the effectiveness of the drug product for its intended use. In addition, the company was required to send to the FDA all adverse reaction reports about the drug product. Pharmaceutical advertisements in medical journals were required to provide complete information about the drug, including its risks. The amendments also required informed consent from subjects who participate in clinical trials.

- *Orphan Drug Act (1983):* This legislation was passed to encourage development of drugs for diseases that only affected small populations by providing financial incentives to pharmaceutical companies to develop such drugs, and provided the sponsor exclusive rights to market these medicines for a period of time as an incentive to develop them. An "orphan" disease is a condition affecting fewer than 200,000 people in the United States; examples are Huntington's disease, Tourette's syndrome, and muscular dystrophy.

- *Drug Price Competition and Patent Term Restoration Act (1984):* This legislation was passed to ensure that less expensive generic versions of approved drugs could be brought to market quickly. A less stringent, abbreviated application process was introduced for approval of generic drug products. In return, patents of new drugs were extended by some of the time lost during their FDA approval process.

- *Prescription Drug User Fee Act (PDUFA, 1992):* This legislation established a system whereby prescription drug manufacturers pay fees to have their new drug and biologic drug applications reviewed by the FDA. This system provided additional funds to help the FDA accelerate its review of applications.

- *Food and Drug Administration Modernization Act (FDAMA; 1997):* This act reauthorized the PDUFA; currently PDUFA III reauthorizes user fees through 2007. It also provided extensions of market exclusivity for pharmaceutical manufacturers who conduct pediatric studies on select prescription drugs, and amended the FD&C and PHS Acts to change the regulatory and approval processes for drugs, biologics, antibiotics, and devices.

Drug Candidate Selection

The process starts with a *sponsor,* usually a pharmaceutical company, seeking to develop a new drug it hopes will be useful to patients and profitable in the market. Extensive initial research goes into studying the disease process and identifying potential targets, such as the ones discussed in Chapter 6, Drugs and Their Targets. A lead compound is identified on the basis of a favorable interaction with the desired drug target. In Chapter 7, Drug Discovery and Optimization, we learned that drugs are not discovered in their final form but go through a process of research and modification to select and make the best possible compound. In this process, the lead is further modified and optimized to make it drug-like (refer to discussion of drug-likeness in Chapter 7), and to increase the probability that the compound will have favorable absorption, distribution, metabolism, and excretion (ADME) properties.

The optimized compound, or a series of promising compounds, is then screened for efficacy in a suitable animal

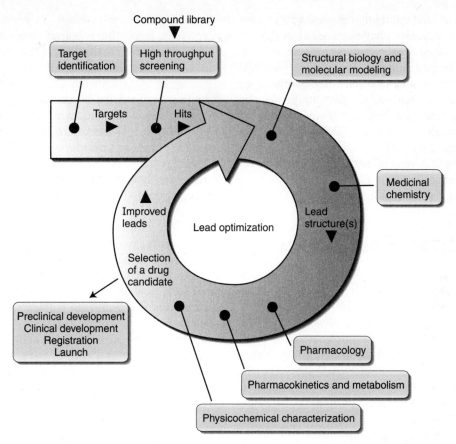

Figure 22.2. The process for lead identification, lead optimization, and selection of a drug candidate for development. The process can take anywhere from 2 to 10 years.

model; the best one, or the best few, is selected for further preclinical studies. The process for selecting a few promising compounds for preclinical testing is illustrated in Figure 22.2.

Preclinical Testing

The goal of early preclinical development is to determine whether a compound is reasonably safe for initial, small-scale clinical studies in humans, and whether it exhibits pharmacological activity in animals that justifies commercial development. Primary activities during the preclinical testing phase are *in vitro* and *in vivo* laboratory animal experiments to evaluate the compound's toxic, pharmacological, and ADME characteristics. The toxicity and ADME of metabolites of the

compound are also investigated at this stage. Additional laboratory investigations include characterization of the chemical structure, purity, and physicochemical properties of the drug compound. A formulation for use in early human trials is designed, and manufacturing processes for the drug compound and dosage forms are developed. Thus, preclinical development encompasses almost all of the concepts we have discussed in earlier chapters.

The major question raised during preclinical testing is whether the drug's behavior in animals will correlate with that in humans; disease processes and drug disposition and action are often different between commonly used laboratory animals and humans. Design and selection of a relevant animal model is a very important consideration in preclinical development.

An animal model that is most appropriate to study the pharmacological action of the drug in a particular disease state is often not suitable for studying ADME behavior, and vice versa. Decisions about extrapolating animal data to justify the first use of a compound in humans are difficult, and testing at this stage can take from 1 to 5 years. Of every 1,000 new drug candidates tested preclinically, on average only one enters clinical trials—a success rate of only 0.1%.

Investigational New Drug

If results from laboratory and animal studies show promise, the sponsor can apply to the FDA to proceed to the next stage of development—testing the drug in humans. At this point, the compound changes legal status and becomes a drug. The Investigational New Drug (IND) application is a proposal from a sponsor to the FDA requesting permission for clinical testing of a drug in humans.

The IND application must contain information in three broad areas:

1. *Animal pharmacology and toxicology studies:* This includes the pharmacological profile of the drug, acute toxicity of the drug in at least two species of animals, and results of short-term toxicity studies ranging from 2 weeks to 3 months, depending on the proposed duration of clinical studies.
2. *Formulation and manufacturing information:* This includes composition of the drug and dosage form, manufacturer, stability, and controls used for manufacturing the drug substance and the drug product. This information is reviewed to ensure that the company can adequately produce and supply consistent batches of the drug product.
3. *Clinical protocols and investigator information:* This includes detailed protocols for conducting clinical trials and analyzing the results, qualifications of clinical investigators, and

commitments to obtain informed consent from the research subjects and to adhere to the investigational new drug regulations.

By law, the FDA has 30 days to review the submitted IND documentation; the IND application is considered approved if the FDA does not disapprove it within 30 days.

However, before human clinical trials can begin, the IND must also be reviewed and approved by an Institutional Review Board (IRB) at the site (e.g., a hospital or medical center) where the proposed clinical studies will be conducted. An IRB is a group that has been formally designated to review and monitor biomedical research involving human subjects. Its primary aim is to ensure the rights and welfare of people participating in clinical trials both before and during their trial participation. The IRB reviews the sponsor's clinical trial protocol, informed consent documents, investigator brochures, and other documents related to the trial. The IRB has the right to approve, disapprove, or require changes to the study.

Clinical Trials

The current system of clinical trials evolved in the early 1960s. To demonstrate safety and efficacy, a new drug must pass through three distinct phases of controlled testing in humans. The phases progressively involve more human subjects tested for longer times. All trial subjects must be provided with sufficient information about the trial and the drug to give informed consent, freely and without coercion, before trial participation.

In a *controlled* clinical trial, subjects are divided into the treatment group (those given the investigational drug) and a control group. Depending on the purpose of the trial, patients in the control group get no treatment, a placebo (an inactive product resembling the investigational drug), another drug known to be effective, or a different dose of the drug under study. Treatment and control groups must be as similar as possible in characteristics that can affect treatment outcome. For example, all patients in both treatment and control groups must have the disease the drug is meant to treat. Treatment and control groups should also be similar in age, weight, general health, and in other characteristics that could affect the outcome of the trial. In a process called *randomization,* subjects are randomly assigned to treatment or control groups rather than deliberately selected for either group. If the sample population is large enough, randomization creates treatment and control groups that are similar in important characteristics.

Along with randomization, another feature known as *blinding* limits bias in the conduct of a clinical study or interpretation of its results. In a *single-blind* study, patients do not know whether they are receiving the investigational drug or a placebo. In a *double-blind* study, patients, investigators, and data analysts do not know which patients received the investigational drug. Only when the assignment code is broken, usually at the end of the trial, is it possible to identify treatment and control patients in a double-blind trial.

Phase I Trials

Phase I is the first series of trials in which an investigational new drug is tested in humans. Single doses of the drug are administered to between 20 and 100 healthy human volunteers, starting at low doses and progressively increasing to higher doses. The emphasis in this phase is the acute safety profile and ADME behavior of the drug in humans. No determination of efficacy is usually possible at this stage. Phase I trials are generally not blinded and take about 1 year to complete.

Phase I studies identify a drug's primary adverse effects and establish a safe dosage range. Volunteers are closely monitored for adverse reactions. Blood, urine, and other biological samples are taken to study how the drug is absorbed, distributed, metabolized, and excreted in humans. If the drug is well tolerated at the end of phase I clinical trials and no major problems such as unacceptable toxicity are encountered, the sponsor can move to phase II clinical testing of the drug.

Phase I trials also provide important information about the ADME of a drug. In particular, data on absorption and bioavailability of the drug product are used to modify the dosage form to improve any deficiencies found. Information about the elimination pathways and pharmacokinetics of the drug in humans is used to design appropriate dosing regimens for the next phase of clinical trials.

Approximately 70% of drug candidates entering phase I are found safe enough to progress to the next phase. The 30% that do not proceed usually fail because they are not well tolerated, or because blood levels are lower than those thought to be necessary for efficacy.

Phase II Trials

In this stage of development, the drug is administered to patients with the target disease or condition to determine efficacy. Another aim of phase II trials is to determine the optimum dose and the most appropriate method of administration. Most phase II trials are double-blinded and randomized; many also have a *crossover* design, in which a second part of the trial has the group initially receiving placebos now receiving the investigational drug, and vice versa. On average, phase II studies involve 100 to 300 patient volunteers and take about 2 years to complete.

Approximately 40% of drugs entering phase II will proceed to the next phase. This occurs if the drug shows efficacy, a safe dose that is therapeutically effective is found, and the drug has acceptable pharmacokinetics for further develop-ment. Information collected at this stage of development is often used to further fine-tune the dosage form for better ab-sorption and bioavailability, and to select an appropriate dosage regimen for phase III trials. Investigational drugs that drop out during phase II are either not suffi-ciently effective or reveal unacceptable side effects not seen in phase I trials.

Phase III Trials

This stage of human clinical trials is sim-ilar to phase II except that a larger (1,000 to 3,000) and more diverse (in age, sex, health, and so forth) group of patients is used to confirm efficacy and safety. Fur-thermore, the trials are conducted at multiple centers and often in a world-wide population. This larger group of diverse patients enables clinicians to identify adverse events that may occur in only one or two patients per thousand, or in one type of patient subgroup. Phase III studies are also longer in duration to pro-vide further reassurance regarding long-term safety. Additional data regarding the risk versus benefit of the drug, dosing regimens, and other information con-tained in the package insert are also ob-tained at this stage.

About 70% of the drugs entering phase III are successful in clearing this hurdle. The failure of an investigational new drug at this stage often opens up new avenues for drug discovery studies. Scientists try to understand why the compound failed in humans, and go back to study other closely related compounds to see whether another analog might be a more viable drug candidate.

New Drug Application and Review

After the successful completion of all three phases of clinical trials, the results are tabulated and analyzed. The sponsor may then file a New Drug Application (NDA) or a Biologics License Application

(BLA) with the FDA. An NDA requests permission from the FDA to market the drug commercially. It details the entire history of the drug product, including preclinical studies, animal studies, human clinical trials, and information about manufacturing and labeling of the drug product. NDAs typically run 100,000 pages or more.

All applications are reviewed by a CDER or CBER review team comprising chemists, pharmacologists, physicians, field inspectors, statisticians, and other experts necessary for a particular drug. This team is responsible for reaching a decision regarding approval of the prod-uct. They examine the NDA carefully to determine whether the results of the well-controlled clinical studies provide substantial evidence of the drug's effec-tiveness, and whether the results show that the product is safe under the condi-tions of use proposed in the labeling. Typical information that must be on a drug product label, usually supplied as a package insert for prescription drugs, is shown in Table 22.1.

Before the review team examines the NDA, it first determines whether the ap-plication should get a standard or fast-track review. The fast-track process was established in the FDA Modernization Act of 1997 to allow faster approval of drugs that address unmet medical needs. A drug that appears to represent an advance over available therapy is given priority with a fast-track review, whereas one that appears to have a ther-apeutic profile similar to those of an already marketed product will get a standard review.

Drug Approval

The FDA's goal is to complete the review of a priority drug and make a decision on the NDA within 6 months after it has been filed; for drugs with a standard des-ignation this time frame is 10 months. However, actual approval times are typi-cally longer.

TABLE 22.1. Typical Information Contained in Drug Product Labeling, Usually Included as a Package Insert With Prescription Drug Products

Boxed warnings
Very serious and potentially life-threatening adverse effects of drug; highlighted in a black box at the top of the package insert

Description
Chemical structure, molecular weight, physicochemical properties of the drug, dosage form, formulation including inactive ingredients, route of administration

Clinical pharmacology
Mechanism of action(s), pharmacokinetics (including bioavailability and ADME information); brief summary of clinical trial results; age, sex, or population differences, if any

Indications
Clinical uses, i.e., indications for which drug is approved; use in special populations; use in pediatric and geriatric patients; genetically linked differences in drug behavior; use in patients with impaired organ function (e.g., hepatic or renal disease)

Contraindications
Situations or patient characteristics in which the drug should not be used, e.g., a prior allergic reaction to a similar class of drugs

Warnings
Serious risks of using the drug; situations in which drug should be discontinued; the most serious of these is in bold black type

Precautions
Actions to be taken during therapy to ensure safety and efficacy; includes consideration of drug interactions, food interactions, hypersensitivity; particular precautions for pregnant women or nursing mothers

Adverse reactions
All significant side effects seen with recommended doses of the drug during clinical trials

Overdosage
LD_{50} of the drug; symptoms of an overdose, recommended actions

Drug abuse and dependence
Potential for abuse, or for psychological or physical dependence

Dosage and administration
Specific age categories for dosing; recommended doses (initial and maximum) and frequency for approved conditions; directions on administration of drug; storage conditions (temperature, protection from light, heat, and air)

How supplied
Route of administration, dosage forms (including descriptions of color, shape, and markings), strengths and units per package

ADME, absorption, distribution, metabolism, and excretion; LD50, dose in animals at which 50% of animals die.

The NDA review team takes one of three actions on the NDA after their review is complete.

1. Approved: This indicates to the sponsor that it may now market the drug product in the United States.
2. Not Approved: This indicates that the product may not be marketed in the United States and provides a detailed explanation of the reasons for the decision.
3. Approvable: This indicates that the FDA is prepared to approve the NDA upon the sponsor satisfying conditions specified in the complete response letter. These drug products may not be marketed until the sponsor has rectified the identified deficiencies as well as other conditions specified by the FDA.

Once the FDA approves an NDA, the pharmaceutical company sponsor can introduce the drug product to the market and make it available for physicians to prescribe. Note that the approval is restricted to the specific drug product (active ingredient, route of administration, dosage form, formulation, strength, manufacturer, and so forth) specified in the NDA. Any changes in these parameters require another FDA review.

FDA Advisory Committees

The FDA or sponsor may request that a non-FDA advisory committee review the information about a drug product to have the benefit of wider national expert input. Advisory committee members are scientific experts such as physicians, statisticians, pharmacologists, and epidemiologists, as well as consumer representatives who represent the patients and the public. This group weighs the available evidence, assesses risk versus benefit, and provides advice on the approval of a drug product. The FDA usually agrees with the advisory committee recommendations, although they are not binding.

Advisory committees play a prominent role at the product approval stage, but may be used earlier in the product development cycle or during postmarketing monitoring.

Accelerated Approval

To speed the approval of promising therapies, the FDA has a special program in which reviewers base the determination of a product's safety and effectiveness on surrogate end points rather than on patient outcomes. A *surrogate end point* can be a laboratory finding or a physical sign that is not in itself a direct measurement of how a patient improves or survives but is likely to predict a drug's therapeutic benefit. For example, tumor shrinkage could be the surrogate end point for efficacy in cancer therapy. The FDA often requires the sponsor to carry out postmarketing studies after accelerated approval to confirm that the drug does produce a clinical benefit such as increased survival.

Early Access

The FDA has designed *early access* programs to allow patients with life-threatening conditions to begin using promising new therapies before formal FDA approval. Under early access, patients may receive investigational drugs that have shown promise in early clinical trials. Patients are informed that they are accepting some risk by using drug products that have not yet received FDA approval, but seriously ill patients are typically willing to accept more risk. Examples of early access are the *treatment IND* and the *parallel track* programs that were designed specifically for individuals with AIDS whose condition prevented them from participating in clinical trials.

Postmarketing Surveillance

After FDA approval, the drug enters the postmarketing surveillance phase that encompasses the entire duration of the product's life on the market. The FDA continues to monitor all drugs that are on the market throughout their lifetime; the Office of Drug Safety (ODS) in the CDER performs this function. The MedWatch Reporting Program of the ODS is a spontaneous method for reporting adverse events and problems with a particular drug product so that significant health hazards can be rapidly identified. It is a voluntary program for health-care practitioners (pharmacists, physicians, nurses) and patients; reporting is mandatory for pharmaceutical companies.

If an adverse event or problem is identified with a marketed drug, the ODS can take any one or more of the following actions:

- Labeling changes: requires manufacturer to add new information to the product's package insert.
- Boxed warnings: addition of a boxed warning to the product package insert.
- Product recalls or withdrawals: these are the most serious FDA actions.

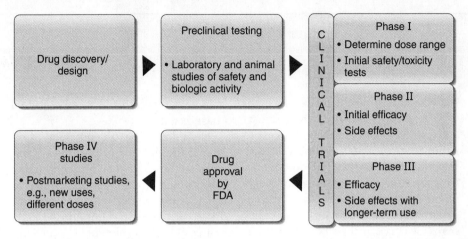

Figure 22.3. The stages of new drug development, starting with preclinical testing and ending with activities monitoring a marketed drug product.

Recalls involve the removal of one or more batches of product from the market; withdrawals require taking the product off the market permanently.

• Medical and safety alerts: the ODS provides important new safety information about the drug product to health professionals, trade, and media organizations.

Figure 22.3 and Table 22.2 summarize the phases of the new drug development process. It is estimated that the average cost of developing a new drug today is about $800 million.

Phase IV Trials

For some drug products, the FDA requires the sponsor to perform additional studies after the drug is in general use (phase IV) to evaluate long-term effects. This is because all possible effects of a drug cannot always be evaluated during phase I, II, and

TABLE 22.2. Activities, Duration, and Success Rates of the Various Stages in the Development of a New Drug				
Activity	*Test Population*	*Duration*	*Purpose*	*Success Rate*
Preclinical	Laboratory studies Animal studies	3–5 years	Effectiveness and safety in animals	5,000 compounds tested
IND				
Phase I	20–100 healthy volunteers	1–1.5 years	Acute safety ADME Dose	5 compounds enter clinical trials
Phase II	100–300 patient volunteers	1.5–2 years	Effectiveness Short-term safety	
Phase III	1,000–3,000 patient volunteers	2–4 years	Long-term safety Confirm effectiveness	
NDA				
FDA review		1–4 years		1 drug approved
NDA Approval				
Phase IV	All patients taking drug	Long-term	Postmarketing surveillance	

ADME, absorption, distribution, metabolism, and excretion; FDA, US Food and Drug Administration; IND, investigational new drug; NDA, new drug application.

Microdosing

The cost of new drug development begins to skyrocket when a pharmaceutical company decides to conduct appropriate preclinical studies to seek IND status for a new compound. This preclinical–clinical interface is also where much risk lies because of the necessity to extrapolate animal data to humans. Several scientists believe that microdosing, or "Phase 0" studies, might provide the answer.

Microdosing involves conducting early human trials in which extremely small subtherapeutic doses of a drug (1/100 or less of the expected therapeutic dose; with a maximum dose of 100 μg) are administered to healthy volunteers. The objective is to collect preliminary ADME and pharmacokinetic information in humans. Microdosing studies are possible because of tremendous advances in analytic techniques so that very small concentrations of a drug can be measured in plasma. The extent of preclinical studies required to conduct microdosing trials in humans will be much less than that required for a conventional phase I trial.

Microdosing has the potential of reducing the number of preclinical (animal) studies essential for conducting early clinical (human) studies, differentiating between good and bad candidate drugs early, and speeding up the early phases of drug development. For example, a number of lead drug candidates with similar structural, pharmacological, and animal ADME properties can be screened during microdosing studies to enable an earlier selection of the best compound to advance into full clinical development. This will enhance not only the probability of success of a drug making it successfully through the clinic and to market, but also potentially save pharmaceutical companies time and money by "killing" unsuitable molecules before time and money are wasted on them.

The concept of human microdosing is currently undergoing debate within the pharmaceutical industry and the FDA.

III clinical trials. An NDA typically includes safety data on several hundred to several thousand patients. If an adverse event occurs in 1 in 5,000 or even 1 in 1,000 users, it could be missed in clinical trials, but could pose a serious safety problem when the drug is used by hundreds of thousands of patients after marketing. Phase IV studies may address a variety of other issues such as drug interactions, alternate dosing schedules, or response in specific patient subpopulations.

Pharmaceutical companies may also conduct postapproval studies to expand the list of approved indications, optimize dosing schedules, or add other new information to product labeling. These studies can provide important marketing information for the product, e.g., fewer adverse effects or better clinical efficacy compared with a competitor drug. Outcomes research is also begun after marketing to measure a drug's cost-effectiveness and therapeutic value compared with other drugs, and with other interventions such as surgery or hospitalization.

FDA Inspections and Compliance

Field investigators of the Office of Regulatory Affairs (ORA) ensure product quality and uniformity throughout the lifetime of each approved drug product. Compliance officers periodically inspect facilities where drug products are manufactured and tested, and work with industry to address product recalls and drug shortage situations. They also address compliance issues involving the import and export of pharmaceutical products, counterfeit drugs, Internet drug fraud, drug diversion, and other illegal activities.

International Harmonization of Drug Development

In the past, the requirements for new drug approval were significantly different from country to country, so that clinical trials and even preclinical studies often had to be repeated in each country before a new drug could be approved and made available to patients. The International Conference on Harmonization (ICH) brought together government regulators and drug industry representatives from the United States, the European Union, and Japan to make the international drug regulatory process more efficient and uniform. The regulatory systems in these regions share the same fundamental concerns for the safety, efficacy, and quality of drug products. The goals of this effort are to:

• Make new drugs available with minimum delay to American consumers and those in other countries
• Minimize unnecessary duplicate testing during the research and development of new drugs
• Develop guidance documents that create consistency in the requirements for new drug approval

Generic Drug Products

An FDA-approved generic drug product is identical to a brand name drug in dosage form, strength, route of administration, quality, performance characteristics, and intended use.

Drug sponsors are required to submit an abbreviated new drug application (ANDA) for approval to market a generic product. The Drug Price Competition and Patent Term Restoration Act of 1984 made ANDAs possible to make less expensive products available to patients quickly after the patent of the innovator expires. The ANDA process allows the generic drug sponsor to skip time-consuming and expensive animal testing and phase I through III clinical trials on active ingredients or dosage forms already approved for safety and effectiveness by the FDA.

The ANDA requirements for approval of a generic drug product are that it must:

• Contain the same active ingredients as the innovator drug; inactive ingredients may vary
• Be identical in strength, dosage form, and route of administration to the innovator drug
• Be bioequivalent to the innovator drug (see definition below)
• Meet the same standards for identity, strength, purity, and quality as the innovator drug product
• Be manufactured under the FDA's good manufacturing practice regulations required for innovator products

If all these conditions are met, it is assumed that the generic product will have the same therapeutic effect as the innovator product, and they can be used interchangeably in most patients.

Two products are considered bioequivalent if the rate of absorption, maximum plasma concentration (C_{max}), extent of absorption, and area under the time–plasma concentration curve (AUC) of the drug from the two products are not statistically different. In other words, bioequivalency means the plasma level curve of the generic and innovator companies are *superimposable*. Bioequivalency is usually demonstrated in single-dose bioequivalency clinical trials in a small (24 to 36) group of healthy volunteers that compares the plasma level curves of generic product against the innovator product. Bioequivalency testing is the only clinical trial requirement for an ANDA.

Certain drug products, such as solutions, and others without a known or potential bioequivalence problem may be eligible for a waiver of *in vivo* bioequivalency study requirements. No clinical studies are necessary for approval of the generic version of such drugs; *in vitro* laboratory studies such as dissolution testing may suffice for demonstration of therapeutic equivalency.

Pharmacogenomics in Drug Development

Chapter 20, Pharmacogenomics, discussed the impact of a patient's genetic information on appropriate therapy choice. Scientists are beginning to use genomic screening techniques early in the drug discovery process to help identify compounds likely to cause serious side effects in a significant number of people.

One example involves screening potential drugs for pathways likely to be involved in their metabolism. Many of these pathways are known to be affected by genetic variants, and people with these variants may not respond well to standard doses of the drug. By early elimination of compounds likely to cause problems, human risk is decreased and efficiency is increased.

The knowledge that genetically determined diversity makes drugs ineffective or toxic in certain individuals is also being exploited in the clinical testing of investigational drugs. Suitable clinical trial participants can be identified by means of genetic tests that provide information on metabolic status, drug target polymorphism, and the presence of specific disease susceptibility genes. Single-

nucleotide polymorphism analysis at an early stage of clinical trials can permit selection of patients who are biochemically able to respond favorably to the drug. Other patients, such as slow metabolizers who are expected to show predictable adverse effects, can be excluded from trials.

The benefits of a pharmacogenomic approach to clinical trial design are listed below.

- Pharmaceutical companies will be able to discover potential therapies more easily using genome targets. Previously failed drug candidates may be revived as they are matched with the niche population in which they work.
- Even small groups of subjects selected in this way can yield statistically significant results. This could reduce the number of patients required for clinical trials of an investigational drug.
- The risk to clinical trial participants will be reduced because individuals with predictable adverse effects will be excluded, and only those persons capable of responding to a drug will be selected.
- The failure rate of drugs in clinical trials will decrease as trials are targeted for specific genetic population groups, providing greater degrees of success.
- The drug review and approval process will be shorter because data from clinical trials will be more uniform and cohesive.
- Therapies for diseases with a small patient population will be more likely to be developed.
- There will be decreases in the number of drugs a patient must try to find an effective therapy; a trial and error approach to therapy will not be the norm.
- An increase in the range of possible drug targets will decrease the overall cost of health care.

Today, a drug that helps only 20% of the subjects in clinical trials would probably not be approved, but a drug that *always* helps 20% of the population with the same genetic marker might be approved for that limited population.

Over-the-Counter Drugs

Over-the-counter (OTC) drugs are medications that do not require a physician's prescription. The first method of developing and marketing an OTC drug product is the process we have already discussed above in which a sponsor company performs research, conducts clinical trials, and so forth, and submits an NDA for an OTC drug.

The second and more frequently used mechanism is the *prescription to OTC switch*. In this process, the sponsor of an approved prescription drug submits to the FDA supplemental application to switch the drug's status from prescription to OTC. The OTC product suggested is usually lower strength than the prescription version. The FDA reviews the drug's performance as a prescription drug, including information obtained during postmarketing surveillance. Toxicity and the risk of side effects are major issues in deciding whether to switch a drug from prescription to OTC status. Another consideration is whether the condition being treated by the drug can be self-diagnosed and recognized without the help of a health-care professional. A third consideration is whether labeling can be developed so that consumers can use the product safely and effectively. This process provides consumers with easy access to safe and effective products without the assistance of a health-care professional.

The third mechanism for marketing OTC drugs is the *OTC drug review process* in which products are marketed without an application as required in the first two mechanisms. Here, the FDA and an advisory panel of experts establish that the active ingredients in a product, rather than the product itself, are safe and effective for OTC use.

KEY CONCEPTS

- In the United States, the Food and Drug Administration (FDA) regulates marketed drugs. In particular, the CDER and the CBER regulate human drugs and biologics.

- Several congressional acts have established and improved drug regulations over the years.

- Preclinical studies (laboratory and animal) on a group of drug candidates select the best compound to move forward into initial testing in humans.

- The IND (Investigational New Drug) application is a proposal from a sponsor to the FDA requesting permission for clinical testing of a drug in humans.

- Phase I trials characterize the acute safety profile and ADME behavior of the drug in healthy human volunteers.

- Phase II trials in patients are designed to investigate efficacy and to determine an appropriate dosing regimen.

- Phase III trials involve a larger and more diverse patient population and are carried out to confirm efficacy and long-term safety.

- The sponsor may file an NDA (New Drug Application) with the FDA after completion of clinical trials. The FDA may deem the drug product approved, not approved, or approvable.

- The FDA's postmarketing surveillance monitors all marketed drugs throughout their lifetime; sponsors may be required to conduct phase IV clinical trials after marketing.

- Generic products may be approved under an ANDA (Abbreviated New Drug Application).

- Clinical trials are now being designed using a pharmacogenomic approach to select the appropriate trial subjects and analyzing data.

ADDITIONAL READING

1. Ng R. Drugs—From Discovery to Approval. Wiley-Liss, 2003.

2. Lee C-J. Development and Evaluation of Drugs from Laboratory Through Licensure to Market, 2nd ed. CRC Press, 2003.

3. Pisano DJ, Mantus D. FDA Regulatory Affairs: A Guide for Prescription Drugs, Medical Devices, and Biologics. CRC Press, 2003.

4. Whitmore E. Development of FDA-Regulated Medical Products: Prescription Drugs, Biologics, and Medical Devices, 2nd ed. ASQ Quality Press, 2003.

REVIEW QUESTIONS

1. What are the specific responsibilities of the CDER and the CBER?
2. What information does the FDA require in an IND application?
3. Why is an IRB review necessary before a clinical trial is begun?
4. Why are clinical studies randomized and blinded? What does single and double blinding mean?

5. What are the goals of phase I, II, and III trials? How many subjects are involved in each, and how long does the process take?

6. What is the purpose of an NDA? What is involved in the review and approval of an NDA?

7. Why is postmarketing surveillance necessary? When and why are phase IV trials conducted?

8. How does an ANDA differ from an NDA? What studies are required for approval of generic drug products?

9. How will a pharmacogenomic approach improve the development of new drugs?

10. What is the difference between a prescription and an OTC drug product? What is the process for switching a drug from prescription-only to OTC status?

Page numbers in *italics* designate figures; page numbers followed by the letter "t" designate tables; page numbers followed by the letter "b" designate text boxes; (*see also*) designates related topics or more detailed subtopics.